Clinical Reasoning in Spine Pain. Volume I

Primary Management of Low Back Disorders Using the CRISP Protocols

Dr. Donald R. Murphy

With

Gary Jacob, DC, LAc, MPH, DipMDT

David R. Seaman, DC, MS

Steven Heffner, DC, Diplomate MDT

Published by: CRISP Education and Research, LLC

Copyright ©2013 Donald R. Murphy

ISBN: 0615888577

ISBN 13: 9780615888576

Library of Congress Control Number: 2013917114

LCCN Imprint Name: Donald R Murphy, Pawtucket, RI

Neither the author nor the publisher assumes any responsibility for injury and/or damage to persons or property resulting from or related to the use of this book or any material contained in it. This publication contains information describing specific treatment protocols that should not be construed as instructions for individual patients. The treatment practitioner is solely responsible for prescribing and applying patient treatment protocols, based on independent clinical expertise and knowledge of the patient.

Published by: CRISP Education and Research, LLC

• DEDICATION •

This book is dedicated, first, to the ladies of my life. My beautiful wife, Laura, without whose support, encouragement and patience this book could not have been possible; and my wonderful daughters Jessica, Alison and Melissa who constantly fill me with a sense of awe with their inner and outer beauty and wonderful perspectives on life.

Second, this book is dedicated to all people who suffer from any spine related disorder. These folks are the very reason this book was created. It is they who provide the spine practitioner with a reason to continually strive for excellence. They are the focus and purpose all spine care. Their welfare is my professional passion.

• CONTRIBUTORS •

Gary Jacob, DC, LAc, MPH, DipMDT
Private Practice
Pacific Palisades, California

David R. Seaman, DC, MS
Professor, Clinical Sciences
National University of Health Sciences
Chiropractic Medicine
Pinellas Park, FL

Steven L Heffner, DC, Diplomate MDT
McKenzie International/USA Faculty

Photography:
Karly Laliberte
Todd Felderstein

Models:
Laura B. Murphy
Jessica L. Murphy
Kattie Bachar

Cover design:
Jessica L. Murphy

• TABLE OF CONTENTS •

• ACKNOWLEDGEMENTS •

This book is the culmination of my experience of nearly 30 years in the spine field. Thus, the number of people who have influenced the creation of this book is so enormous that listing them all would require a whole separate book. I will focus primarily on those individuals who have provided me with the information, inspiration, encouragement, perspective and insight that has made this book possible.

I would first like to thank my contributing authors, Gary Jacob, DC, LAc, MPH and David Seaman, DC, MS. They not only contributed key sections of this book, but served as advisors, guides, sounding boards and, when they needed to be, sources of harassment for me as I struggled to communicate the information and perspectives regarding primary spine care and the CRISP™ protocols in the clearest way possible.

I would particularly like to thank Gary, who continually forced me out of my comfort zone and to reach deep inside to find my own clarity as to what I wanted to say and how I wanted to say it.

I would also like to thank the individuals who reviewed chapters or sections of chapters and gave me valuable input on the content and presentation of the information. These individuals include Brian Justice, DC, John Ventura, DC and Gary Ierna, DC.

I would like to thank all those who have been an influence on my writing, particularly my late father, Charles A. Murphy, who helped me so much in the early stages of my writing career and my brother, Charles J. Murphy, who helped with editorial assistance with this book and many of my articles. I would also like to thank my mother, Loyola M. Murphy, for her support and encouragement throughout my career.

In addition, I would to thank Dana Lawrence, DC who provided me with advice on issues of grammar and syntax.

I would like to thank those colleagues and mentors who have inspired, supported and informed me over the years and as a result have helped me become the primary spine physician that I am, particularly

Gary Jacob, DC, LAc, MPH; Michael Schneider, DC, PhD; Stephen Perle, DC, MS; David Seaman, DC, MS; Gary Ierna, DC; Robin McKenzie, CNZM, OBE; Mark Laslett, FNZCP, PhD; Scott Haldeman, DC, MD, PhD; Gordon Waddell, MD; John J. Triano, DC, PhD; Vladimir Janda, MD; Karel Lewit, MD; Gwendolyn Jull, PT, PhD; Craig Liebenson, DC; Janet Travell, MD; Kristy Dalrymple, PhD; Diane Lee, PT; John Mennell, MD; Joseph Ferezy, DC; Jennifer Christian, MD, MPH; Anthony Onorato, DC; Warren Hammer, DC; Lillian Ford, DC; Hunter Mollin, DC; Paul Dougherty, DC; Richard Vincent, DC; Craig Nelson, DC, MS; Roger Nelson, PT, PhD; Paul Beattie, PT, PhD; Kim Humphreys, DC, PhD; Cindy Peterson, DC; Ericka McGovern, DC; Josh Randall, MSPT, Amy Gregory, DC; and Charles Rybeck, DC.

I would particularly like to thank Scott Haldeman, DC, MD, PhD who has been an inspiration and guide to me as well as one of the greatest champions of the cause of primary spine care.

Special thanks go to Eric Hurwitz, DC, PhD whose dedication, insight and intelligence have allowed me to embark on so many research projects that would otherwise have been completely out of my reach

Special thanks also go to the West Hartford Group for advancing the cause of primary spine care.

Finally, extra special thanks go to my *compañeros* in Spine Care Partners and the Primary Spine Practitioner Network: Brian Justice, DC, John Ventura, DC, Ian Paskowski, DC, MBA and Thomas Neuner, DC, JD who invited me to take part in the little task of revolutionizing spine care by bringing clinical excellence, efficiency and value to the care of patients with spine related disorders.

Finally, I would like to thank God for Being.

Donald R. Murphy, DC, DACAN

30 August 2013

· INTRODUCTION ·
Primary Spine Care and Low Back Disorders

Low back disorders (LBDs) are among the most common and debilitating conditions in Western society. They cause untold pain, disability and suffering for millions of people. In addition, the financial burden LBDs place on society is tremendous. This financial burden includes costs for diagnosis and treatment as well as work loss, productivity loss and disability payments. Diagnostic and treatment costs have been estimated to be upwards of $12.2 to $90.6 billion per year in the United States alone, with disability costs further adding to the burden to society. Of course, the costs in terms of human suffering are immeasurable.

In some areas of health care, high cost is the price that is paid for high quality care. Even in other areas of life, it is often said that "you get what you pay for." However, what is tragic about the care of LBDs is that, although costs for diagnosis and treatment have skyrocketed in recent decades, the outcome of care has steadily *worsened*. A staggering amount of money has been spent on this group of disorders and yet we have seen increased pain, disability and suffering.

Where does this leave the patient with LBD? In 2008 Haldeman and Dagenais (see Recommended Reading list) published a paper outlining the "Supermarket Approach" to understanding the predicament of patients navigating the LBD treatment landscape. They analogized this with someone visiting a foreign supermarket in which a wide variety of products are offered with no guidance regarding what are the most beneficial and cost-effective options. Another image that can be used to represent the world of LBDs is that of an open-air market in which the patient is faced with a large number of different vendors (health care practitioners, device companies, nutrition and exercise vendors) each offering a solution to the problem, and trying to entice the patient to purchase his or her product, service or device. Often, this enticement is based on marketing and salesmanship rather than good science, clinical reasoning and patient-centeredness.

Clearly, a different direction is needed regarding how society takes care of patients with LBDs.

Part of the difficulty presented by LBDs is that, as will be seen throughout this book, this group of disorders is multifactorial, and the factors that contribute to patients' pain, disability and suffering are varied and relate to different domains of "personhood." In most cases, the approach offered by each of the many types of professionals in the "supermarket" attempts to address one or another of the contributing factors, but fails to consider the person as a whole.

The groups of professionals that have claimed effectiveness in patients with LBDs include chiropractors, physical therapists, orthopedic surgeons, neurosurgeons, physiatrists, anesthesiologists, osteopaths, internists, family practice physicians, occupational medicine physicians, neurologists, rheumatologists, acupuncturists and psychologists. In addition, a number of non-"doctor" professionals claim to be helpful in the care of patients with LBDs, including massage therapists, Reiki practitioners, Rolfers, Alexander technique instructors, Feldenkrais instructors and yoga instructors. It is likely that many of these professional groups have something of value to offer patients, however, because of the "supermarket" environment, confusion rather than clarity typically results.

This book responds to the confusion by integrating the disparate information found in the vast literature on LBDs, combined with my clinical experience, the clinical experience of my contributing authors and that of the many great individuals we have interacted with professionally over the years. It brings this all together to form a cohesive clinical approach. This approach involves the application of Clinical Reasoning in Spine Pain™ (CRISP™). CRISP™ is a process that I have developed that enables the spine practitioner to use sound clinical reasoning, based on the evidence regarding the pathophysiology, diagnosis and treatment of LBDs, in formulating a working diagnosis. From this working diagnosis, management decisions can be made in helping the patient overcome the problem.

In addition, this book builds upon, and provides a clinical blueprint for, the establishment of a new type of health care professional – the primary spine practitioner (PSP) (see Chapter 1 and Murphy, et al in Recommended Reading list). Why does society need yet another professional claiming to be helpful to patients with spine related disorders (SRDs)? Because the supermarket approach has not worked. It has resulted in dramatically increased costs and diminished outcomes for patients. Therefore, what is needed is a primary care practitioner for patients with SRDs. The job of the PSP is to sort out the miasma of theories and methods available and to function as the first-contact practitioner who can *manage the majority of patients without the need for referral*, as well as coordinate the activities of any other players who have something to offer the SRD patient.

There are other individuals, most notably Scott Haldeman, DC, MD, PhD, who have taken up the primary spine care cause (see Recommended Reading list). I see primary spine care as an idea whose time has come, one that will lead to a major shift in the efficiency and effectiveness of spine care delivery in Western society.

This book can be seen as the "how-to" workbook for training the PSP. However, it is not exclusive to this category of practitioner. There are many practitioners who see patients with LBDs but also see patients with a variety of other types of musculoskeletal problems; indeed, even the PSP will likely be consulted by a variety of patients with non-spine problems. Any health care practitioner who sees patients with LBDs will benefit from the information, methods and approaches provided in these pages. In addition, the book is applicable to practitioners who see themselves as "specialists" rather than primary practitioners. Anyone who sees patients with LBDs on any level will likely find something of value in this book.

Together, we can revolutionize one of the most expensive, inefficient and ineffective areas in all of health care. This is a large task that will require will, determination, expertise, skill and innovative thinking. The purpose of this book is to help provide the clinical tools needed to advance the cause of primary spine care.

How to Get the Most out of This Book

For the PSP, PSP-in-training or anyone who sees patients with LBDs on a regular basis, this book should be read cover-to-cover. The reason for this is that chapter by chapter I have built: 1) a working model for conceptualizing LBDs (or, to state it more accurately, the patient with a LBD); 2) a clinical reasoning process by which the practitioner can organize the clinical information about each patient in arriving at a diagnosis; 3) a decision making process by which treatment can be determined; 4) an evidence-based means of monitoring progress and; 5) guidance in making management and referral decisions. Thus, the whole of this book is far greater than the sum of its parts. The real value comes from the integration of the information. The individual diagnostic and treatment techniques have, for the most part, known reliability, validity and efficacy. But the key to their usefulness is the context in which they are applied within the CRISP™ thought process.

In each chapter rather than use the standard reference format, I chose to include a "Recommended Reading" list. There are two key reasons for this. First, this is a clinical workbook rather than a textbook;

as such, it is intended for the reader to absorb and utilize the information without getting bogged down by lots of reference numbers. Second, my purpose with this book is to integrate all the information and methodology I have learned, acquired and developed over nearly 30 years in the spine field and to bring it together into a whole package. This book represents the clinical approach that I apply with patients every day in the clinic. It is the culmination of years of reading various textbooks, articles and research papers, taking seminars and workshops, attending conferences and speaking with colleagues from around the world, combined with my own critical observations and clinical research. The information presented in this book cannot be reduced to a group of references. I wanted to make this book as clinically applicable as possible. Writing the book this way rather than having to constantly think "OK, is there a specific reference for that insight?" allowed me to free myself to provide knowledge and clinical perspectives in a way that would have been very difficult, if not impossible, in the traditional scholarly "reference every statement you make" format.

The Recommended Reading list at the end of each chapter is designed to, first, present the source of certain specific statements of fact that I make in each chapter, second, direct the reader to sources of additional information so a deeper insight into each topic can be pursued and third, give attribution to those scientists and clinicians who have contributed to the development of my clinical approach. The Recommended Reading lists are not meant to be exhaustive and it is incumbent upon the reader to seek as much knowledge as possible regarding LBDs.

The presentation of the hands-on methods in this book should not be seen as a replacement for actual formal training in the principles and methods of primary spine care. This is a workbook that is designed to be an adjunct to formal training. I highly encourage the reader to obtain such training. Anyone interested in the PSP movement, particularly regarding the training program to become a certified PSP can find information at:

www.primaryspineprovider.com

However once the practitioner has obtained adequate training and has reached a level of mastery in primary spine care, this book can serve as a reference for information and methods of diagnosis and treatment. The book can supplement the practitioner's existing knowledge base, serve as a refresher, or build upon the practitioner's established skill set.

This book is "Volume I" of a two-volume set on diagnosis and management of patients with SRDs. This volume specifically relates to low back disorders. Volume II will cover cervical related disorders.

The Origin of CRISP™

Many people ask me how I came up with the clinical approach that I previously referred to as the Diagnosis-Based Clinical Decision Guide and that I now term Clinical Reasoning in Spine Pain™ (CRISP™). This diagnostic and management model evolved out of my desire to provide the absolute best care for my patients by taking a rational, evidence-based approach that considers not just the "spine disorder", but the *patient who is experiencing the disorder.* This desire was coupled with my frustration that my chiropractic education and the scientific literature failed to provide adequate guidance regarding how to best go about this. In chiropractic school I learned a great deal about anatomy, physiology, histology, biochemistry, microbiology, pathology, radiography and diagnosis. I had a large number of "technique" courses that taught me to be excellent at the art of spinal manipulation and other manual treatments. But at no point did I learn how to assess the *whole* patient, find out what he or she was *really* suffering from, and then help the patient *overcome the problem.*

There were attempts in school to take a "comprehensive" view of patients. I recall one class in which the instructor described in detail a postural analysis in which we were taught to look first at the foot, assessing for abnormal positioning, then to look at how that positioning affected the position of the knee, followed by the hip. We were then taught to assess the effect this had on pelvic positioning and ultimately the impact all this had on the spine. I raised my hand and asked, "After we have completed this comprehensive assessment, what do we do about it?" The answer was the same as the answers to virtually all of my previous pesky questions to this instructor: "Palpate the spine, find the subluxation and adjust it." So that is it? No matter what you look for, no matter how comprehensively you assess the patient, all you end up doing is finding the subluxation and adjusting it? Do you ever treat beyond the individual spinal segment? Do you ever talk to the patient? Does the patient ever have anything to offer in the search for what ails him or her?

In the years following graduation, in working with students and interns from various chiropractic schools I saw that the situation improved gradually, but not nearly to the extent I was looking for. In fairness, in this time I also taught a large number of medical students and residents in various medical specialties and found that these students actually learn less than chiropractic students about the optimum evaluation and management of patients with non-surgical spine problems. My experience with various other health professional schools revealed a similar predicament.

I turned to the scientific literature. I thought for sure that the vast research in the spine field would enlighten me. I found a large number of articles that attempted to investigate the causes of SRDs.

Various pathoanatomic processes were discussed such as "disc degeneration", "facet arthrosis", "ligament failure" and the "pain-spasm-pain cycle." But the further I looked into these pathoanatomical explanations for patient suffering the more I realized that these were red herrings – the evidence did not support a purely pathoanatomical model of SRDs.

I also encountered plenty of randomized, controlled trials examining this or that treatment for SRDs, and systematic reviews of those trials and even systematic reviews of the systematic reviews. In nearly all cases, these studies were of single treatments applied to an entire population of patients without regard for the individual diagnostic features in each case, and without regard for the multidimensional nature of SRDs. Rarely, if ever, did a study examine an approach that considered all of the potential contributing factors in the development and perpetuation of SRDs. The predictable conclusion of virtually all of these studies was that no treatment helped very much.

I continued my search. I heard and read a great deal about the so-called "biopsychosocial (BPS) model" of understanding SRDs. I read many articles and heard numerous lectures about how we need to view this group of disorders as involving biological, psychological and social factors, all contributing to the clinical picture. I also traveled the world taking seminars and workshops in the US, Canada and Europe. I studied the work of Janda, Lewit, McKenzie, Waddell, Travell, Jull, Hodges, Faye, Lee, Hammer and numerous other bright, sincere, dedicated, learned and visionary individuals and absorbed all I could from each of them. I thought, "This BPS model is a nice concept, but what does this *really* mean? What *are* the specific biological factors, psychological factors and social factors that contribute to the pain, disability and suffering experience my patients are having? Furthermore, how do I detect these individual factors and, most important of all, how can I help my patients overcome them?"

I saw that the BPS model provided an excellent framework for the development of a clinical approach to patients with SRDs. I realized that I had learned a tremendous amount regarding particular aspects of the diagnosis and management of patients with SRDs but it seemed that no one ever really got to the essence of the BPS model in a comprehensive way that could be practically applied to individual patients, addressing each patient's unique needs.

I felt as if I had been learning from the metaphorical "blind men and the elephant." In John Godfrey Saxe's poem, six blind men feel various parts of an elephant, each interpreting what they are perceiving as vastly different objects (a wall, spear, snake, tree, fan or rope), none of them realizing that it was an elephant. Individuals had gained an understanding of one aspect of the spine pain experience or another, but no one had identified the full "elephant." As Saxe concluded in his poem, "Though each was partly in the right…all were in the wrong!"

There was no process I could find that organized all the disparate information available regarding SRDs into a cohesive clinical approach that could be applied in a busy practice environment. I had encountered a great number of sources that provided useful information about individual components of the pain, disability and suffering experience, but no one ever put it all together and prioritized it for me.

I had reached a fork in the road. I was at a decision point. I could just give up on my pursuit and do what so many others have done – treat patients the way that they have always been treated by applying various "modalities" regardless of whether they are beneficial. Or I could take, to paraphrase another poet, Robert Frost, "the road less travelled by."

The correct choice was clear.

Then I had what is often called an "a-ha moment." I encountered a patient who had been suffering from chronic low back pain for years. She had seen a large number of practitioners from various different disciplines without relief. She had heard that I knew a great deal about the detection and treatment of "faulty movement patterns" that I had learned in Europe, and sought my help. I assessed her using several movement tests and, sure enough, she had several movement patterns (patterns of contraction of muscles during movement tests) that did not conform to what I had learned was "normal." With my eyes and hands, and without having to listen to the patient, I had discovered why she had chronic back pain! All I had to do was correct her movement patterns and she would be free of pain. I applied skilled treatments and exercise approaches over the course of a few weeks. And they worked beautifully. All of the movement patterns that had previously been "faulty" became "normal." My treatment had worked! But there was one problem. When I asked the patient how she was feeling, she told me the pain was exactly the same. Her suffering had not changed a bit.

How could this be? I had used the best of my skills in applying the work of brilliant mentors. I had found several areas of "dysfunction" and had corrected all of them. Where did I go wrong?

Then I remembered something my dear friend (and contributor to this book) Gary Jacob had taught me at a McKenzie seminar: "Do not put the pathoanatomical cart before the empirical horse." I realized that I had been so caught up in looking for the anatomical "dysfunction" that was "causing" the problem that I never actually connected with the patient and *found out from her experience what the problem actually was*!

I sat down with the patient and asked what I have increasingly come to realize is one of the most important and fundamental questions a spine practitioner can ask a patient, "what would you like to be able to do in life that you can't do, or are afraid to try, because of this problem?" She told me, "I would just like to be able to stand up straight. Perhaps even bend backward. I can't do that now." I discussed with her extensively what her experience was in trying to stand up straight and trying to bend backward. I found out what she felt when she tried to do this – not just in terms of pain but emotionally. "Why don't you just go ahead and stand up straight?" I asked. "I don't dare because it hurts too much!" was the reply. "So what if we were to work on that – gradually move your spine toward the direction of upright stance, and perhaps even backward, and see how it goes?" I asked. And that is what we did. We explored together what we needed to do to help her regain what she had lost – the ability to stand up straight and to stretch backward.

How we went about this is irrelevant to the story (the reader will learn this throughout the remainder of this book). The point is that I realized from this that one of the keys to helping patients overcome SRDs is to *communicate with them*! To get to know them and to find out *from them* what they are suffering from. I discovered that when I can figure out what a patient is suffering from I am in a much better position to really help. I also realized that another key to helping patients overcome SRDs is to change my focus from what *I* think should be "normal" to what the patient needs. That is, I realized that I was trained in the same practitioner-centered model as virtually all health care practitioners. One in which the practitioner knows what is "normal" and it is up to the practitioner to determine whether the patient fits the "norm" or not. The patient does not have a say in the matter and simply does what he or she is told. But perhaps the patient has more of a role to play than I thought. Perhaps (Heaven forbid!) the patient is actually more important than I am in this whole process. Perhaps listening to and developing a healing relationship with the patient puts me in the best position to be helpful. Once the healing relationship is established I can apply my medical knowledge and skills to help the patient overcome the problem – *after* I have a clear understanding as to what the problem actually is!

I also realized that if I was going to take an approach that considered all the disparate information on the BPS nature of spine pain, and the many treatment methods that have been developed, I would have to create it myself. So I did. I developed and began applying what I now refer to as the CRISP™ protocols and I found (and have published – see Recommended Reading list) that the outcomes of this approach are quite good. People benefit from CRISP™. So I decided that I had to share this with others; if I was to be able to help as many patients with SRDs as possible, I needed to disseminate the CRISP™ model in a way that practitioners could apply to their own patients.

From this process of soul searching, studying, world travel and my "a-ha moment" arose this book as well as the training and certification program that I, together with my partners in the Primary Spine Practitioner Network, have developed. My passion lies in providing the absolute best primary spine care for my patients but also bringing clinical excellence in primary spine care to as many patients suffering from SRDs as possible, by training practitioners to become high-quality PSPs. Details can be found at www.primaryspineprovidernetwork.com.

It is my sincere hope that this book and the Primary Spine Care courses not only inform but inspire spine practitioners of all types to become passionate about helping patients overcome SRDs, converting the disabled into the "enabled" and showing the way toward functional independence, self-efficacy and freedom from the shackles of pain. If my long journey leads to improving the lives of patients who otherwise would be trapped in the downward spiral of pain, disability and suffering, it will have been well worth the effort.

Recommended Reading

Haldeman S. Looking forward. In: Phillips RB. The Journey of Scott Haldeman. Spine Care Specialist and Researcher. National Chiropractic Mutual Holding Company, 2009: 447-462.

Haldeman S, Dagenais S. A supermarket approach to the evidence-informed management of chronic low back pain. Spine J 2008;8(1):1-7.

Murphy DR, Justice BD, Paskowski IC, Perle SM, Schneider MJ. The Establishment of a primary spine practitioner and its Benefits to Health Care Reform in the United States. Chiropr Man Therap 2011;19(1):17.

Murphy DR, Hurwitz EL. Management of patients with sacroiliac joint pain: a prospective observational cohort study. Platform presentation at the Research Agenda Conference, Washington, DC. March 15-16, 2013.

Murphy DR, Hurwitz EL. Application of a Diagnosis-Based Clinical Decision Guide in Patients with Low Back Pain. Chiropr Man Therap 2011;19(1):26.

Murphy DR, Hurwitz EL: Application of a Diagnosis-Based Clinical Decision Guide in Patients with Neck Pain. Chiropr Man Therap 2011;19(1):19.

Murphy DR, Hurwitz EL, McGovern EE. A non-surgical approach to the management of patients with lumbar radiculopathy secondary to herniated disc: A prospective observational cohort study with follow up. J Manipulative Physiol Ther 2009;32(9):723-33.

Murphy DR, Hurwitz EL, McGovern EE. Outcome of pregnancy related lumbopelvic pain treated according to a diagnosis-based decision rule: A prospective observational cohort study. J Manipulative Physiol Ther 2009;32(8):616-24.

Murphy DR, Hurwitz EL, Gregory AA, Clary R. A nonsurgical approach to the management of patients with cervical radiculopathy: a prospective observational cohort study. J Manipulative Physiol Ther 2006;29(4):279-287.

Murphy DR, Hurwitz EL, Gregory AA, Clary R. A non-surgical approach to the management of patients with lumbar spinal stenosis. Biomed Central Musculoskel 2006;7:16.

Section I:
Background

• CHAPTER 1 •

Principles of Primary Spine Care

This chapter introduces the general principles of the management of patients with low back disorders (LBDs). The approach to LBDs taken in this book is Clinical Reasoning in Spine Pain™ (the CRISP™ protocols). This approach is informed by the biopsychosocial (BPS) model (see Chapter 2). The BPS model has been written and talked about a great deal but is very poorly, if ever, applied in the actual care of patients. Considering the attention that has been paid to the BPS model it is remarkable how there has not been widespread application for the millions of patients who suffer from LBDs. The purpose of this book is to change that.

Also introduced in this chapter is the concept of *Primary Spine Care*. In the Western world, spine care is disjointed, inefficient and largely ineffective. It has increasingly become dominated by specialists and specialized procedures, usually applied in isolation, with little or no communication, organization or cooperation. A solution is desperately needed. Certainly, specialists and specialized procedures play an important role in spine care – in those situations in which they are necessary. But what the health care system needs is a primary-level practitioner who has the knowledge, expertise and skill to serve at the front line, managing the majority of patients without the need for referral, triaging those relatively few patients who require special tests or specialty consults, and coordinating the efforts of others who may be involved in the care of the spine patient. This individual is the *primary spine practitioner*. This book can be seen as the operations manual for primary spine care.

Finally, the conceptual framework for the approach to LBDs that will be taken throughout this book is presented. The remainder of the book will build on this conceptual framework and ultimately help the spine practitioner to take a targeted but comprehensive approach to patients with LBDs.

Low Back Disorders

This book is about the diagnosis and management of patients with low back disorders (LBDs). For the purpose of this book, LBDs include any problem that can cause symptoms referable to the thoracolumbar spine, lumbar spine or pelvis, with or without symptoms in the lower extremity. LBDs include uncommon but potentially serious disorders such as infection or cancer as well as common "sprains and strains" and lumbar radiculopathy. They include problems that begin following injury or trauma as well as those of insidious onset. This group of disorders is among the most common in all of health care and often causes untold pain, disability and suffering amongst individuals of all ages, nationalities, ethnicities, occupations, lifestyles and geographic locations, as well as both genders. For the purpose of this book, the term LBD, rather than low back pain (LBP), is used. This is for two reasons. First, this book is about any symptom related to the thoracolumbar and lumbopelvic spine. The most common symptom is pain but also included are symptoms such as numbness, paresthesia and motor loss related to neurologic disorders in this area. More importantly, however, the term LBD is used rather than LBP because this book focuses not just on pain but on *pain, disability and suffering*. It is critically important for the reader to keep this in mind and this theme will be developed and repeated throughout the book.

This book is meant to provide the spine practitioner with the perspective, knowledge and methodology needed to provide the highest quality non-surgical spine care. It is particularly directed to the primary spine practitioner (PSP), i.e., that practitioner who serves as first contact for the management of patients with spine related disorders (SRDs). However, any practitioner who sees this group of patients will benefit from the teachings in this book.

Primary Spine Care

Over the years, care for spine related disorders has become increasingly specialist-focused, procedure-oriented and dependent on special tests. As a result, it has become extremely expensive. This situation might be acceptable if it were associated with a corresponding improvement in outcomes related to pain, disability and suffering or any other patient-centered measure. However, exactly the opposite is the case. While society has spent billions on the diagnosis and treatment of spine related disorders, the pain, disability and suffering related to these disorders have steadily and dramatically increased. This situation is untenable and must change.

In 2011 the principle author of this book (DRM) and several colleagues wrote a paper entitled, "The Establishment of a Primary Spine Practitioner and its Benefits to Health Care Reform in the United States" (see Recommended Reading list). Proposed and detailed in that paper was the designation of a new category of health care practitioner - the PSP. The benefits to patients, society and the health care system were discussed and the specific skill set required of this category of practitioner was presented. This book is designed to provide specific instruction in the skills required for functioning as a high quality PSP. As mentioned earlier, the book is not to be taken as a substitute for the extensive and personalized clinical training required to become a high quality PSP. Rather it is designed to augment this training and to serve as a workbook for instructors and learners in the diagnosis and management of patients with LBDs.

For the purpose of presenting the primary spine care model, excerpts from the 2011 paper are reproduced here, with kind permission of the co-authors of that paper:

"Primary care" is defined in part by the American Academy of Family Physicians (AAFP) as "that care provided by physicians specifically trained for and skilled in comprehensive first contact and continuing care for persons with any undiagnosed sign, symptom, or health concern (the "undifferentiated" patient) not limited by problem origin (biological, behavioral, or social), organ system, or diagnosis" [http://www.aafp.org/online/en/home/policy/policies/p/primarycare.htm accessed 18 January 2013]. The role of the traditional primary care practitioner (PCP) is to apply comprehensive knowledge about the differential diagnosis of conditions that might arise in *any* bodily system, including the spine and musculoskeletal system. However, recent studies have shown that traditional PCPs are not well trained in the differential diagnosis and management of musculoskeletal disorders, probably due to the heavy emphasis on internal diseases in medical school education and in primary care residency programs. Even those traditional PCPs who profess to have a special interest in SRDs tend to have anachronistic beliefs about best practices for managing these disorders. And guidelines do little to change practitioners' beliefs and practice. The traditional PCP is not likely to be the best choice in the primary care of SRDs.

The term *primary care* is not being used here in the context of a generalist who provides medical care for any condition involving virtually any organ system. The term *primary spine care* is being used in the context of a focused practitioner who provides clinical care for all patients with problems related to a specific organ system – the spine. This model is analogous to the general dentist, who provides "primary care" for oral health. To paraphrase the AAFP definition for this purpose, "primary spine care" can be defined as "that care provided by practitioners specifically trained for and skilled in comprehensive first contact and continuing care for persons with any undiagnosed sign, symptom, or health concern (the "undifferentiated" patient) not limited by problem origin (biological, behavioral, or social), *involving the spine*."

Primary spine care would be provided by practitioners who are specifically trained to diagnose and manage the majority of patients with SRDs with the most evidence-based methods. They would also coordinate the referral and follow up of the minority of SRD patients who might require special tests (e.g. radiographs, MRI or electrodiagnostic testing) or more intensive (e.g. multidisciplinary rehabilitation) or invasive (e.g. injection and surgery) procedures.

The PSP would function as the first contact for patients with SRDs, i.e. the first practitioner that a patient consults when he or she develops a spine problem. The PSP could also function as a resource for traditional PCPs (family practice physicians, general internal medicine physicians, pediatricians, etc) to refer patients who present with SRDs.

The Necessary Skill Set of the Primary Spine Practitioner

The PSP would require several important characteristics in order to provide maximum value to society. Some of these characteristics include:

Skills in differential diagnosis: Serious pathology as a cause of spinal pain occurs in only 1% of patients. However this means that the busy PSP could potentially see at least one case every couple of months. Thus, skill in the recognition of serious pathology is essential, as many of these disorders require immediate investigation or treatment. This includes an understanding of what diagnostic tests to order when certain "red flags" are present. Also essential in this regard is an understanding of when diagnostic testing is *not* necessary as efficiency and cost-effectiveness would be an essential aspect of primary spine care.

Skills in the management of the majority of patients with spine pain: Any primary level practitioner should ideally be able to manage the majority of patients he or she sees without the need for referral. The first-line treatments that the PSP would employ would include those methods shown to be evidence-based, minimally invasive and cost-effective. There is a variety of such treatment methods that have been found to be effective and have broad application which include manual therapies, particularly manipulation and mobilization, the McKenzie method, neural mobilization techniques, various forms of exercise, patient-specific, evidence-based education, non-steroidal anti-inflammatory and non-opioid analgesics (most of which are available over the counter) and nutritional approaches. The PSP would be required to be knowledgeable and skilled in the application of these strategies without the need for referral.

A wide ranging understanding of spinal pain: SRDs are currently understood to be a complex mixture of biopsychosocial phenomena. It is increasingly being recognized that the experience of spinal pain and its related disability involves a combination of biological and psychological processes that occur within a certain social context. The PSP would require a keen understanding of these disparate but interrelated processes. Patient satisfaction in spine care is closely tied to the practitioner providing a clear explanation of the problem. Therefore, the PSP would be required to clearly articulate the complexities of spine pain to patients in simple terms. The ability to recognize the many facets of some complex SRDs, educate the patient about his or her condition, its natural history and the patient's role in recovery, and then motivate the patient to actively participate in care are all necessary, but quite refined, skills that the competent spine provider must have.

The ability to detect and manage psychological factors: It is increasing recognized the psychological factors play an important, and in many cases the most important, role in the perpetuation of pain, disability and suffering in patients with SRDs. The PSP would have to be knowledgeable and skilled in the detection of processes such as fear-avoidance, catastrophizing, passive coping, poor self-efficacy, cognitive fusion and depression and to be able to address these as part of the overall management strategy. As a purely psychological approach may not be effective it is essential that management of these factors is incorporated by the PSP into the management of the somatic factors.

An appreciation of minimalism in spine care: The PSP would have to understand that often in spine care "less is more." That is, an approach that focuses on education regarding the natural history of SRDs, maximizes patient empowerment and minimizes practitioner-driven intervention is likely to be most beneficial. This would allow the practitioner to focus on the *value* of care (i.e. outcome per unit cost) which would not only benefit patients with SRDs but also the health care system and society as a whole by helping control costs while expediting early return to a productive life. This approach would also minimize the growing problem in spine care of patient dependency, whether on pharmaceuticals, interventional procedures, passive modalities or other practitioner-provided services.

An understanding of the methods, techniques and indications of intensive rehabilitation, interventional treatments and surgical procedures: It would be the responsibility of the PSP to coordinate the referral and follow up for the minority of patients who need secondary and tertiary level treatment. This would require knowledge and experience regarding the appropriate indications for these interventions, an ability to explain them to patients and an ability to follow up with these patients after the intervention to monitor the progress and outcome.

An understanding of the unique features of work-related SRDs: SRDs that begin in the workplace have particular features that differentiate them from those that are not perceived as work-related. Many physicians, particularly traditional PCPs, are uncomfortable with work-related back pain and have misperceptions about the important role that early return to work and return to other normal activities plays in recovery. The PSP would be required to understand the nuances of work-related SRDs and the unique aspects of management that are required to effectively care for this patient population.

An understanding of the unique features of SRDs related to motor vehicle collisions: Similar to work-related SRDs, those related to motor vehicle collisions (particularly whiplash associated disorders) have particular features that require specialized knowledge. The PSP would require an understanding of issues that are unique to this type of patient such as injury mechanisms, patterns of injury, risk factors for chronicity, medicolegal reporting and the delicate balance between the need for early, aggressive treatment and the potential role this can play in chronicity.

Public health perspective: The PSP would require a broad perspective regarding how spine problems and spine care fits in the grander scheme of public health. For example, many of the health conditions that are the focus of public health education and promotion campaigns are associated with SRDs as complicating factors. These include: smoking, obesity, type II diabetes, lack of physical exercise, and mental health disorders. Public health campaigns regarding SRDs are in the early stages and it can be expected that further public health efforts regarding this widespread set of problems will be undertaken and will require input from primary-level practitioners with expertise in this area.

The ability to coordinate the efforts of a variety of practitioners: As we stated earlier, a high-quality PSP should be able to manage the majority of patients with SRDs without the need for referral. However, in those patients who require specialized services, the PSP would have to be skilled in the coordination of these services and in follow up to ensure that maximum benefit is derived.

The ability to follow patients over the long term: As SRDs typically take on a recurrent course that is life-long the PSP would have to be skilled in the long-term follow-up of patients to monitor recurrences, teach patients how to effectively interpret and self-manage the majority of these recurrences, and provide management of those recurrences for which self-management is not effective.

The Primary Spine Practitioner: potential benefits for patients

Any patient benefits that may result from a focused management strategy with a well trained PSP would have to be investigated through a rigorous research effort. However, based on the current understanding of SRDs, we would anticipate a number of such benefits. Some examples include:

Faster recovery: By providing targeted, evidence-based care the well-trained PSP would avoid unnecessary treatment, promote active care plans and patient empowerment and appropriately triage when necessary. This can be expected to facilitate maximal outcomes in the shortest time.

Cost savings: The PSP could save patients considerable time and money both at the point of encounter and in the future by ordering diagnostic tests only when necessary, applying evidence-based treatments, avoiding unnecessary treatment and taking a "less is more" approach through education and motivation in self-directed care.

Avoiding iatrogenic disability: Judicious use of imaging and appropriate communication of findings may also help avoid the iatrogenic disability that can arise as a result of the medicalization of imaging findings that are of questionable clinical significance, such as "disc degeneration." Inappropriate communication of diagnostic test results can lead to unnecessary catastrophizing of benign spine pain that may result in prolonged disability and unnecessary invasive procedures. Having a PSP who understands when advanced imaging is necessary and when it is not necessary, and who can put into the proper perspective the findings of these tests, can help to reverse the costly imaging- and specialist-dominated culture that has developed in the area of SRDs.

Increased productivity: Encouragement to remain active, particularly with work-related SRDs and engaging in a targeted stay at work/ return to work strategy would lessen the likelihood of work loss and its resultant economic hardship.

Decreased likelihood of becoming a "chronic pain sufferer": Appropriate care plans that focus on active care and patient empowerment are likely to help the patient avoid becoming a chronic pain sufferer. The recognition of "yellow flags" of psychosocial involvement can lead to early intervention, before these factors lead patients down the path of prolonged disability.

High patient satisfaction: In the age of consumer-driven health care, the importance of the patient's overall experience of health care is of great importance. Cost effective and clinically effective care provided by a practitioner who has good communication skills to educate, motivate and empower the patient will likely lead to high levels of satisfaction.

Shared decision making: The PSP would have a wide-ranging understanding of the various diagnostic and management strategies available to patients with SRDs and thus could provide information, resources and support in making decisions regarding their care.

Focus on prevention: While no program of prevention of future SRDs has been shown to be completely successful, it has been demonstrated that taking a preventative approach can help limit disability related to SRDs and well as reduce the frequency of future episodes.

The Primary Spine Practitioner: potential benefits to society

As with patient benefits, research would be required to determine any societal benefits that may result from the institution of a PSP. However we anticipate that there are many potential benefits to society of having a practitioner who is charged with providing primary care for patients with SRDs. Some examples include:

1. *Knowledgeable care coordinator:* A wide variety of practitioners is currently involved in the management of SRDs with little coordination of their efforts. This leads to inefficiency and compromises value. In our view it would be much more efficient and valuable to create teams of professionals with expertise in SRDs working together to provide efficient and effective patient care. The PSP could play the role of "team captain" by organizing and supervising the work of the various disciplines that may be contributing to the management of any particular patient. This could be expected to improve outcomes by turning what is oftentimes a disjointed effort into a coordinated effort. It would also be likely to help control costs by having a single person in charge of monitoring a particular treatment to determine if it is bringing about meaningful improvement and should continue or is not bringing about meaningful improvement and should be altered or stopped.

2. *SRDs as a public health initiative:* Increased recognition is being given to the potential of a public health approach to SRDs. The PSP can spearhead efforts in this area to facilitate and implement such public health campaigns as well as reinforce public health messages on an individual level with patients. Community-wide approaches to back pain have been successful in the past. These programs involve a consistent evidence-based approach by primary contact providers coupled with community-wide education programs to inform the public on how to prevent disability related to SRDs and what to do if spine pain occurs. The success of these programs requires an understanding on the part of the PSP of the essential public health messages regarding SRDs. A community-wide public health initiative regarding SRDs has the potential to save millions of dollars and to prevent needless human suffering.

3. *Improved worker productivity:* SRDs trigger significant amounts of absenteeism and "presenteeism" (the worker being present at the workplace but with significant losses in work productivity). The economic impact of these losses to a community is substantial. The establishment of a PSP could potentially lead to significant community-wide savings in both direct and indirect costs of SRDs.

4. *Less long term disability:* A significant portion of health care costs related to SRDs goes toward the management of chronic and recurrent conditions. Appropriate initial evaluation and treatment can significantly reduce the number of acute pain patients who become chronic, and to reduce the cost of medical care, lost productivity and disability. A "culture of disability" can spread through a family or business or community, creating emotional and financial hardship for society. Having a PSP who is skilled in disability management could potentially help reduce the risk of long term disability by acting at the early stages of a SRD episode.

The Primary Spine Practitioner: potential benefits for the health care system

At present the delivery of health care to patients with SRDs is incredibly inefficient and expensive. Having a primary spine care provider to manage patients with SRDs may benefit the health care system in a number of ways, including:

Controlling costs: By having a PSP who has the skills to manage the majority of patients with SRDs without the need for special tests or referral to specialists or other practitioners, a dramatic decrease in the cost of SRDs could be realized.

Unburdening traditional PCPs: The traditional PCP has the responsibility of managing the overall health needs of his or her patients. This includes, in many cases, multiple co-morbidities. The PSP would handle a significant portion of the traditional PCP's current case load, increasing the PCP's availability to the numerous other responsibilities of these practitioners. Thus, traditional PCPs would benefit by being relieved of the burden of caring for a large group of patient complaints for which they have little training. This could also potentially result in a decrease in the projected PCP shortfall. Having a PSP to whom traditional PCPs can refer patients with SRDs, or whom these patients can consult directly without having to see their PCP (a more efficient pathway), would remove from the already-overbooked schedule of traditional PCPs those conditions (SRDs) for which they have minimal training in diagnosis and management. This will allow them to focus on what they do best.

More strategic specialist referrals: Specialists who care for patients with SRDs would benefit for a similar reason as would traditional PCPs. Many patients with SRDs who see specialists such as orthopedic surgeons, neurosurgeons, interventional physiatrists or pain management physicians have no indications for surgery, injections or other invasive procedures. In addition, it has been found that in many cases these specialists do not have a keen understanding of the management of non-surgical SRDs. This is likely because the bulk of the training of these specialists is focused on the application of interventional and surgical procedures in complex cases. By having all SRD patients see the PSP, who is trained to recognize those who require more invasive procedures, only those patients who need such procedures would be channeled to the surgical or interventional specialist. This would allow these specialist practitioners to focus their practice on doing what they do best – applying skilled surgical or interventional procedures.

Disruptive innovation: The establishment of practitioners who can provide primary spine care would represent a significant "disruptive innovation" in health care. According to Christensen et al (see Recommended Reading list), disruptive innovation is the process in which complex, expensive products and services are transformed into simple, affordable ones. Disruptive innovation in any industry occurs when a company, a group of individuals, or a profession comes along with new ideas and a new approach that leads to the transformation of the industry so that products and services become dramatically more affordable and accessible. This happened in the 1970s when Toyota disrupted the auto industry and in the early 1980s when Apple disrupted the computer industry. We suggest that the introduction of the PSP can serve as a disruption in the delivery of spine care services that could potentially lead to dramatic improvements in the delivery, accessibility, cost and outcomes of this care. This viewpoint is supported by the example of the Spine Care Program at Jordan Hospital in Plymouth, Massachusetts where the PSP model has been implemented in an ACO-style environment. Preliminary evidence indicates that this program has been successful in the areas of outcomes, patient satisfaction and cost efficiency. In addition, 80% of the patients in this program are referred by traditional PCPs supporting our viewpoint that the PSP model would be helpful in reducing the burden on these practitioners.

Standardization of care: Inconsistent clinical decision-making, unnecessary ordering of imaging studies, overutilization of invasive procedures, over-prescription of pharmaceuticals and excessive reliance on passive care approaches all trigger huge health care losses both in money and time. A standardized, evidence based patient care pathway followed by knowledgeable practitioners has the potential to greatly minimize these costs.

New evidence and technologies: Currently, new treatment approaches or technologies regarding SRDs are often driven into the health care system more by marketing efforts than by good science. With the introduction of a single group of PSPs throughout the health care system, quality, evidence-based technologies and procedures could more quickly and efficiently be introduced.

Obstacles to the implementation of the primary spine care model

There are a number of hurdles to overcome for the successful implementation of a primary care of spine model. These obstacles include:

Educational changes: Currently, none of the major health care educational institutions are consistently graduating providers who meet all the criteria necessary to be successful PSPs. However with some basic fundamental changes, and a commitment from state and federal governments, trade organizations and school administrators and faculty, this obstacle can be overcome. Institutions of chiropractic medicine, for example, provide training that is focused primarily on the spine. Many of the skills required of the PSP are already taught at these schools. By instituting some specific changes, that are already being discussed within this health care profession, these institutions can become at least one source of appropriately trained PSPs. Other disciplines that include some level of spine care training within their respective curricula are institutions of osteopathic medicine and physical therapy. The primary focus of most osteopathic programs in the US is the diagnosis and treatment of internal disorders with a majority of osteopathic physicians working in the field of family medicine. Physical therapy education does contain some spine-related coursework, but is more broadly focused on musculoskeletal, neuromuscular, cardiopulmonary, and wound care. Thus, significant changes in these curricula would be required if they are to successfully train PSPs.

Incentivizing value: Traditionally, in the area of SRDs and as in other areas of health care, providers have typically been paid by the procedure, thus incentivizing more procedures. This would have to change for successful implementation of primary spine care services into the health care system. PSPs would have to be adequately paid for activities such as patient education, coordination of care and stay at work/ return to work strategies. In addition, they would have to be financially incentivized to take a "less is more" approach. There are signs that this is starting to occur, however. As the health care system moves from fee for service toward a shared risk management model, providers and care pathways that add value to the system will be the leaders, thus increasing the support of their programs and services. The concept of the PSP fits well into this model, allowing a "less is more" approach that involves fewer procedures and greater patient empowerment to replace the present inefficiencies in the care of patients with SRDs.

Overcoming prejudice: It is likely that the best candidates to be groomed to become primary care spine providers may not come from the allopathic medical profession. This may be resisted in some aspects of the medical community. It would be important that a competent, appropriately trained provider be accepted regardless of the degree after his or her name. The institution of new models of health care in general, including primary spine care, will require non-traditional ways of thinking about which provider will become the "team captain" for any particular medical condition.

The detrimental effect on those invested in current model of spine care: For health care practitioners who currently see a large volume of patients with SRDs and who remain invested in the current incentive system in which more procedures are emphasized without regard for outcome or value, the institution of a PSP could be detrimental. If a system in which value rather than volume is rewarded, some practitioners will be negatively impacted and some may even go out of business. Thus, the disruption of the health care system that the institution of a PSP will be a part of will undoubtedly be resisted by some individuals or groups who are unable or unwilling to embrace this change. However, such resistance has occurred in response to major disruptions of other industries and we would anticipate that the benefits of the disruption we are suggesting will overcome any opposition that will inevitably arise.

Resistance from within the profession(s) that could potentially be the source of PSPs: For whatever profession or professions that respond to the need for a PSP, this will be a significant disruption to the traditional practice patterns or self-image of these professions. As a result, the role that we are introducing here will be actively resisted. However, given the fact that SRDs affect virtually 100% of the population, it can be expected that whatever profession accepts the role of PSP will likely dramatically increase the volume of patients that seeks its services.

Implementation: The implementation of primary spine care services will require support from several areas of the health care system, including the profession(s) from which the non-surgical spine care practitioner will arise, third party payors, who will have to provide the financial incentive to bring value to spine care, regulatory and legislative bodies that may have to institute changes in allowing this area of health care to fully realize its societal benefits and other members of the health care system who will have to support and accept the implementation of primary spine care services. Again, disruptive innovations in other industries have required such changes and we would anticipate that the same can occur in response to the primary spine care innovation.

Sustainability: Any disruptive innovation has to be sustained in order for society to fully realize its benefits. Because of the great need we have presented here for high-quality, low-cost (i.e., valuable) spine care, we feel that this need, and the benefits realized as a result of the institution of primary spine care services, will drive the sustainability of these services. However, this sustainability will also be dependent on the consistent supply of practitioners who are appropriately skilled in providing primary spine care. As we indicated earlier, this will require commitment on the part of whatever health care profession(s) elects to supply the system with appropriately trained practitioners.

Value in Spine Care

As of the time period in which this book was written, very little attention had been paid in most health care systems to the importance of *value*. However, this has begun to change. It has been increasingly recognized in recent years that the cost of health care has skyrocketed to unsustainable levels. Western societies have dramatically increased spending on health services. This spending increase particularly applies to the diagnosis and management of LBDs. Disappointingly, the benefit to patients has not increased commensurate with costs. In fact, as discussed earlier, exactly the opposite has occurred, i.e., despite the incredible amount of money that has been spent on LBDs, we have seen increased levels of pain, disability and suffering on the part of patients.

Value in health care is defined as outcome per unit cost (see Porter in Recommended Reading list). High value means the best possible outcome in terms of improved health and satisfactory patient experience at the least possible cost. Value is an essential element of all industries. For any product, service, company or business entity to be effective, it must provide value to whomever it serves. That is, providing the greatest benefit for the least possible cost is what creates a successful business proposition. It is essential that spine practitioners pay close attention not only to whether the care they provide to patients is beneficial, but also whether that care provides *value* to society. Therefore, in designing care pathways for an institution as well as individual care plans for patients, the over-arching question must be "how can this pathway or care plan provide maximal benefit to the patient at the least cost necessary?" This will serve as a guide to the development of the most efficient and effective approach.

Efficiency in Spine Care

When it comes to spine care, the axiom "less is more" applies. That is, the best care for patients with LBDs is that which utilizes as little practitioner-driven activity as possible and which places the greatest focus on patient-driven activity. This includes not only exercise and self-care strategies but also involves the spine practitioner encouraging and guiding patients to take responsibility for their health, helping them improve their self-efficacy, (i.e., their confidence in their ability to overcome the LBD and maintain good spine health). It also includes helping patients become mindful of their cognitions and beliefs about LBDs so they can challenge any preconceived notions that may be self-limiting. This also helps patients gain an understanding of the spine that promotes functional independence. Helpful in this regard is to draw out of patients their most deeply held values regarding their health and how they would like to conduct their life.

Throughout this book we will be discussing a variety of methods and techniques of both diagnosis and treatment that require the efforts of a highly skilled and experienced professional. But patients can only overcome LBDs when they are empowered to perceive themselves as being in charge of life, rather than the LBD being in charge. In achieving this, practitioner-driven procedures are merely a stepping stone, a means to an end, with the end being the patient becoming functionally independent from pain.

In the business world, efficiency is often described as the ratio of expenses to revenue. A more efficient business is one in which this ratio is relatively low, i.e., the lower expenses are in relation to revenue, the more efficient the business. In the context of spine care, efficiency is the ratio between practitioner activity and functional outcome for the patient. In other words, more efficient spine care is that which obtains greater patient-oriented outcome with less activity on the part of the spine practitioner and the remainder of the health care system. Therefore, the most valuable spine care is that which achieves the greatest patient benefit with the least intervention, both diagnostic and therapeutic.

In spine care it is often seen that more effort on the part of practitioners and the health care system can actually lead to less favorable functional outcomes for patients (e.g., see Cote, et al in the Recommended Reading list). So in spine care it is often the case that "less is more." That is, the most effective, and efficient (and thus valuable), spine care is that which takes a targeted approach; only the most essential diagnostic and treatment activities are utilized and maximal focus is placed on helping patients to help themselves.

Throughout this book, a great many procedures will be presented that are useful in the diagnosis and management of LBDs. However, it must always be kept in mind that it is not the procedures themselves that are most important but the role each procedure plays in overall patient management. Therefore it is incumbent on the spine practitioner to always be mindful of whether a given procedure is maximally useful in a given situation or whether the procedure is unnecessary, superfluous or should be avoided. This allows the practitioner to establish a strategy that maximizes efficiency and value, which will translate into maximal benefit for the patient and for society.

From Practitioner-Centered Care to Patient-Centered Care to Relationship-Centered Care

An evolution is taking place in the approach to health care in general, and spine care in particular, that has the potential to dramatically impact the quality of the care patients receive. In the past, the typical approach has been practitioner-centered, in which the primary focus of the health care encounter is the practitioner. With this, who the practitioner is and what the practitioner does is most important. In practitioner-centered care the patient delegates responsibility and power to the practitioner and, often unquestioningly, *receives* treatment *from* the practitioner, who has knowledge and skills the patient does not possess. The practitioner is the authority figure and the patient is subservient to the practitioner.

More recently, transition away from the practitioner-centered approach toward a patient-centered model has begun, in which the patient becomes the primary focus of the encounter. This is certainly a step in the right direction as it recognizes that the needs of the patient should be seen as the most important purpose of the encounter.

However it must be recognized that there are two human beings involved in the practitioner-patient encounter (and often, as will be seen, multiple human beings). It is in the *relationship between* the practitioner and the patient where "healing" takes place.

Any encounter between a practitioner and a patient is one in which not only is a diagnosis *applied to* the patient, leading to treatment being "*done to*" the patient, but a relationship is formed. The healing encounter is a partnership between the practitioner and the patient. Each individual has a role to play and, while there is disparity in expertise and skill in this partnership, each partner is an "equal." As with patient-centered care, the primary purpose is to help the patient overcome whatever problem he or she is seeking help for, and to live as healthy, fulfilling and productive a life as possible. The benefit to the practitioner results from the quality and value that he or she brings to the encounter.

However, while patient benefit is the primary purpose of the encounter, it should be viewed in a broader context. Each individual in the practitioner-patient relationship brings to the encounter his or her entire life experience and worldview – cognitions, beliefs, fears, joys and perspectives that are highly individual but are part of the shared human experience. These cannot be separated from any other aspect of the healing encounter. The practitioner should not attempt to ignore or "push out" these things. Rather, it is the job of the practitioner to be mindful of all the normal human "stuff" he or she brings to the encounter, to allow the "stuff" to be there, and then to place maximal focus on being helpful to the patient. This may mean leaving behind any "stuff" that is not useful in helping the patient. This will be discussed further in Chapter 8.

Part of relationship-centered care is the relationship between all other members of the team, including family members and other loved ones, medical professionals, case managers, attorneys, office staff and hospital personnel. It is essential to cultivate a healthy working relationship amongst these individuals that has one primary purpose – to help the patient overcome the LBD and to live a healthy, fulfilling and productive life to the greatest extent possible.

Particularly for those who play the role of PSP, there is an opportunity to take the lead in establishing a relationship amongst all those involved in the care pathway that maximizes benefit to the patient. The PSP can do this by, first, setting an example of one who is cognizant of the importance of a healthy working relationship and, second, placing the focus of the relationship between all parties on the primary purpose, i.e., the welfare of the patient. That is, serving as "captain of the spine care team" involves setting the tone of the relationship between all parties as one of cooperatively working together toward the common goal of helping the patient.

Helping Patients *Overcome* LBDs

The reader will notice that this book will repeatedly refer to "helping patients *overcome* LBDs." This terminology has been chosen carefully because this should be the goal of all care for LBDs. It is different from "treating LBDs" or "getting rid of the pain." By placing our focus on "treating LBDs", we place the practitioner at the center of the process. After all, it is the practitioner who does the "treating." This is very temping for anyone. There is a natural tendency for all human beings to want to be the primary focus of any effort; to be at the center of attention. In addition, it is natural to want to "do things to the patient" and have those "things" be the reason for the positive outcome. However, to be of maximal benefit to patients, it is essential for the practitioner to observe and acknowledge this tendency, and to be ever mindful that the purpose of the practitioner-patient encounter is to be as beneficial to the patient as possible.

Placing focus on "getting rid of the pain" puts the pain at the center of the process. This focus is not conducive to achieving the ultimate goal – helping the patient live life in a way that is most consistent with his or her most deeply held values, without being hampered by a LBD. Reducing the intensity of the pain or eliminating it completely can be very helpful in the process, and should be pursued. However there are circumstances in which completely getting rid of the pain is not possible. In addition, the nature of back pain is that it tends to return. By placing focus on "getting rid of the pain" the practitioner promotes the idea that the only way to live life to the fullest is to be completely pain-free at all times. This is not only untrue, it is not realistic. What is more, it teaches the patient to focus on the wrong thing – the pain – rather than having a more valuable focus – on living life in a way that is most consistent with the patient's goals and values.

No one can live life pain-free, but nearly everyone can live a life free of pain. What this means is that occasional pain is a normal part of life for everyone. But it is not necessary to be in a pain-free state to live a fulfilling life. Nearly everyone can be happy, healthy and productive independent of whether at any given time there happens to be a nociceptive stimulus somewhere in the body that reaches the patient's awareness.

Management in a Cognitive-Behavioral, Acceptance-Commitment Context

Central to the application of the BPS model is for all patient care to be applied in a cognitive-behavioral, acceptance-commitment (C-B, A-C) context. That is, to establish a framework in which every interaction between the practitioner and the patient occurs in an environment that constructively influences the patient's thinking about the nature of spine pain. In addition, the environment must be one that helps the patient experience the pain as an objective observer and to get in touch with his or her deepest held values. From the moment the practitioner greets the patient, positive messages about LBDs should be incorporated in the practitioner-patient communication. These messages may be provided directly through verbal communication and physical demonstration or indirectly through the practitioner leading by example. For this to be effective the spine practitioner must have a clear understanding of the nature of LBDs, the meaning of physical sensations and imaging findings and the role activity may or may not play in the causation, perpetuation and management of LBDs.

It is important to apply the principle of "meeting the patient where he or she is." That is, the communication process should begin from the patient's perspective, rather than from the practitioner's perspective. It is not helpful to hit the patient over the head with C-B, A-C messages. This will only be met with resistance. Rather, by acknowledging where the patient is now in his or her thinking the practitioner can start challenging the patient's thinking and provide empowerment messages. Again, C-B, A-C messages can be provided directly through verbal counseling of the patient. However, the most powerful application of C-B, A-C principles is for these ideas to be a part of every aspect of the practitioner-patient interaction. That is, these messages must be so ingrained in the practitioner that everything that is said and done during every encounter exudes C-B, A-C principles. The key messages and methodology of the C-B, A-C approach will be discussed in Chapters 8 and 11.

Research in Spine Related Disorders and the Problem of Diagnosis

Outcomes research in the area of spine related disorders typically involves the application a single treatment to all patients, as if all patients had identical etiologies and needs and there was only one treatment that was required in each case. The randomized, controlled trial (RCT) is widely considered in medicine as the "Gold Standard" of clinical research. With the RCT, patients with a certain disorder are randomly assigned to various groups. One group receives a certain treatment while the other group(s) receives an alternate treatment or a placebo or are placed in an untreated control group. Importantly, it is assumed that all patients included in an RCT have the same condition, and thus are comparable. The RCT is an appropriate design in studying well-defined conditions and unidimensional treatments. However in the area of SRDs, while RCTs have provided some general information about "what works and what doesn't", they have failed to provide clinicians with clear direction regarding how best to help their patients. This is because, first, in the majority of RCTs patients with "low back pain" or "neck pain" are lumped together as if they all have the same diagnosis and they all need only one treatment modality. The purpose is to identify whether that one treatment is effective. Second, the effectiveness of the study treatment is only assessed *on average across the entire population of patients*. Whether any individual patient or patients in the study benefitted from the treatment cannot be determined.

Spratt (see Recommended Reading list) provided a wonderful analogy that illustrates the problem in relying on RCTs to study treatments for patients with SRDs. He presented a hypothetical study that attempts to determine the effectiveness of nitroglycerine and antacids for patients with chest pain. Patients with "chest pain" are randomized to receive nitroglycerine, antacid or placebo, with no attempt to determine the cause of the chest pain. Because there is no attempt to make a diagnosis in these "chest pain" patients, some individuals, (those with a cardiac cause of their chest pain) will respond very well to the nitroglycerine, whereas a number of patients (those with a non-cardiac cause of their chest pain) will not respond at all. Likewise, some individuals (those whose pain was arising from acidic irritation to the esophagus) will respond well to antacid, whereas others (those whose pain was not acid-related) will not. In all likelihood, when looked at statistically across the groups, neither nitroglycerine nor antacid will "perform" much better than placebo. The "logical" conclusion would be that because of the meager effectiveness of these medications their use cannot be justified in patients with "chest pain".

However what if the same study were repeated with a slight alteration? This time those patients whose chest pain was determined to be related to coronary artery pathology were identified and randomized to receive either nitroglycerine or placebo. It is likely that the nitroglycerine would "become" an effective treatment. Likewise, if patients whose pain related to acid reflux were identified and randomized to receive antacids or placebo, antacid would "become" an effective treatment for this group of patients.

So identifying a diagnosis prior to attempting an RCT improves the value of the study. However there is another problem with using the RCT design to study the management of SRDs. While the RCT works well with conditions such as coronary artery disease or acid reflux, in which there is a single identifiable lesion that his causing the symptom, it still is problematic in patients suffering from a condition that is multifactorial and cannot be reduced to a single "lesion."

Thus, the RCT, at least in the way it has been used in spine research thus far, is an inadequate design in studying the management of patients with SRDs. Hundreds of RCTs and systematic reviews of RCTs have been conducted, costing millions of dollars and hours and hours of valuable time of some brilliant scientists and all there is to show for it is "nothing seems to work – or at least not well." It is time for a moratorium on all RCTs and systematic reviews of treatments for patients with SRDs. New, innovative methods of studying this unique, multifactorial problem are needed.

In clinical practice, it is very commonly seen that the treatment a patient with a low back or neck disorder receives is often determined by the type of practitioner he or she sees, rather than by the specific needs of each patient. For example, if a practitioner's primary treatment modality is manipulation, that is the treatment virtually all patients will receive. If another practitioner primarily uses injections, virtually all patients will receive injections. It will be likewise with medications, passive physiotherapy modalities and surgery. This phenomenon is particularly acute when the practitioner is financially incentivized to perform certain procedures irrespective of patient needs.

Identifying specific characteristics in patients with SRDs has been deemed critically important for some time. This has led to efforts to try to "subgroup" SRD patients. These attempts at subgrouping include dividing patients into "syndromes" (e.g. the McKenzie Method) and developing treatment-based "clinical prediction rules." A great deal of insight and some high-quality research by intelligent scientists were behind these efforts. However one problem with attempting to subgroup patients is that this approach does not satisfactorily consider the multidimensional nature of SRDs. As will be discussed throughout this book, there are a number of factors (many known, others yet to be discovered) that have the potential to contribute to the SRD experience. Some factors are present in certain individuals and other factors in others. In addition, the extent to which one or another factor contributes is different in different patients. One patient may have facet joint pain that is contributing a small amount to the overall experience, while in another the facet pain may constitute virtually the entire clinical picture. Another patient may have no facet pain at all but may have a painful disc. However in one patient with disc pain the disc itself may be a relatively minor factor and their fear and catastrophizing is contributing more significantly to their pain, disability and suffering experience. Another patient with disc pain may not have a great deal of fear and catastrophizing but dynamic instability is leading to recurrent episodes.

Thus it can be seen, and it will become clearer throughout this book, that the SRD experience is unique to each individual. Each patient experiences the pain, disability and suffering of an SRD in his or her own way. In essence, there are some 7,000,000,000 potential subgroups!

Diagnosis in patients with SRDs is extremely challenging. There are three chief reasons for the difficulty with diagnosis in SRDs:

1. SRDs are multifactorial, biopsychosocial phenomena – as discussed in this chapter and throughout the book, there are a number of different factors that contribute to the SRD experience. Thus, the diagnosis cannot be reduced to a single "lesion."

2. The diagnostic factors encompass various domains of "personhood" - the pain, disability and suffering experience on the part of SRD patients can involve somatic, neurophysiological and psychological factors that all contribute to a greater or lesser extent. These all occur in the unique social context in which each patient lives.

3. The spine practitioner cannot rely on objective tests – for the majority of the diagnostic factors that contribute to the SRD experience there currently are no objective tests that definitively identifies their presence.

As a result of these challenges, being a high-quality spine practitioner requires a unique skill set that not only allows him or her to identify certain diagnostic characteristics, but also to be comfortable with "gray areas." SRDs are rarely "black and white" and it is in the "gray areas" that a true understanding of the pain, disability and suffering of the SRD patient can be found. Therefore an evidence-based *clinical reasoning process* must be employed that considers all of the potential contributing factors that may be involved in each patient. The clinical reasoning process must utilize diagnostic procedures that, whenever possible, have been demonstrated to provide meaningful diagnostic information when skillfully applied and interpreted.

But the diagnosis of SRDs does not result purely from the application of a group of examination procedures and diagnostic tests, although, as will be seen, these things play a critical role. It arises from the *relationship between the practitioner and the patient*. That is, the specific characteristics that are contributing to each patient's pain, disability and suffering experience are best identified in the context of the practitioner-patient interaction. It is through this relationship that the spine practitioner can truly understand the patient and thus derive a multifactorial diagnosis, develop a patient-specific management strategy and monitor the outcome of that strategy in a way that is *meaningful to the patient*.

Clinical Reasoning in Spine Pain™ - the CRISP™ Protocols

The CRISP™ protocols were developed by the primary author of this book (DRM) for the purpose of helping the spine practitioner apply the BPS model in patient care. The CRISP™ protocols were referred to in previous publications as the Diagnosis-Based Clinical Decision Rule or the Diagnosis-Based Clinical Decision Guide (see Recommended Reading list). The CRISP™ protocols integrate the best clinical and scientific evidence regarding the various BPS components of the LBD experience into a clinical reasoning process. The CRISP™ protocols enable the practitioner to develop a working diagnosis and to make treatment decisions. The CRISP™ approach is based on the "Three Questions of Diagnosis":

1. Do the presenting symptoms reflect a visceral disorder, or a serious or potentially life-threatening illness?

2. Where is the pain coming from?

3. What is happening with this person as a whole that would cause the pain experience to develop and persist?

We will look at these questions briefly here and delve into them in great detail throughout the remainder of the book, particularly in Chapters 4, 5 and 6.

The first question of diagnosis ("Are the symptoms with which the patient is presenting reflective of a visceral disorder, or a serious or potentially life-threatening illness?") is one in which we consider pathological processes other than those that create common, "everyday" LBDs. This is often referred to as "ruling out red flags" but diagnostic question #1 not only considers the typical "red flag" conditions such as cancer or infection, but any non-musculoskeletal cause of the presenting symptoms. Diseases such as primary or metastatic cancer, benign tumor, spine infection, fracture and certain visceral disorders can cause low back pain with or without leg pain. The first question of diagnosis allows the spine practitioner to determine whether there are historical factors, symptoms or examination findings that suggest the presence of one of these disorders. A "yes" answer to diagnostic question #1 should only be expected in approximately 1-3% of patients. However this means that a busy spine practitioner is likely to encounter this on a fairly regular basis. Therefore, it is imperative for the spine practitioner to remain alert to the possibility that a visceral disorder or a potentially serious or life-threatening condition may underlie a patient's LBD.

With the second question of diagnosis ("Where is the pain coming from?"), we are essentially asking, "Are there characteristics of the pain generating tissue or tissues that can be identified and that allow treatment decisions to be made?" It is well known that in the majority of patients with LBD there is no way to be absolutely certain of the specific tissue that is generating the pain. This is because in the majority patients there is no objective test that definitively identifies the involved tissue. However, as we will see, there often are characteristics that can be detected on history and examination that at least provide clues regarding the pain generating tissue. This then allows the practitioner to provide a reasonable explanation to the patient as well as to decide which treatment or treatments to try first. As with a variety of other conditions throughout medicine, a SRD is very much a "clinical diagnosis."

The third question of diagnosis ("What is happening with this person as a whole that would cause the pain experience to develop and persist?") is one in which we consider perpetuating factors, that is, factors that serve to contribute to an ongoing pain, disability and suffering experience. There are various somatic, neurophysiological and psychological problems that can serve as perpetuating factors in patients with LBD. One or more of these factors may be significant in any given patient.

An algorithmic representation of the diagnostic aspect of the CRISP™ protocols can be found in Fig. 1-1. The coming chapters will clarify each point in the algorithm as well as the integration of all the clinical information gathered with the three questions of diagnosis.

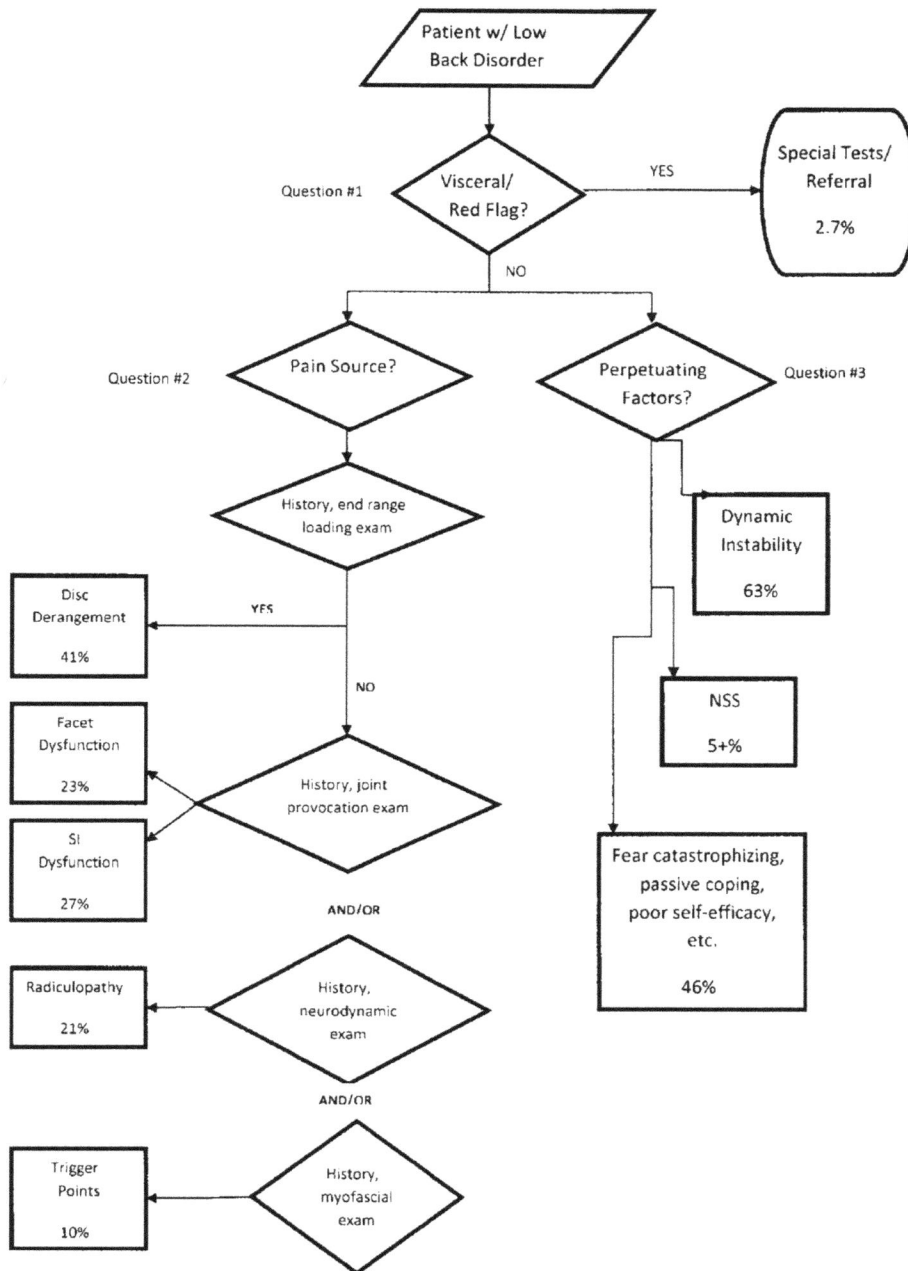

Figure 1-1. Algorithm for three questions of diagnosis using the CRISP™ protocols. The percentages reflect the frequency with which each finding was detected in a study of the CRISP™ protocols in patients with low back disorders (Murphy DR, Hurwitz EL. Application of a Diagnosis-Based Clinical Decision Guide in Patients with Low Back Pain. Chiropr Man Therap. 2011 Oct 21;19(1):26.)

Based on the answers to the three questions of diagnosis, management decisions can be made that address the key diagnostic features identified in each patient. Because of the multifactorial nature of LBDs, the management strategy will typically be multi-modal. That is, each patient will likely require a combination of treatment approaches. Critically important to the effective management of patients with LBDs, however, is the context in which the management strategy is conducted. This is addressed in great detail in Chapter 8.

An algorithmic representation of the management aspect of the CRISP™ protocols can be found in Fig. 1-2.

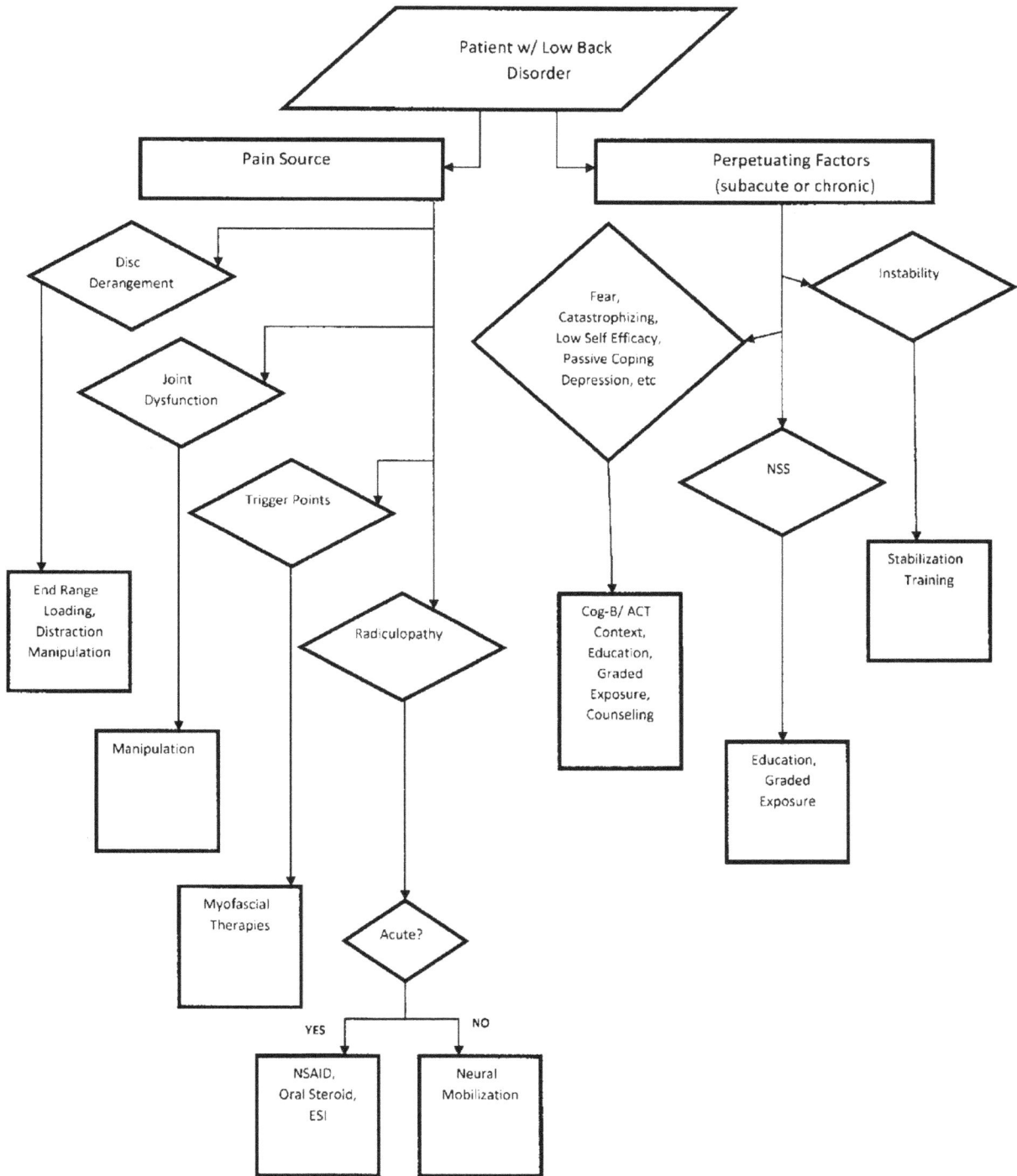

Figure 1-2. Algorithm for management decisions in response to the three questions of diagnosis.

There have been previous admirable attempts to integrate information on the diagnosis and treatment of LBDs into an approach that can help the spine practitioner move beyond generic designations such as "non-specific low back pain." Particularly interesting was the work of Laslett and van Wijman (see Recommended Reading list). These authors based their classification system on some of same scientific literature that has helped inform the CRISP™ protocols, although there are clear and striking differences in the two systems. As will be seen, the work of Laslett has been very important in the development of the CRISP™ protocols, particularly with regard to diagnostic question #2.

This book presents a practical application of the BPS model to patients with LBDs. The approach taken in the book, based on the CRISP™ protocols, is a major departure from the "supermarket" approach that is currently so common in the world of SRDs. It enables the spine practitioner to see the patient as a whole person and integrate all the various factors that can contribute to the pain, disability and suffering experience into an evidence-based clinical reasoning process. This will help lead to improved outcomes, improved patient satisfaction and improved value that is so desperately needed in the spine care world. The coming chapters will build upon the foundation established in this chapter to help the spine practitioner take an evidence-based, relationship-centered approach to the care of patients with LBDs.

Recommended Reading

Christensen CM, Grossman JH, Hwang J. The Innovator's Prescription: A Disruptive Solution for Health Care. New York: McGraw-Hill; 2009.

Cote P, Hogg-Johnson S, Cassidy JD, Carroll L, Frank JW, Bombardier C. Early aggressive care and delayed recovery from whiplash: Isolated finding or reproducible result? Arthritis Rheum 2007;57(5):861-8.

Cote P, Hogg-Johnson, S, Cassidy, D, Carroll, L, Frank, JW, Bombardier, C. Initial patterns of clinical care and recovery from whiplash injuries. Arch Intern Med 2005;165:2257-63.

Deyo RA, Mirza SK, Turner JA, Martin BI. Overtreating chronic back pain: time to back off? J Am Board Fam Med 2009;22(1):62-8.

Haldeman S. Looking forward. In: Phillips RB. The Journey of Scott Haldeman. Spine Care Specialist and Researcher. National Chiropractic Mutual Holding Company, 2009: 447-462.

Hancock MJ, Maher CG, Laslett M, Hay E, Koes B. Discussion paper: what happened to the 'bio' in the bio-psycho-social model of low back pain? Eur Spine J 2011;20(12):2105-10.

Hurwitz EL. Commentary: Exercise and spinal manipulative therapy for chronic low back pain: time to call for a moratorium on future randomized trials? Spine J 2011;11(7):599-600.

Laslett M, van Wijman P. Low back and referred pain: diagnosis and a proposed new system of classification. New Zealand J Physiother 1999;27:5-14.

Murphy DR, Hurwitz EL. Application of a Diagnosis-Based Clinical Decision Guide in Patients with Neck Pain. Chiropr Man Therap 2011;19(1):19.

Murphy DR, Hurwitz EL. Application of a Diagnosis-Based Clinical Decision Guide in Patients with Low Back Pain. Chiropr Man Therap 2011;19(1):26.

Murphy DR, Justice BD, Paskowski IC, Perle SM, Schneider MJ. The Establishment of a Primary Spine Practitioner and its Benefits to Health Care Reform in the United States. Chiropr Man Therap 2011;19(1):17.

Porter ME, Teisberg EO: Redefining Health Care: Creating Value-Based Competition on Results Boston, MA: Harvard Business School Press; 2006.

Spratt KF. Statistical relevance. In: Fardon DF, editor. Orthopaedic Knowledge Update Spine 2. Rosemont, IL: The American Academy of Orthopaedic Surgeons; 2005. p. 497-505.

Suchman AL, Sluyter DJ, Williamson PR. Leading Change in Healthcare: Transforming Organizations Using Complexity, Positive Psychology and Relationship-Centered Care. London; Radcliffe Publishing, 2011.

· CHAPTER 2 ·

The Etiology of Low Back Disorders –
The Biopsychosocial Model

While a great deal is known about the nature of low back disorders (LBDs), much still remains to be discovered regarding how they develop, what tissues become painful and why, and what perpetuates the ongoing pain, disability and suffering experience of patients with chronic LBDs. This is an area of continued research. Presented here is the theoretical model of the etiology of LBDs, upon which the CRISP™ protocols are based. This model is consistent with the current understanding of the somatic, neurophysiological, psychological and social factors that contribute to LBDs. The purpose of this chapter is to present an overview of these factors; for a more in-depth exploration, the reader is directed to the Recommended Reading list.

The Biopsychosocial Model of Understanding LBDs

The understanding of LBDs has evolved markedly over the years from a biomedical model, which attempts to explain LBDs from the standpoint of tissue pathology, with medical treatments directed to the involved tissue, to a biopsychosocial (BPS) model, which attempts to understand not just the LBD itself, but the patient who is experiencing the LBD. That is, the BPS model is one that recognizes that LBDs cannot be explained simply on the basis of an injured tissue sending nociceptive signals to the central nervous system, leading to the perception of pain. The BPS model recognizes that there is much more to the pain, disability and suffering experience than just nociception, although nociception is certainly an important part of the BPS model.

There are several factors that contribute to the pain, disability and suffering experience for which a patient seeks help. Somatic factors, neurophysiologic factors and psychological factors all contribute to the LBD experience to varying degrees. The degree to which each contributes is unique to the individual. The contributing factors all occur in the social context in which the patient lives (Fig. 2-1).

The BPS model dictates that we consider all the components, individually and as a group, in seeking an understanding of the LBD experience.

The application of the BPS model to patients with LBDs is the purpose of this book. The clinical aspects of this will be described in the coming chapters. This chapter presents what is known about the specific individual BPS factors that can be involved in the pain, disability and suffering experience related to LBDs. It is important to be aware that for explanatory purposes the BPS nature of LBDs is broken down to its individual components. But in clinical reality there is no sharp delineation between the biological, psychological and social factors that produce the LBD experience. Any combination of these components may be present in any individual patient, and these factors interact to produce the clinical picture the spine practitioner encounters.

It is also important to be aware that the contributing factors to LBDs have proven to be extremely difficult to study. So while there are working models that help in the understanding of what happens to spinal tissues that leads to pain, and what causes perpetuation of pain beyond the period of tissue healing, there are currently no definitive answers. This chapter, and the entirety of this book, focuses on "doing the best we can with what we know at present."

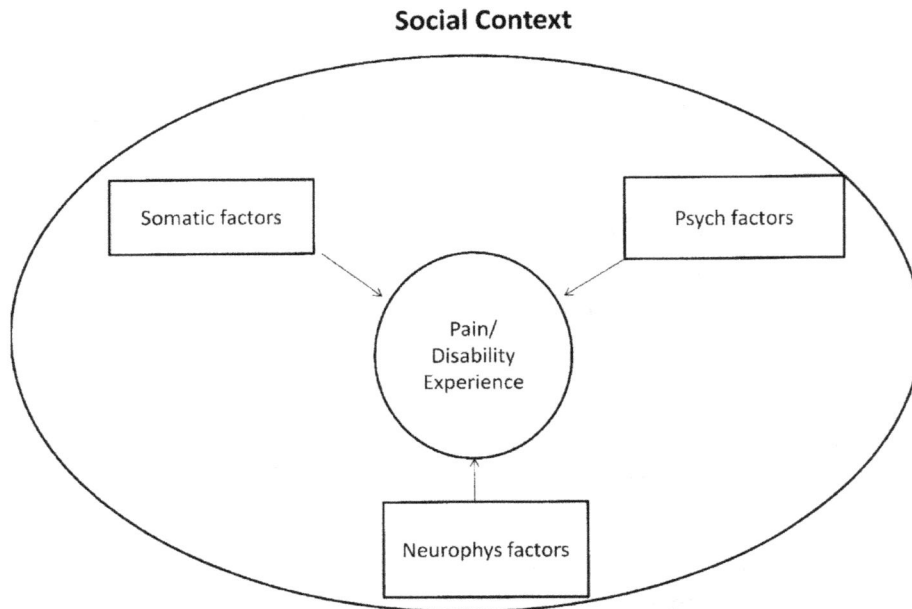

Figure 2-1. The Biopsychosocial model of low back disorders

Pathophysiologic and diagnostic labels are used to represent the various factors that are thought to contribute to LBDs. These labels are used for communication purposes however it is extremely important that the spine practitioner *avoid becoming attached to any particular label*. Again, the labels represent working models, based on the current understanding of spine pain. These labels may change over time as the research in this area evolves.

As detailed below the BPS model consists of somatic and neurophysiological factors (the "bio") and psychological factors (the "psycho") all occurring the social context in which the patient lives (the "social"). As discussed earlier, somatic factors have traditionally received the greatest attention in the spine field. Neurophysiological, psychological and social factors been appreciated more recently. It is important for the spine practitioner to understand that the LBD experience arises from the combined effect of the individual BPS components.

It is also important to understand that the somatic pain generating tissues – the peripheral sources of nociception – only create the potential for the development of a pain, disability and suffering experience. Whether the nociception that is arising from a certain tissue is actually experienced by the patient, and the impact the nociception has on the patient's life, is determined in the central nervous system (CNS). Discs, joints, nerve roots and muscles do not feel pain. Human beings feel pain. And when a human being feels pain, the impact the pain has on his or her life will depend on a number of factors, neurophysiological and psychological, that occur within the CNS. It is important for the spine practitioner to keep this in mind in studying spine related disorders (SRDs), as this will help maintain an appropriate perspective that will be passed on to patients.

The "Bio"

The biological factors that contribute to LBDs come in two forms – somatic factors and neurophysiological factors.

Somatic factors

Disc derangement

This is the diagnostic label that is applied to pain that arises from the intervertebral disc. It is important to distinguish disc pain from nerve root pain that results from a disc herniation (detailed below).

In the latter case, the nerve root is the pain generating tissue, though in most cases of radiculopathy secondary to disc herniation the disc itself also contributes to the pain.

Disc derangement is believed to arise from tears that develop in the annulus fibrosis that allow migration of nuclear material into the periphery of the disc. Circumferential tears develop in the annulus fibrosis that can later coalesce to form radial tears. The radial tears gradually become larger and may extend from the periphery of the annulus to the nucleus. Disc derangement results from nuclear material migrating into a radial tear (Fig. 2-2). It is believed that because of the chemical makeup of the nuclear material the presence of this material in the periphery of the disc causes an inflammatory reaction, leading to pain. Disc derangement is caused by repetitive flexion movements. It is thought that tens of thousands of cycles of flexion is required to produce derangement. If compression is added to these cycles, fewer total cycles are required. It is possible that torsion, resulting from rotational movements, also contributes.

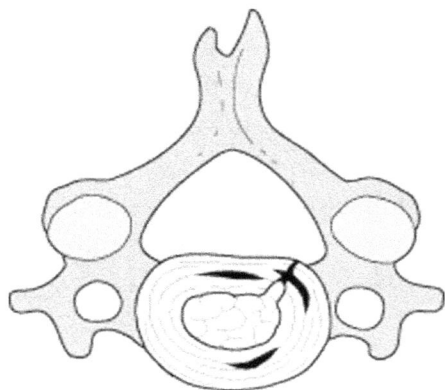

Figure 2-2. Migration of nuclear material into a radial tear creating a disc derangement. Note that this is a cervical segment and not a lumbar segment. Reprinted with permission from Murphy DR, ed. Conservative Management of Cervical Spine Syndromes. New York: McGraw-Hill, 2000.

If the nuclear migration into a radial tear is sudden, it may be symptomatic, creating an acute disc derangement. However, if the migration occurs gradually, it may be well accommodated and thus can be asymptomatic. When the tear becomes nearly complete, it may require only a mild flexion/compression force to break though the remaining annular fibers and allow the nucleus to enter the lateral canal, resulting in disc herniation. This can cause radiculopathy (see below).

Joint dysfunction

Joint dysfunction has traditionally been identified in the chiropractic profession by the term "subluxation." Many in the chiropractic profession continue to use this term. Other terms have been used by various practitioners and practitioner groups such as "somatic dysfunction", "joint blockage" and "joint fixation." The prevailing theory for the development and perpetuation of joint pain in the spine is that of "dysafferentation", a term coined by Seaman and Winterstein (see Recommended Reading list).

In order to understand the theory of dysafferentation it is important to understand the role that mechanoreceptors play in the inhibition of nociceptive input. There are two general classes of neurologic receptors embedded in peripheral tissues - mechanoreceptors and nociceptors. Mechanoreceptors respond to mechanical events such as touch, stretch or tension. Nociceptors respond to noxious stimulation, which can potentially lead to the experience of pain.

As can be seen in Fig. 2-3 when nociceptive signals arise from any peripheral tissue (not only a joint), they are transmitted by small diameter afferent fibers to the dorsal horn. In the dorsal horn the nociceptive afferent axon synapses, either directly or indirectly through an interneuron, to a projection neuron that then projects the nociceptive signal to the thalamus. From the thalamus the signal is relayed to several areas in the cerebral cortex, where the experience of pain is created.

One of the functions of afferent input from mechanoreceptors is to presynaptically inhibit the projection neuron, directly via synapse with the projection neuron and indirectly through the same interneuron network that contributed to the transmission of nociceptive input. This serves the purpose of modulating the projection of nociceptive information to the thalamus, and ultimately to the cortex. A pain-free

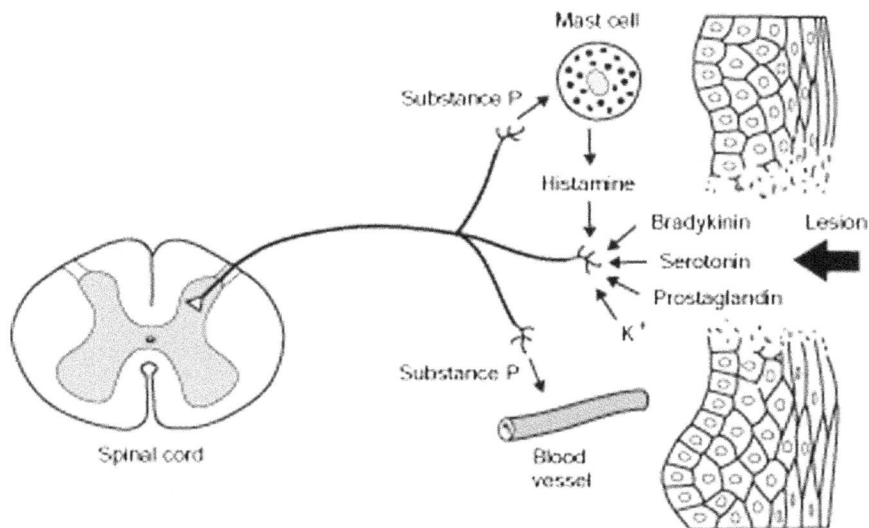

Figure 2-3. Transmission of nociceptive signals to the do rsal horn. Reprinted with permission from Murphy DR, ed. Conservative Management of Cervical Spine Syndromes. New York: McGraw-Hill, 2000.

state of a joint is determined, in part, by appropriate balance between nociceptive input and mechano-receptive input. This process is depicted in Fig. 2-4.

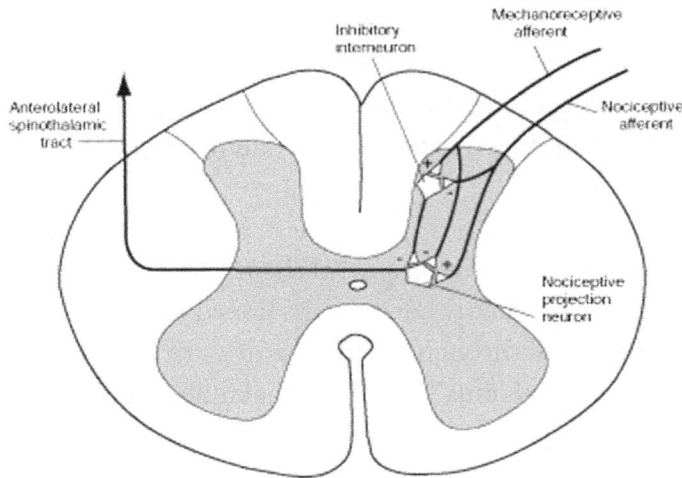

Figure 2-4. Presynaptic inhibition of the nociceptive projection neuron in the dorsal horn as a result of mechanoreceptive input. Reprinted with permission from Murphy DR, ed. Conservative Management of Cervical Spine Syndromes. New York: McGraw-Hill, 2000.

According to dysafferentation theory, an abnormality in the movement of a joint results in imbalance between the input from the mechanoreceptors related to the joint (particularly joint mechanoreceptors and muscle spindles) and the nociceptors related to the joint. This imbalance occurs in the form of a relative decrease in the input from mechanoreceptors and a relative increase in the input from nociceptors. This disruption in the balance between mechanoreceptive and nociceptive input decreases the presynaptic inhibition of the nociceptive projection neuron in the dorsal horn. This, in turn, leads to increased likelihood that the individual will experience pain from the involved joint.

The presence of dysafferentation does not necessarily guarantee that the individual will experience pain. This is because, as will be seen later in this chapter, there is much more that determines the experience of pain than nociceptive input alone.

Radiculopathy

Radiculopathy is a pathologic process involving a nerve root. It is a commonly misused term as it is often used for any condition in which pain from the back radiates into the lower extremity. Therefore it is important that the spine practitioner only use this term when clinical findings implicate the nerve root as a generator of pain or other symptoms and signs. The most common causes of radiculopathy are *spinal stenosis* and *disc herniation*.

Spinal stenosis is a process in which, due to degenerative changes that occur with ageing, osteophytes form on the vertebral body and facet joints and the ligamentum flavum hypertrophies. Depending on the extent and location of these degenerative changes, bony or ligamentous encroachment can occur in the lateral canal or lateral recess (lateral stenosis - see Fig. 2-5) or in the central canal (central stenosis – see Fig. 2-6).

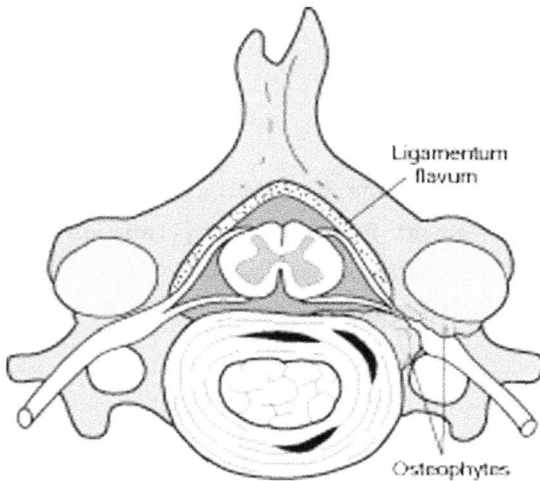

Figure 2-5. Lateral stenosis. Note that this is a cervical segment and not a lumbar segment. Reprinted with permission from Murphy DR, ed. Conservative Management of Cervical Spine Syndromes. New York: McGraw-Hill, 2000.

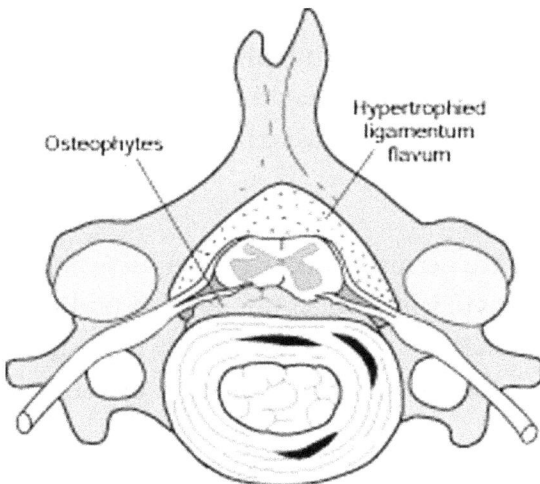

Figure 2-6. Central stenosis. Note that this is a cervical segment and not a lumbar segment. Reprinted with permission from Murphy DR, ed. Conservative Management of Cervical Spine Syndromes. New York: McGraw-Hill, 2000.

Disc herniation is a process in which a portion of the nuclear material inside the disc herniates through the annulus. If the nuclear material approximates the outermost annular fibers, it can lead to a focal outpocketing (*protrusion*). The nuclear material can rupture completely through the outer annular fibers, resulting in an *extrusion* (Fig. 2-7). Uncommonly a piece of the nuclear material can become displaced from the remainder of the nucleus, resulting in a *sequestration*.

Any of these types of disc herniation can cause chemical irritation and/or compression of the nerve root.

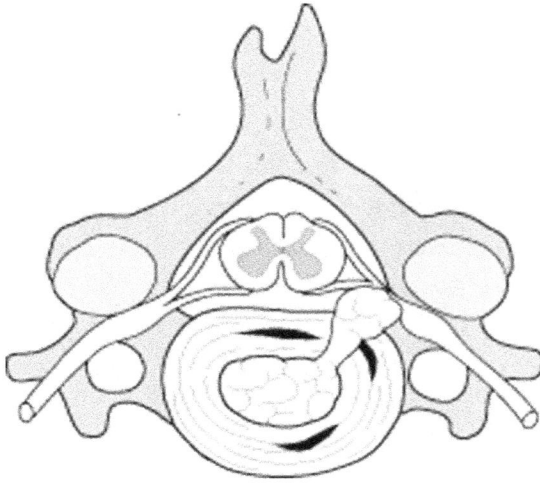

Figure 2-7. Disc extrusion. Note that this is a cervical segment and not a lumbar segment. Reprinted with permission from Murphy DR, ed. Conservative Management of Cervical Spine Syndromes. New York: McGraw-Hill, 2000.

The mechanism of pain generation with acute radiculopathy primarily relates to inflammation, i.e., the pain is largely chemical in nature. Acute radiculopathy most commonly results from disc herniation. The presence of nuclear material in the lateral recess or lateral canal leads to the release inflammatory cytokines such as interleukin-1 beta, interleukin-6, tumor necrosis factor, and other chemicals that cause the nerve root to become painful.

Eventually, the acute inflammatory process resolves. In addition, the herniated nuclear material eventually desiccates, as a result becoming smaller in size. But there are times in which adhesions develop, leading to adherence of the nerve root to the herniated material. If these adhesions reduce the mobility of the nerve root, tension and/or compression of the nerve root can occur during movement of the lower extremity.

The mechanism of chronic radiculopathy is one of congestion and adhesions (although there is likely some residual inflammatory process as well). This can result either from spinal stenosis or from long-standing disc herniation. Encroachment on the nerve root from bone, ligament and/or disc material can lead to vascular congestion, ischemia, and intraneural edema which in turn leads to periradicular fibrosis. As with the adhesions that can develop after acute radiculopathy from disc herniation, the periradicular fibrosis can cause reduction of nerve root mobility during movement of the lower extremity. It is likely that this is at least one of the mechanisms of neurogenic claudication, the classic symptom of radiculopathy related to spinal stenosis.

Myofascial Pain

Myofascial pain is thought to arise from myofascial trigger points. Simons, et al (see Recommended Reading list) define a myofascial trigger point (TrP) as "a hyperirritable spot in a skeletal muscle that is associated with a hypersensitive palpable nodule in a taut band. The spot is painful on compression and can give rise to characteristic referred pain, referred tenderness, motor dysfunction and autonomic phenomena."

The development of a TrP begins with a localized shortening of a fascicle of muscle fibers in which a group of sarcomeres remain in a state of contracture rather than returning to their normal resting length (Fig. 2-8). This contracture can be palpated as a "taut band." TrPs result from the development of a focal area of metabolic distress in which the shortening of sarcomeres causes disruption of vascular supply to the area. This leads to a chemical cascade resulting in the depolarization of nociceptors in that part of the muscle.

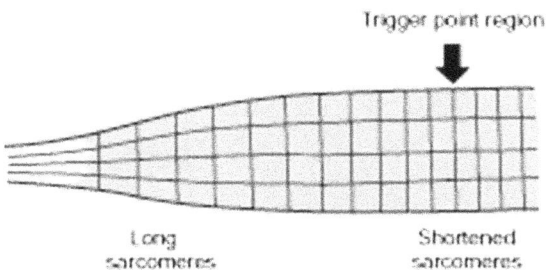

Figure 2-8. A myofascial trigger point. Reprinted with permission from Murphy DR, ed. Conservative Management of Cervical Spine Syndromes. New York: McGraw-Hill, 2000. Adapted from Simons DG. Myofascial pain syndrome due to trigger points. In: Goodgold J, ed. Rehabilitation Medicine. St. Louis: Mosby; 1988:686-723.

Neurophysiological factors

Dynamic and passive instability

Spine stability results from a combination of passive and dynamic mechanisms. The purpose of these mechanisms is to provide protection to the spine in response to the common perturbations that result from daily activities. In peripheral joints such as the shoulder and knee, passive mechanisms are most important in providing stability. However the spine is different from these peripheral joints in that it is surrounded by a vast array of muscles. Thus, dynamic mechanisms take on much greater importance in stabilizing the spine.

According to Panjabi (see Recommended Reading list) there are three subsystems that interact to provide the spine with the necessary stability to avoid injury (Fig. 2-9). These are:

1. The active subsystem: Spinal muscles.

2. The control subsystem: Mechanoreceptors in the ligaments, joint capsules and muscles of the spine along with the neural control centers in the CNS.

3. The passive subsystem: Ligaments, joint capsules, bones, facet joints, discs and the passive mechanical properties of muscles.

The active and neural control subsystems provide dynamic stability, i.e. dynamic responses to forces that act on the spine and that have the potential to cause injury. The passive subsystem provides passive stability, i.e. preventing excessive motion at end range in much the same way as occurs in peripheral joints.

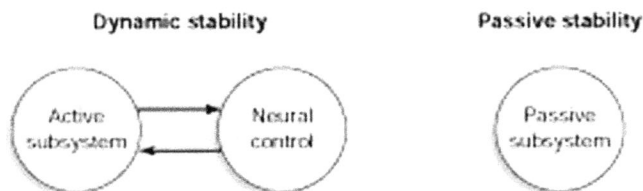

Figure 2-9. The three subsystems of spine stability. Reprinted with permission from Murphy DR, ed. Conservative Management of Cervical Spine Syndromes. New York: McGraw-Hill, 2000. Adapted from Panjabi MM. The stabilizing system of the spine. Part I. Function, dysfunction, adaptation and enhancement. J Spinal Disord 1992; 5(4):383-389.

The manner in which the dynamic stabilization system works is depicted in Fig. 2-10. When the spine is subjected to a perturbation that may have the potential to cause injury, this is detected by the mechanoreceptors in the tissues involved and information regarding the amplitude and acceleration of that perturbation is sent into the neural control center (the CNS). Based on this information the neural control center makes a determination as to what pattern of muscle contraction is required by the spinal muscles to respond appropriately to the perturbation, to provide protection to the spine. The muscles then report back to the neural control center regarding what action was taken. This, of course, all happens in a fraction of a second; any delay in this response may subject the spine to injury.

Dynamic instability

If the dynamic stability mechanism functions efficiently, the spine remains well protected against most common perturbations. However, dysfunction in this system reduces the efficiency of the response, leading to *dynamic instability*. Dynamic instability may then serve as a perpetuating factor to the generation of pain from the discs, joints, nerve roots or muscles as a result of inadequate protection of these tissues against repetitive microtrauma.

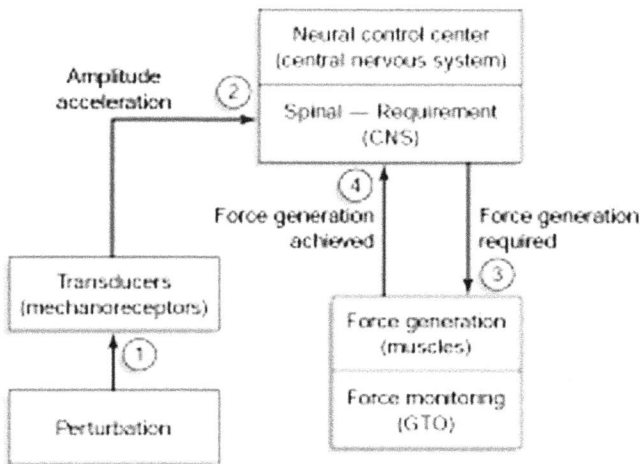

Figure 2-10. The mechanism of dynamic stability of the spine. Reprinted with permission from Murphy DR, ed. Conservative Management of Cervical Spine Syndromes. New York: McGraw-Hill, 2000. Adapted from Panjabi MM. The stabilizing system of the spine. Part I. Function, dysfunction, adaptation and enhancement. J Spinal Disord 1992; 5(4):383-389.

For reasons that currently are unknown, the pattern of dysfunction that appears to occur with dynamic instability in the lumbar spine commonly involves inhibition of the transverse abdominis and multifidis muscles, i.e., delayed and diminished activation of these muscles. Some have misinterpreted this as indicating that these muscles are more important in dynamic stability mechanisms and rehabilitation than the other spinal muscles. However, this is a mistake. All spinal muscles play important individual roles in providing dynamic stability. Ultimately it is the harmonious action of the entire dynamic stability system is the key. However, as will be discussed in Chapter 11, particular attention must be paid to the transverse abdominis and multifidis muscles in the early stages of rehabilitation because of the inhibition of these muscles that occurs with dynamic instability.

Passive instability

The passive subsystem plays a lesser role in the spine than in extremity joints in which there generally are no muscle bellies that directly cross the joint to provide dynamic stability. However, in uncommon cases, particularly when acute, severe ligamentous injury or profound degenerative changes have compromised the holding capacity of the passive structures, *passive instability* can occur. Passive instability can be equated with what is sometimes referred to as "ligamentous instability." With passive instability the passive subsystem fails, resulting in excessive movement at end range or excessive translation of the spinal segment.

Nociceptive system sensitization

Nociceptive system sensitization (NSS) is a condition in which the nociceptive system becomes hypersensitive, thus intensifying the patient's experience of pain. There are several mechanisms by which this state develops and these mechanisms gradually evolve over time.

Acute spinal pain is initiated in the periphery as a result of injury and inflammation of one or more tissues (Fig. 2-3). When a certain tissue in the spine is injured or irritated, be it disc, joint capsule, nerve root or muscle, a variety of chemicals are released from the injured tissue and from the nociceptive receptors that innervated the tissue. These chemicals include substance P, bradykinin, serotonin, prostaglandin E2, potassium ions and histamine. The chemicals cause sensitization and depolarization of small diameter fibers (i.e. nociception). As discussed above with regard to joint dysfunction, the nociceptive signal is transmitted to the dorsal horn and projected to the thalamus to be relayed to higher centers where it may or may not be experienced as pain.

This acute chemical phenomenon generally resolves over time by natural history. In most cases, once this process resolves the pain ceases. However there are some patients in whom chronic pain develops that cannot be explained purely the basis of peripheral tissue injury. This occurs, in part, as a result of NSS.

NSS results from changes in both the peripheral and central nervous system.

Peripheral mechanisms of NSS

1. The awakening of "silent nociceptors": These are receptors that lie within the joint capsule that do not normally respond to mechanical stimulation. In the presence of chemical sensitization resulting from tissue damage and inflammation, they can "awaken" and become responsive, even to normal movement.

2. "Hyperalgesic priming" of nociceptive receptors: This also results from the acute inflammatory process. It involves the presence of protein kinase C, which "primes" the nociceptive afferent

fiber to be increasingly responsive to subsequent nociceptive input, even that which would ordinarily not be experienced as painful.

Central mechanisms of NSS

1. Sensitization of dorsal horn neurons: Sensitization of neurons is a process by which an increase in membrane excitability and synaptic efficacy, along with reduced inhibition, results in facilitation, potentiation, augmentation and amplification of nociceptive signals. This can result either from an acute bombardment of nociceptive signals, such as can occur with acute trauma, or from lower intensity but persistent nociceptive input. The dorsal horn neurons that receive nociceptive signals and project them to higher centers can become sensitized; they become increasingly responsive to subsequent nociceptive input. In some cases these neurons, once sensitized, will also start transmitting non-nociceptive input (i.e. mechanoreceptive input) as if it were nociceptive, potentially causing normal movements to be perceived as painful.

2. Sensitization of thalamic neurons: It was once thought that the thalamus was simply a passive relay station, where all sensory information from the periphery (with the exception of the sense of smell) was received and relayed to various areas of the cerebral cortex. However recent evidence suggests that thalamic neurons can also become sensitized as a result of intense or persistent nociceptive input. When this occurs these neurons amplify nociceptive signals prior to relaying them to the cortex. This causes the nociceptive information received by cortical centers to be of significantly higher intensity than that originally projected to the thalamus.

3. Sensitization of cortical neurons: Ronald Melzack (see Recommended Reading list) introduced the concept of the "neuromatrix", the network of neurons in various cortical centers that are involved in the perception and localization of pain as well as the determination of the emotional and behavioral response to pain. As with the other neurons involved in the experience of pain, these neurons can become sensitized in response to an acute pain episode or persistent nociceptive input. The sensitization of these neurons leads to a heightened pain experience as well as intensification of emotional responses and pain behavior.

4. Cortical reorganization: In patients with chronic LBDs reorganization of the cortical representation of the low back in the somatosensory cortex can take place. The representation of the low back expands to occupy a wider area of the somatosensory cortex and shifts to the left to invade the area that represents the lower extremity.

5. Structural changes in the brain: This includes a decrease of gray matter in the cingulate cortex, orbitofrontal cortex, insula and dorsal pons.

6. Dysfunction of descending inhibitory mechanisms: There are descending pathways from higher centers that serve to modulate nociceptive transmission and maintain a pain free state. This descending influence arises from a variety of centers but the central focus of this system is the periaqueductal gray area (PAG) of the midbrain. This system is illustrated in Fig. 2-12.

7. Expansion of receptive fields: Intense and/or persistent nociceptive input can also cause increase in the receptive fields of dorsal horn cells. As a result, these cells become capable of responding to input from a greater number of incoming afferent fibers, and a greater variety of types of stimuli. This leads to the development of referred pain. A normal dorsal horn neuron contains a receptive field for a certain area of the body. But as a result of intense and/or persistent nociceptive input, previously dormant receptive fields of that neuron can awaken to tissues that may be remote from the neuron's normal receptive field. Thus the patient can experience pain that appears to be arising from the remote tissue.

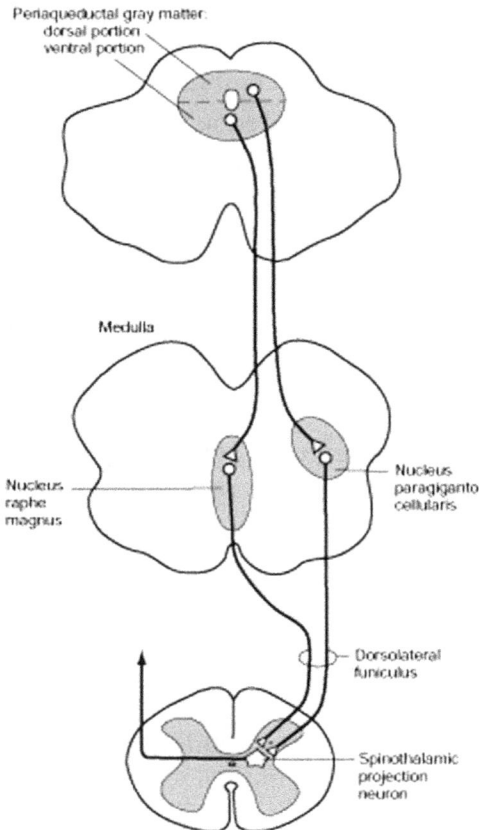

Figure 2-11. The descending nociceptive inhibitory system. Reprinted with permission from Murphy DR, ed. Conservative Management of Cervical Spine Syndromes. New York: McGraw-Hill, 2000.

Both the peripheral and central mechanisms of NSS require ongoing nociceptive input from the periphery in order to maintain the chronic pain state. This ongoing input arises from persistent nociceptive signals from the primary pain generator (disc derangement, joint dysfunction, radiculopathy, TrPs) as well as from circulating pro-inflammatory cytokines in the blood.

It is important to note that there is great interaction between NSS and the psychological factors, discussed in the next section, that serve to perpetuate the ongoing pain experience. Psychological distress reinforces and exacerbates the sensitization of the CNS neurons involved in the experience of pain as well as dysfunction of the descending nociceptive inhibitory system. In addition, focusing on pain relief in lieu of improvement of functional abilities actually reinforces NSS. This critical point will be discussed further in the next section as well as in Chapters 5 and 8. It should also be pointed out that chronic use of narcotic and opioid medications can facilitate NSS.

It is likely that in any patient in whom pain continues beyond the duration of time required for tissue healing (i.e., the patient whose condition becomes subacute or chronic) has some degree of NSS. However there are varying degrees of severity of NSS, depending on the case.

NSS leaves the patient in a state in which the pain experience is disproportionate to the intensity of the nociceptive stimulus arising from the spine. As patients generally have no reason not to "believe" what their nociceptive system is "telling" them, their interpretation of the significance of the pain is similarly disproportionate to the actual physical condition. NSS can contribute to fear and catastrophizing (see below) as, particularly when the NSS is severe, the nociceptive system is essentially "telling" the patient that he or she has ongoing severe tissue damage, which the patient naturally interprets as a fearsome catastrophe.

The "Psycho"

A variety of psychological factors have been recognized as playing an important role in the perpetuation of the pain, disability and suffering experience of patients with SRDs. These are sometimes referred to as "yellow flags." The understanding of these processes and the role they play is essential in helping patients overcome LBDs. A detailed discussion of every factor that can contribute is beyond the scope of this book. Presented here is the essential information regarding the key factors that the spine practitioner must be aware of. It is important to note that these factors are not necessarily "black or white." That is, one or more of these factors can be present to a greater or lesser degree in any particular patient and at any point in time. Also, there is great overlap and interaction between these psychological factors and it is essential for the spine practitioner to understand the role that these factors play in the overall clinical picture. In addition, as stated earlier, there is often a significant relationship between the presence of NSS and these psychological factors. Finally, a certain amount of distress in a LBD patient is normal and appropriate. It is only when emotional and psychological processes become maladaptive or interfere with recover that they become a problem to be addressed.

The following factors represent the "Big 5" psychological factors in LBD patients:

1. Fear

2. Catastrophizing

3. Passive coping

4. Poor self-efficacy

5. Depression

Fear

This is sometimes referred to as fear-avoidance and is a process in which the patient develops beliefs about the pain that lead him or her to become fearful, particularly regarding movement and activity. Fear is a natural emotion that can be useful at times, but in some situations it can be maladaptive. LBD patients often develop inaccurate or unrealistic beliefs about their pain and its relation to movement and activity. Often the fear revolves around the belief that if the patient were to engage in normal movements or activities he or she would "worsen" the "damage" in the spine. This is certainly an understandable and natural fear but, first, in the vast majority of cases it is inaccurate and, second, the fear itself can interfere with recovery.

Fear leads to avoidance of normal activities of daily living, as well as activities that would be helpful in overcoming the LBD. This leads to the development of chronic pain, disability and suffering and also leads to depression, as will be discussed later. Further, fear imparts upon the pain a power that it would not otherwise possess. Giving it such power causes the pain, disability and suffering experience to become more intense and all-encompassing, further reinforcing the fear and causing the LBD to appear to be a catastrophic problem.

Catastrophizing

Catastrophizing occurs when the patient dwells on the most negative possible outcomes of the LBD. In the case of patients with LBD this means dwelling on the thought that the presence of pain in the spine is an indication that something is seriously wrong and that the patient is doomed to suffer continuously because of the disorder.

If a patient believes that the LBD is a catastrophe, it is likely that this will be his or her experience. The patient will tend to experience everything related to the pain through that lens, with each experience reinforcing the belief. This leads to chronic pain, depression (see below) and further avoidance of activities.

Passive coping

There are different methods or styles that people use to cope with any problem. In the case of LBDs, patients can either cope in a relatively active manner or a relatively passive manner. An active coping strategy is one in which the patient actively confronts the pain. With active coping the patient seeks to maintain as normal a level of function as possible despite the presence of pain, distracts him- or herself from the pain by engaging in meaningful activities and seeks to return to a normal level of activity. A passive coping strategy is one in which the patient tries to avoid discomfort, depends on others for pain control, engages in behaviors that reflect seeking relief of pain in lieu of restoration of function and allows the pain to dictate behavior by avoiding any activity that may be perceived as having the potential to cause "harm."

Passive coping strategies lead to the development of chronicity by reinforcing the belief on the part of the patient that the only solution to the suffering is to reduce and/or eliminate the pain. So the pain (or at least the patient's interpretation of it), rather than functional abilities, becomes the major focus. As was discussed regarding fear, this puts the pain in a position of power that it would not otherwise posses because, in the patient's mind, the ability to function is determined by the presence or absence of pain, and thus is not in his or her control. Furthermore, passive coping actually *increases* pain perception by enhancing certain aspects of NSS. In addition, by avoiding activities that may provoke the pain the patient becomes deconditioned, further perpetuating chronic pain.

Poor self-efficacy

Self-efficacy is the confidence that one has in one's ability to perform a task or overcome a problem. In the case of the patient with a LBD, it is the confidence that he or she has in overcoming the disorder.

This may be the most important of the psychological processes discussed here. It is important to note that self-efficacy is not a fixed character trait. That is, a person can have a great deal of self-efficacy with regard to his or her ability to perform a certain task or overcome a certain problem, but very little self-efficacy with regard to performing another task or overcoming another problem. So a LBD patient may have very little self-efficacy when it comes to overcoming the LBD but may have a great deal of self-efficacy regarding, say, his or her ability to repair an automobile that is not running properly or to prepare a six course meal. This is important because it illustrates the fact that poor self-efficacy related to overcoming a LBD is not a character flaw and can improve with the proper experiential "training" and practice.

Naturally, a great deal of confidence in dealing with a problem increases the likelihood of success in overcoming that problem. In the LBD patient, poor self-efficacy with regard to the ability to overcome the LBD and return to normal activities perpetuates the pain, suffering and disability experience because it results in feelings of helplessness and hopelessness, depression and fear-avoidance. It also reinforces the cognition that the LBD is a fearsome catastrophe. After all if it were not, the patient would have confidence in overcoming the problem.

Depression

Depression, in general, is a mood disturbance in which the patient feels a sense of despair and hopelessness in the face of the LBD, resulting in a negative affect and a negative outlook regarding the problem. Depression can lead to decreased motivation, passivity and social withdrawal, all of which perpetuate the LBD.

However, in the context of LBDs depression is more complex than the other psychological perpetuating factors discussed here. Like the other factors, depression can be a part of the psychological and emotional reaction to the pain, i.e., a maladaptive response that, while understandable and "normal", can interfere with recovery. But depression can also be a diagnosable health condition that is often part of a more general pattern of ill-health that can include other chronic illnesses such as obesity, metabolic syndrome, hypertension (along with other risk factors for cardiovascular disease and stroke), type 2 diabetes and chronic LBD.

In addition to the "Big 5", there are other psychological processes of importance in intensifying and perpetuating the pain, disability and suffering experience.

Perceived injustice

This construct is one in which the patient perceives that their basic human rights have been unfairly violated, irreparable loss has occurred, people do not understand how severe the suffering is and, importantly, that this injustice is *someone else's fault*. It is particularly relevant in the subset of patients whose pain began following a work-related incident, a motor vehicle collision (in which another driver is considered "at fault") or a slip-and-fall incident that occurs on someone else's property. Perceived injustice is closely related to catastrophizing and likely compounds catastrophizing in that, in the mind of the patient, it is bad enough to be experiencing a catastrophe but, to make matters worse, "someone did this to me."

Perceived injustice leads to heightened disability in part due to its association with catastrophizing but also in part because in patients affected, disability may be perceived as the only "power" of retribution they have against the perceived perpetrator of the injustice.

Cognitive fusion

This occurs when one's assumptions, beliefs and cognitions about the world become "fused" with one's experience of reality. Applied to the patient with LBD, this is a phenomenon in which, rather than experiencing the pain as an objective fact, the patient views it through the lens of his or her assumptions about the pain ("the pain is an indication of something seriously wrong"), beliefs about the nature of pain in general ("pain is always a reason to stop activity") and cognitions about the pain ("it feels like something is being pinched in my back"). As a result, the patient's experience of the "reality" of the LBD is consistent with these assumptions, beliefs and cognitions. This is an important process in the LBD patient because even if these assumptions, beliefs and cognitions are completely inconsistent with the true nature of the problem, as far as the patient's experience is concerned, the LBD will be as catastrophically painful and disabling as the mind has decided.

Hypervigilance for symptoms

This occurs when the patient focuses on the pain, as filtered through the patient's assumptions, beliefs and cognitions, along with on those things in the environment that the patient perceives as a threat. Further, the patient cognitively prioritizes sensations he or she perceives as being related to the pain so that an experience or sensation that would normally be perceived in a neutral fashion becomes anxiety-provoking. Critical with regard to this is the fact that continually seeking pain relief in lieu of increasing functional abilities actually intensifies the pain by enhancing NSS, as discussed earlier, and by encouraging hypervigilance. This will be discussed further in Chapters 5 and 8.

Anxiety

This is similar to fear except that it relates to the future and is less specific than fear. For the LBD patient anxiety relates to emotional distress about potential future threats to the patient's well-being. This is tied in with hypervigilance as the patient tends to scan the environment for threatening stimuli. Like fear, anxiety leads to avoidance, which temporarily relieves the anxiety but ultimately leads to intensification of the pain experience because, first, avoidance leads to disuse and deconditioning, second the patient does not give him- or herself an opportunity to desensitize to environmental stimuli (see Chapter 11) and, third, the patient confirms in his or her mind that the pain is reflective of a fearsome catastrophe – otherwise why would the patient have to avoid normal activities?

The "Social"

The "social" aspect of the BPS model consists of the social context in which the LBD occurs and the effect this has on the pain, disability and suffering experience that results. These factors are sometimes referred to as "blue flags" and "black flags." There are several important aspects of the social context that have a potential impact on recovery or perpetuation of the problem.

Work

Work is an important part of life. It is not only a means by which people can support themselves and their families, it is essential for health and well being. Involvement in meaningful and fulfilling work has a positive impact on psychological and physical health. This is true for a number of reasons. Meaningful work provides:

- A sense of purpose and meaning to a person's daily life

- A sense of financial security

- An opportunity to pursue, as Pink has described (see Recommended Reading list) autonomy, mastery and purpose

- Physical and mental activity

- A sense of identity

- Structure

- An opportunity to be creative

- A source of social interaction and support

On the other hand, lack of meaningful work can have detrimental effects on health. Being out of work, or working in an environment that is unsatisfying and does not provide the opportunity for autonomy, mastery and purpose, places patients at risk of developing chronic pain. This is one of the reasons, as will be discussed in later chapters, that early and rapid return to work is so important in patients with LBDs, particularly in cases in which the problem started at work.

Issues related to work have an important impact on recovery from a LBD. These include high physical demands of the job, low job satisfaction, lack of communication with coworkers and the perception that the job is very "stressful." Perhaps the most important work related factors, particularly in patients who are out of work due to a LBD, are low expectation or confidence in being able to return to work and lack of job accommodations or modified work.

Needless disability

It is common for patients with LBDs to be "put on disability" despite the fact that they are capable of engaging in meaningful work. This is often the result of well-meaning health care providers or others who recommend that work be avoided in order to prevent the problem from getting worse. The recommendation to avoid work is often based on erroneous assumptions about the spine, particularly in light of benign imaging findings such as "disc bulge" or "disc degeneration." These erroneous assumptions are often imparted on the patient. This can not only contribute to needless disability but also to fear, catastrophizing, poor self-efficacy and passive coping (see the discussion of "iatrogenic imaging disability" in Chapter 9).

Needless disability is one of the most powerful risk factors for the development of chronic LBDs. The vast majority of patients with LBDs can engage in some form of work. Even if a patient is temporarily unable to perform his or her normal job duties, there are almost always modifications that can be made. It is important for patients to be given the opportunity to experience the benefits of meaningful work while avoiding irritating a (temporarily) inflamed tissue.

Home life

A difficult home life can arise from problems with spousal or child relationships, financial pressures or a multitude of other factors. These can have a negative impact on health due to the stress that it produces as well as by taking the patient's focus away from addressing the LBD. In addition, social support (see below) is important in overcoming a LBD and the most important source of social support is one's life partner.

Social support

The social support system can include family, friends, work superiors and coworkers. Social support provides people with a means to confide in someone, to share problems and concerns and to receive feedback on potential solutions. The lack of effective social support can be of great detriment in overcoming any problem of life, particularly a health problem such as a LBD.

The "Pain Partner"

There are times when a significant other, such as a spouse, can be a crucial source of social support that helps the patient cope effectively with, and ultimately overcome, a LBD. However there are also times in which the significant other can interfere with recovery by, on the one hand, being excessively punitive about a patient's pain and pain behavior or, on the other, excessively reinforcing pain behavior as well as the sick role.

Lack of meaningful relationships

In some cases the LBD patient may be lacking in meaningful relationships. These patients do not have a strong social support system. They also do not have someone who can provided assistance with home and work activities, exercises and self-care strategies and health care visits. Meaningful relationships include not only personal relationships such as those with a spouse and other family members but also with friends and coworkers.

Litigation

It is common for patients with LBDs to be involved in some form of litigation. These are often cases in which the LBD began during the course of employment, from a motor vehicle collision or from a slip-and-fall incident. These patients are often dismissed as having issues of "secondary gain" and at times are even labeled "malingerers." While there are rare cases in which an individual literally fakes an injury for the purpose of making money, in the vast majority of cases the patient's pain is real. However, the litigation process brings a level of complexity and suspicion to the case that is not present in non-litigated situations.

Patients who are involved in litigation often feel as if they are put in a position to have to "prove" they are really in pain. This almost invariably increases pain behavior, which in turn can increase the intensity of the pain, disability and suffering experience. If a patient is receiving disability payments, this brings an addition level of fear (in addition to the fear of "re-injury") to the return-to-work process because patients are often nervous about giving up these payments when they are unsure of their ability to successfully transition back to work.

The litigation process is, almost by definition, adversarial. It forces the patient to consider the LBD as being someone else's "fault." This often leads to perceived injustice on the part of the patient, i.e., that he or she would not be suffering if it were not for the negligence of the other party. Justified or not, this can have a large detrimental effect on recovery.

Some of the social factors discussed here are not diagnostic *per se*. These factors may not be within the spine practitioner's ability to influence. However, it is important to understand all of the contributing factors in the context of the patient's social environment in order to fully understand the patient and the pain, disability and suffering experience.

Chronic LBD as Part of a Generalized Pattern of Ill Health

It is becoming clear that LBDs, particularly when they become chronic, do not necessarily occur in isolation but are often a part of a larger picture of ill health. The coexistence and interaction between chronic LBDs and other chronic problems such as depression and obesity as well as arthritis, headache and other chronic pain complaints makes it clear that LBDs must be viewed in a more global context than previously appreciated. Consideration of common factors linking these various disorders, such as chronic inflammation, poor nutrition and sleep, inactivity and a generalized unhealthy lifestyle must be a part of the conceptualization of LBDs and their management. This is discussed further in Chapter 9.

It can be seen that LBDs are a complex mix of somatic, psychological and social factors that converge to produce the pain, disability and suffering experience of each patient. However, as was stated at the beginning of this chapter, it is important to see LBDs not as a collection of individual factors that occur in isolation but rather as an integrated whole. The different BPS factors interrelate to produce the particular LBD that any individual experiences. Thus it is essential that the practitioner "think globally and act locally" when it comes to patient management. That is, the particular therapeutic processes that the practitioner undergoes in helping the patient overcome the LBD may be directed toward individual components of the problem, but the "big picture" that is provided by the BPS model must always be kept in mind.

The coming chapters will go into detail as to how the spine practitioner can identify and address each of the individual diagnostic factors in patients with LBDs while maintaining an awareness of the role each component plays in the overall picture.

Recommended Reading:

Adams M, Bogduk N, Burton K, Dolan P. The Biomechanics of Back Pain. Edinburgh: Churchill Livingstone, 2002.

Adams MA, Hutton WC. Prolapsed intervertebral disc. A hyperflexion injury 1981 Volvo Award in Basic Science. *Spine (Phila Pa 1976)* 1982;7(3):184-91.

Bove GM, Seaman DR. Subclassification of radicular pain using neurophysiology and embryology. Proceedings of the 7th Interdisciplinary World Congress on Low Back & Pelvic Pain. November 9-12, 2010. Los Angeles. P.155-159.

Callaghan JP, McGill SM. Intervertebral disc herniation: studies on a porcine model exposed to highly repetitive flexion/extension motion with compressive force. Clin Biomech (Bristol, Avon) 2001;16(1):28-37.

DeLeo JA. Basic science of pain. J Bone Joint Surg 2006;88-A(Suppl 2):58-62.

Hancock MJ, Maher CG, Laslett M, Hay E, Koes B. Discussion paper: what happened to the 'bio' in the bio-psycho-social model of low back pain? Eur Spine J 2011;20(12):2105-10.

Hides J, Stanton W, Mendis MD, Sexton M. The relationship of transversus abdominis and lumbar multifidus clinical muscle tests in patients with chronic low back pain. Man Ther 2011;16(6):573-7.

Kendall NAS, Burton AK, Main CJ, Watson PJ, on behalf of the Flags Think-Tank. Tackling musculoskeletal problems: a guide for the clinic and workplace - identifying obstacles using the psychosocial flags framework. London, The Stationery Office, 2009. www.tsoshop.co.uk/flags [accessed 16 April 2013]

Langevin HM, Sherman KJ. Pathophysiological model for chronic low back pain integrating connective tissue and nervous system mechanisms. Med Hypotheses 2007;68(1):74-80.

Latremoliere A, Woolf CJ. Central sensitization: a generator of pain hypersensitivity by central neural plasticity. J Pain 2009;10(9):895-926.

Leone A, Guglielmi G, Cassar-Pullicino VN, Bonomo L. Lumbar intervertebral instability: a review. Radiology. 2007;245(1):62-77.

Lloyd D, Findlay G, Roberts N, Nurmikko T. Differences in low back pain behavior are reflected in the cerebral response to tactile stimulation of the lower back. Spine 2008;33(12):1372-7.

Main CJ, Foster N, Buchbinder R. How important are back pain beliefs and expectations for satisfactory recovery from back pain? Best Pract Res Clin Rheumatol 2010;24(2):205-17.

May A. Chronic pain may change the structure of the brain. Pain 2008;137(1):7-15.

Melzack R. Evolution of the neuromatrix theory of pain. Pain Pract 2005;5(2):85-94.

Omoigui S. The biochemical origin of pain: the origin of all pain is inflammation and the inflammatory response. Part 2 of 3 - inflammatory profile of pain syndromes. Med Hypotheses 2007;69(6):1169-78.

Omoigui S. The biochemical origin of pain-proposing a new law of pain: the origin of all pain is inflammation and the inflammatory response. Part 1 of 3--a unifying law of pain. Med Hypotheses 2007;69(1):70-82.

Panjabi MM. A hypothesis of chronic back pain: ligament subfailure injuries lead to muscle control dysfunction. Eur Spine J 2006;15(5):668-76.

Pink DH. Drive: The Surprising Truth About What Motivates Us. New York: Riverhead Books, 2009.

Reichling DB, Levine JD. Critical role of nociceptor plasticity in chronic pain. Trends Neurosci 2009;32(12):611-8.

Seaman DR, Winterstein JF. Dysafferentation: a novel term to describe the neuropathophysiological effects of joint complex dysfunction. A look at likely mechanisms of symptom generation. J Manipulative Physiol Ther 1998;21(4):267-80.

Simons DG, Travell JG, Simons LS. Myofascial Pain and Dysfunction: The Trigger Point Manual. Volume 1. Baltimore: Williams and Wilkens; 1999.

Sullivan MJ, Scott W, Trost Z. Perceived injustice: a risk factor for problematic pain outcomes. Clin J Pain. 2012;28(6):484-8.

Veres SP, Robertson PA, Broom ND. The influence of torsion on disc herniation when combined with flexion. Eur Spine J 2010;19(9):1468-78.

Waddell G. The Back Pain Revolution. 2nd ed. Edinburgh: Churchill Livingstone, 2004.

Wand BM, Parkitny L, O'Connell NE, Luomajoki H, McAuley JH, Thacker M, Moseley GL: Cortical changes in chronic low back pain: current state of the art and implications for clinical practice. Manual therapy 2011;16(1):15-20.

Section II:
Diagnosis Using the Clinical Reasoning in Spine Pain™ Protocols

· CHAPTER 3 ·

Taking a Thorough and Efficient History

The challenge for the spine practitioner in formulating a diagnosis and management strategy is balancing the need, on the one hand, to be thorough in gathering information with, on the other hand, the pressures of time that naturally arise in a busy clinic environment. For this reason, efficiency is of the utmost importance. When it comes to taking the history, it is essential for the spine practitioner to focus on eliciting key information while at the same time cultivating a healing relationship and helping the patient feel valued and "listened to."

Presented in this chapter is a brief overview of history taking. The historical factors that are most useful in establishing a diagnosis will be presented in the next three chapters.

Relationship Building

Some of the material in this section was adapted from the fine work of Catherine Dubé, EdD from the Centers for Behavioral and Preventive Medicine of Warren Alpert Medical School of Brown University. Her permission to use this material is greatly appreciated.

One of the purposes of taking a history is to gather information that may be useful in establishing a differential diagnosis. However, history taking is not merely a data-gathering mission. Another purpose of history taking is to establish a working relationship with the patient that will form the foundation for healing. The latter purpose is often overlooked and is a key factor in successful patient management. The process of applying the biopsychosocial (BPS) model in a cognitive-behavioral, acceptance-commitment context, as discussed in Chapter 1, starts from the first time the practitioner greets the patient. Making eye contact, listening attentively and acknowledging and having empathy for the distress the patient is expressing are essential communication tools that can be applied from the very start.

The five most important skills in establishing an effective practitioner-patient relationship can be remembered by the acronym "SLRRP":

Support: The practitioner should make it clear to the patient that his or her purpose in the encounter is to be as helpful as possible.

Legitimation: Express to the patient that his or her emotional response to the problem is understandable. Here it is important to "meet the patient where he or she is." That is, even if the patient expresses an emotion that is irrational or unfounded (such as being afraid to engage in a relatively benign activity for fear of "damaging" the back), it is essential for the practitioner to understand the fear from the patient's perspective. In this way the practitioner can legitimize the emotion and be in a better position to effectively educate the patient, and to challenge any notions about LBDs that are self-defeating. An example would be "Given the fact that your back pain started when you were using that machine at work, it is certainly understandable that you would be afraid to go back to the same machine."

Reflection: Repeat back to the patient the emotions that are being expressed, e.g., "it sounds like you are worried about whether you will ever be able to play with your children."

Respect: Compliment the patient on how he or she has handled the problem up to this point, e.g., "I am impressed with how well you have coped with this given how much pain you have been in."

Partnership: Include the patient in any decision-making process, emphasizing that the practitioner and the patient are members of a team whose purpose is to help the patient overcome the LBD.

Some general principles of history taking that can greatly enhance the process are:

Open to closed cone questioning: Start with questions that are as open as possible (e.g., "What brings you to the office today?") then gradually narrow the focus as the narrative of the history develops. The practitioner may already have a significant amount of specific information from the intake form the patient will have completed prior to the practitioner-patient encounter, but it is important to avoid jumping into the details before the patient has had a chance to express his or her overall feelings about the problem.

Allow the patient to tell his or her story: As stated earlier, rapport and trust are essential elements of the therapeutic encounter and these are greatly enhanced when the patient feels that the practitioner fully understands the problem and its impact.

Interrupt to redirect: In allowing the patient to tell the story it is sometimes necessary to keep him or her on the narrative path so that the story can be understood without missing important details. This must be done in a manner that allows the patient to feel he or she is being treated with respect. Saying things like "I am sorry to interrupt but you said something important that I think we should get back to. Tell me again about how heavy the object was that you lifted" can be an effective way of respectfully interrupting to steer the patient back to the main storyline.

Use facilitation methods: Little things like making eye contact, leaning toward the patient and having an open posture, using affirmative gestures such as nodding the head frequently or occasionally say "mm-hm" can help make the patient feel more comfortable in being forthcoming with information.

Repeat back to the patient the key aspects of the history – this is one of the most powerful ways to assure the patient that you not only care enough to give full attention, but that you understand the problem and all its elements. It is important not only to repeat back to the patient the facts of the history but also the emotional aspects. An example would be, "Your pain is exacerbated every time you ride your bike, which is something you love to do, and you are afraid you will have to give this up."

Information Gathering

In addition to establishing rapport and a quality working relationship with the patient, the purpose of history taking is to gather information to help answer the three questions of diagnosis.

History of the present illness

In general, when eliciting information regarding the history of the present illness, the commonly used pneumonic "LMNOPQRST-AS" is useful.

L = Location – this involves having the patient specifically identify the location of the pain. This can be done via a pain drawing that the patient can complete prior to seeing the practitioner. Then during history taking the practitioner should have the patient identify with one finger the entire area of pain. The patient's description should be consistent with the pain drawing.

M = Mechanism – this identifies how the problem began. In some cases there may be a specific incident that initiated the symptoms. In other cases the onset will be insidious. In cases in which there is no specific mechanism of onset, it is useful to ask the patient if he or she has any theories as to how the problem started. The patient's theories may or may not be accurate, but asking about this can help the practitioner gain an understanding of the patient's beliefs and perceptions about the pain.

N = New or chronic – this identifies whether the patient has had the problem for a long time or whether it began recently.

O = Onset – this includes when the symptoms began, whether they have been continuous or intermittent and whether the patient has ever had the same or similar symptoms. It should also include what practitioners the patient has seen for these symptoms, what tests have been performed, any treatments the patient has received and the results of those treatments.

P = Provoking and Palliative factors – this involves asking the patient what causes the symptoms to increase in intensity and what causes them to decrease in intensity. This includes movements, activities and positions as well as attempts at self-treatment. As we will see, this can be essential in gaining clues with regard to the answers to the three questions of diagnosis.

Q = Quality of the pain – while this has been classically included as a part of history taking, it has limited usefulness in establishing a diagnosis.

R = Radiation or Referral – this allows the practitioner to inquire as to whether the symptoms extend into the buttock or leg, and in what pattern. Contrary to popular belief, nerve root pain from all levels except S1 should not be expected to follow a specific dermatome; however, in general, posterior lower extremity pain that extends below the knee is more likely of nerve root origin than pain that remains above the knee. Anterior thigh pain of upper- to mid-lumbar origin will generally remain above the knee (see Chapter 5).

S = Severity – this relates to how severe the symptoms have been from the patient's perspective. This can be done using a Numeric Rating Scale (see Chapter 7).

T = Timing – this relates to the times of the day or night the symptoms are at their worst and their best.

AS = Associated Symptoms – it is important to ask the patient whether there are any other symptoms that may be related to the pain such as numbness, paresthesia, motor loss, gastrointestinal or genitourinary symptoms, fever, chills, constitutional symptoms or unexplained weight loss.

Functional history

This includes the patient's present work status and current activity level, particularly as it applies to the LBD. An essential question in the functional history is, "what would you normally be doing that you can't do or avoid doing because of this problem?"

Past medical history

Exploration of the patient's past medical history can be done with the initial intake form, but it is important to review this with the patient so that a complete understanding of the health history can be obtained. It is also important to find out what medications the patient is taking. Patients will occasionally forget to bring up certain conditions until you discover that they are taking medications for a disease that they had not revealed during history taking. So be sure to review the medication list carefully and inquire about any medications that are not consistent with the health history they provided.

Review of systems

With this, the practitioner surveys various systems, asking about any recent problems the patient has been having. Any system in which the patient reports symptoms or difficulties, particularly those that have not been evaluated by the patient's primary care provider or another practitioner, can be explored. The review of systems should be comprehensive enough to cover all body systems without being overly cumbersome to the patient. Some practitioners may choose to have the patient complete a form in which symptoms are checked off, and then to review these checked items during history taking. Others may choose to ask each patient about these symptoms themselves. An example of a checklist for review of systems can be found in Table 1.

Table 1. The review of systems

General:
___Wt. change
___ Fever
___ Chills
___ Night Sweats
___ Weakness
___ Fatigue
___ Headache

Eyes:
___ Vision
___ Pain
___ Discharge

Ears:
___ Hearing
___ Ringing
___ Pain
___ Discharge

Nose:
___ Pain
___ Bleeding
___ Taste

Mouth/Throat:
___ Sores
___ Bleeding
___ Taste

Skin:
___ Rash
___ Itching
___ Hair Changes
___ Nail Changes
___ Cough

Neurologic:
___ Blue Extremities
___ Dizziness
___ Convulsions
___ Mass

G-I:
___ Appetite
___ Abdominal Pain
___ Vomiting
___ Diarrhea
___ Constipation
___ Depression
___ Moods

G-U:
___ Frequent Urination
___ Painful Urination
___ Incontinence
___ Upper Extremities
___ Lower Extremities

Cardio:
___ Murmur
___ Chest Pain
___ Palpitations
___ Difficulty Breathing
___ Wheezing
___ Swollen Extremities
___ Fainting

Breasts:
___ Pain
___ Discharge
___ Self-exam

Psychologic:
___ Anxiety
___ Memory

Musculoskeletal
___ Neck
___ Upper Back
___ Lower Back

Additional Data: _____
_____

Social history

This includes the patient's marital or partner status, number of children and any other people the patient lives with. The social history should also include health habits such as tobacco and alcohol use and exercise. It is important to be specific with these, including the number of cigarettes and/or alcoholic beverages consumed per day or week and specifically what types of exercise activities the patient engages in, along with the frequency and duration of exercise. Nutritional habits can also be included in the section although some practitioners may prefer to undergo a separate, more formal nutritional analysis.

Family history

This should include major diseases such as hypertension, cancer, diabetes, heart disease and stroke and should focus on immediate family members, i.e., parents, siblings and children.

In most cases, the practitioner should have one or several possible diagnoses in mind by the end of the history. Examination is then carried out for the purpose of exploring these possibilities.

History taking gives the spine practitioner an opportunity to establish rapport, empathy and a productive healing relationship. Much can be learned about the patient's beliefs and cognitions about the pain during history taking. In addition, careful questioning can reveal important diagnostic information that can then inform the physical examination. Details with regard to the examination will be explored in the next three chapters.

Recommended Reading

Henschke N, Maher CG, Refshauge KM, Herbert RD, Cumming RG, Bleasel J, et al. Prevalence of and screening for serious spinal pathology in patients presenting to primary care settings with acute low back pain. Arthritis Rheum 2009;60(10):3072-80.

Murphy DR, Hurwitz EL, Gerrard JK, Clary R. Pain patterns and descriptions in patients with radicular pain: Does the pain necessarily follow a specific dermatome? Chiropr Osteopat 2009;17(1):9.

Wu WH, Meijer OG, Mens JMA, van Dieen JH, Wuisman PIJM, Ostgarrd HC. Pregnancy-related pelvic girdle pain (PPP) I: Terminology, clinical presentation and prevalence. Eur Spine J 2004;13:575-89.

· CHAPTER 4 ·

Diagnostic Question #1: Are the symptoms with which this patient is presenting reflective of a visceral problem or a potentially serious or life-threatening illness?

There are certain visceral disorders or potentially serious illnesses for which low back pain may be one of the initial symptoms. The patient may seek care for the low back pain and it is necessary to ask the appropriate questions and perform the appropriate examination procedures in making a differential diagnosis. In the application of the Clinical Reasoning in Spine Pain™ (CRISP™) protocols, the first question of diagnosis investigates symptoms and signs that may suggest the presence of one of these disorders, possibly warranting referral or further investigation.

In general, the conditions being evaluated with the first question of diagnosis are:

- Cancer

- Infection

- Benign tumor

- Fracture

- Aortic aneurism

- Cauda equina syndrome

- Gastrointestinal disease

- Genitourinary disease

- Spondyloarthropathy

Table 4-1 provides the most important conditions covered by diagnostic question #1 and their detection.

Table 4-1. Conditions that are considered under diagnostic question #1 and their detection

Disorder	Detected by
Cancer	History of cancer No position of relief Fever Constitutional symptoms Unexplained weight loss Blood in the stool Pain in multiple sites
Benign tumor	Local severe pain No position of relief Relief with NSAID Pain on percussion
Infection	History of fever or chills Febrile (but often afebrile) Point tenderness Immunocompromised individual History of diabetes
Fracture	History of trauma History of osteopenia or osteoporosis Pain on percussion

Dissected or ruptured AAA	Over 50
	History of hypertension
	History of smoking
	Syncope
	Sudden, severe onset
	Abdominal pain
	Abdominal pulsation
GI disease	GI complaints
	Pain with food
	Positive abdominal exam
GU Disease	GU complaints
	Bleeding
	Spotting
	Discharge
	Positive GU exam
Cauda Equina Syndrome	Bowel/ bladder dysfunction
	Saddle anesthesia
	Decreased anal sphincter tone

The investigation of diagnostic question #1 is carried out through careful history and examination.

History of the Present Illness

The "LMNOPQRST-AS" questions presented in Chapter 3, are useful in soliciting information that may lead the practitioner to ask more pointed questions in seeking the answer to diagnostic question #1:

1. Have you had numbness, tingling or pins and needles in your legs or feet? In your groin area?

A "yes" answer to this question suggests the presence of radiculopathy. Numbness or paresthesia in the groin area ("saddle anesthesia") suggests cauda equina syndrome. However, these symptoms could possibly reflect some other neurologic disorder.

2. Have you had weakness in your legs or have you noticed one or both feet dragging when you walk?

A "yes" answer to this question also suggests radiculopathy or another type of neurologic disorder with motor involvement. The weakness can be reflective of an upper- or lower motor neuron problem and does not, in and of itself, distinguish between the two. This question is important because, as will be discussed, motor loss has a greater influence on surgical decisions than sensory loss.

3. Is there any position of relief?

In a patient who reports no position of relief, cancer, infection, dissecting aortic aneurism or visceral disease such as renal calculus should be suspected. Of course, there will be some patients with an acute low back disorder (LBD) who do not have any of these conditions but who will still initially report no position that provides relief. Therefore, it is important to be meticulous in questioning the patient regarding whether he or she is truly in pain at all times, regardless of position. Often the patient will identify one or more positions in which the pain is relieved once asked to be specific. However, if the patient is not able to identify any position at all that is comfortable, suspicion is warranted.

Often, patients with GI or GU disease or dissecting aneurism will pace around and not be able to sit still. This is in stark contrast to the patient acute disc or nerve root pain, who will generally try to avoid movement.

4. Have you had abdominal pains, gassiness, belching? Does your pain change after or before eating?

A "yes" answer to the question suggests the presence of a gastrointestinal disorder.

5. Are you generally stiff in the morning?

Generalized stiffness suggests the possibility of a generalized inflammatory arthritide. Localized stiffness in the low back may be suggestive of spondyloarthropathy however morning stiffness is a common symptom of disc derangement (see Chapter 5). With disc derangement patients the stiffness typically resolves shortly after the patient has been moving around. Therefore, morning stiffness that lasts at least 30 to 45 minutes should raise the concern for spondyloarthropathy.

6. Have you had difficulty with urination, painful urination or blood in your urine?

A "yes" answer to this suggests the possibility of either cauda equina syndrome (in the case of urinary retention or incontinence) or a disorder of the kidney or urinary system.

Cauda equina syndrome can be of the incomplete type or the complete type. With incomplete cauda equina syndrome the patient will have urinary difficulties such as altered urinary sensation, loss of desire to urinate, weak urinary stream or will require great effort to empty the bladder. The patient typically will have unilateral or partial saddle anesthesia and may have normal sensation on testing.

With complete cauda equina syndrome the patient typically has urinary retention (inability to void) as well as overflow incontinence (inability to sense fullness of the bladder, leading to "leaking" or "dribbling"). The patient typically will have complete saddle anesthesia. It is important to detect cauda equina syndrome early, as the incomplete type carries a better surgical prognosis than the complete type.

7. Have you had fever or chills? Have you generally been feeling ill?

A "yes" answer is suggestive of the presence of cancer or infection.

8. Have you had unexplained weight loss?

A "yes" answer is suggestive of cancer.

9. In female patients who are pregnant or of child-bearing age: Have you had bleeding, spotting, bouts of diarrhea or unusual discharge?

A "yes" answer raises the suspicion of ectopic pregnancy or miscarriage.

10. Is your pain worse at night?

A "yes" answer raises the suspicion of cancer however it should be noted that the specificity of this finding is likely to be very low. That is, there will be many patients who do not have cancer who have increased pain at night. Therefore, this factor should particularly be of concern in the presence of other "red flags" for cancer.

Past Medical History, Review of Systems, Social History, Family History.

There may be certain factors in the past medical history that provide potentially important clues in seeking the answer to diagnostic question #1:

Cancer: This raises the possibility of metastatic disease. Of course, the majority of patients with LBD who have a history of cancer will not have "mets." But with those who do have such a history, it is important to be on the lookout for other signs and/ or symptoms that may contribute further to this suspicion. Find out the type of cancer and the tissue that was involved, as certain tissues of origin have a predilection for metastasis to bone, particularly to the spine. These are provided in Table 4-2. The likelihood of metastasis decreases over time but never disappears. So it is important to consider the possibility of metastatic disease in any patient with a history of malignancy.

Factors that may cause immunosuppression: These raise the possibility of infection such as epidural abscess. Risk factors for immunosuppression include cirrhosis, AIDS, long-term steroid use and diabetes, (particularly if the patient self-injects insulin)

Risk factors for infection: These also raise the possibility of infection such as epidural abscess and include recent bowel perforation, IV drug use and recent surgery, injection, infusion therapy or dental work.

Hypertension and/or diabetes: Especially if they are not well controlled, these conditions are risk factors for abdominal aortic aneurism.

Disorders associated with spondyloarthropathy: These include psoriasis (in a patient with psoriasis it is important to ask about related arthritis), Crohn's disease and inflammatory bowel disease.

Medications that may predispose patients to certain disorders that can cause back pain: These include anticoagulant medications, which are a risk factor for subdural hematoma, and statin medications, which may be predispose the patient to muscle pain or myopathy.

Risk factors for deep vein thrombosis: These are important in patients with leg pain and include recent paralysis or prolonged immobilization, recent major surgery (within four weeks) and a strong family history (≥2 first degree relatives) of deep vein thrombosis.

Smoking: This is a risk factor for a number of diseases including lung cancer (which can metastasize to the spine) and abdominal aortic aneurism.

Table 4-2. Primary cancers that have a predilection for bone.
Those that have particular predilection for the spine are indicated by an *.

*Breast	Thyroid
*Lung	Bladder
*Prostate	Endometrium
*Kidney	Cervix
Melanoma	

Following the history, examination is carried out in an attempt to gain more information. The specifics of the examination may be determined by the history. For example, in a patient who reports GI complaints, an abdominal examination can be carried out. A careful neurologic exam should be conducted which should at a minimum include a sensory, motor and reflex examination of the lower extremities. Depending on the outcome of the history, a complete neurologic screening examination may be necessary.

Vital Signs

The typical vital sign examination consists of blood pressure, temperature, pulse rate and respirations. Temperature is particularly useful as fever may be suggestive of spine infection such as epidural abscess.

The Screening Neurologic Examination

With practice, the entire central and peripheral nervous system can be screened in less than four minutes (see Table 4-3). There are a number of excellent sources of information regarding how to properly conduct a neurologic examination, particularly the book by Blumenfeld that can be found in the Recommended Reading list. Presented here is an efficient flow that can be applied to the screening neurologic examination.

Patient Standing

Heel, toe and tandem walking and standing in Romberg's position with eyes closed

The patient is asked to rise on the toes and take a few steps. Difficulty with this on one or both sides suggests the possibility of neurologic weakness involving the S1 or perhaps S2 nerve roots. With subtle weakness it may be necessary to have the patient lift one foot of the floor and then rise on the other toe. If the patient expresses difficulty, it is important to ask whether this is due to pain or weakness.

The patient is then asked to raise the forefeet off the floor and take a few steps. Difficulty on one or both sides suggests the possibility of neurologic weakness involving the L4 or L5 nerve roots. However, difficulty with heel walking can also be an early sign of upper motor neuron weakness as well.

Next, the patient is asked to walk with one foot directly in front of the other as if walking on a tight-rope. Difficulty with this may reflect a problem in a number of areas including the cerebellum, posterior columns and motor system. However, it must be noted that many older patients will have difficulty with tandem walking.

Finally, the patient is asked to stand with the feet together with eyes closed (Romberg's position). The practitioner should stand close by in case of loss of balance. If the patient starts to fall or sways widely, this suggests the possibility of a problem with the posterior columns or vestibular system, or lower extremity peripheral polyneuropathy.

Patient sitting

Cranial nerve (CN) examination

In the screening neurologic examination, all cranial nerves are tested with the exception of CN I (which would be tested by the patient's ability to smell) and CN X (which would be tested with the gag reflex) although CN X is tested in part by assessing the patient's speech during history taking by listening for dysphagia.

CN III, IV and VI: The patient visually follows an object such as the examiner's finger, moving only the eyes. The object is moved in the form of the letter "H." Convergence is then tested by the practitioner slowly moving the finger toward the patient's nose.

CN II: The visual fields are assessed by the practitioner holding up a finger of each hand in each field of vision, asking whether the patient can see both fingers. CN II can be examined directly via the opthalmoscopic exam. Particularly important for the spine practitioner is assessing for papilledema in patients with headache.

CN II and III can also be tested by assessing the pupillary response to light. A light is shone alternately into each eye, assessing both the direct (the eye in which the light is shining) and indirect (the opposite eye) pupillary response.

CN V: The practitioner lightly touches the patient's face in each of the divisions of the trigeminal nerve. The practitioner then palpates the contraction of the masseter muscles while the patient clenches the teeth.

CN VII: The patient is asked to raise the eyebrows, close the eyes tightly and smile.

CN VIII: The practitioner rustles the fingers alternately next to each of the patient's ears and asks if the patient can hear the sound.

CN IX and XII: The patient is asked to stick the tongue straight out, then move it left and right. The patient is then asked to stick the tongue straight out, open the mouth and say "Ahh." The practitioner observes the elevation of the palate.

CN XI: The practitioner holds the patient's head steady while the patient tries to turn the head left and right. The patient then elevates the shoulders and the practitioner presses downward on the shoulders while the patient resists this pressure.

Muscle stretch reflexes (deep tendon reflexes)

Using a reflex hammer (a disc-top reflex hammer is preferable to a "tomahawk" or other type of hammer), the practitioner tests the biceps (primarily C5 and C6), brachioradialis (primarily C6), triceps (primarily C7), patellar (primarily L4) and Achilles (primarily S1 and S2) reflexes. These should be graded according to the following scale:

0: Absent

1+: Present but depressed

2+: Normal

3+: Increased

4+: Clonus

If reinforcement (i.e., the *"Jendrassik* maneuver,") is required to elicit the reflex, it should be graded in the same way but with the addition of "…with reinforcement."

In patients with nerve root or peripheral nerve dysfunction, there may be asymmetric diminishment of one or more of these reflexes (except in the case of bilateral radiculopathy). In patients with an upper motor neuron lesion there may be a unilateral or bilateral increase in the reflexes below the level of the lesion.

Motor strength

This is tested manually in the sitting position and individual muscles are tested separately (to the extent possible) in an attempt to identify focal deficit.

Testing the tibialis anterior and gastrosoleus via heel and toe walking was discussed earlier. The tibialis anterior can also be tested in the sitting position but the gastrosoleus is too strong to gain useful information through manual muscle testing. It is useful to start the motor strength exam from the top and work downward. In sequence the deltoids (primarily C5), biceps (primarily C5 and C6), triceps (primarily C7), wrist extensors (primarily C6), wrist flexors (primarily C6 and C7), finger flexors (primarily C8) and finger abductors (primarily T1) are tested. The motor strength exam then moves to the lower extremities where the hip flexors (L2-L4), quadriceps, (primarily L3 and L4), hamstrings (primarily S1), tibialis anterior (L4 and L5), extensor hallucis longus (primarily L5) and peroneus muscles (L5, S1) are tested. It is important to note that the tibialis anterior is a particularly strong muscle so considerable force must be applied by the examiner to elicit subtle weakness.

Motor strength should be graded according to the following scale:

0/5: No contraction

1/5: Flicker but no movement

2/5: Movement possible but not against gravity

3/5: Movement possible against gravity but the patient cannot resist examiner pressure

4-/5: Slight movement against resistance

4/5: Moderate movement against resistance

4+/5: Submaximal movement against resistance

5/5: Normal

Sensory testing

As part of the general neurologic screening examination, sensory testing is best performed with pin-prick. It is important to ask the patient if the pinprick feels the same on each side or if it feels markedly different on one side compared to the other. The sensory examination is very subjective and abnormal sensation should only documented if the patient states that he or she cannot feel the sharpness at all. If the patient states that the sensation feels sharp on both sides but that one side is less sharp, this should not be considered abnormal in most cases. Because this is a screening neurologic examination specifically for patients with LBDs, the lower extremity dermatomes should be examined individually. The upper extremity can be screened by simply testing the hand in general.

The neurologic screening examination can be completed in the seated position by testing rapid alternating movements (alternately tapping the hand with the palmar and dorsal surfance), heel-to-shin movements (placing one heel on the opposite knee, then slowly running the heel downward along the tibia), pronator drift (with the patient holding the arms extended in front with palms up and eyes closed) and finger-to-nose movements (from the pronator drift position rapidly touching the nose with each index finger with eyes closed).

The neurologic screening examination is designed to give the practitioner an overview of the function of the central and peripheral nervous system. If significant positive findings are noted in one or more parts of the screening examination, more detailed examination procedures may be indicated.

Table 4-3. The neurologic screening examination

Standing	Seated
Heel walking	• Cranial nerve examination • Visual fields • Pursuit EOM • Sensory • Motor • Tongue • Palate • Fundoscopy
Toe walking	Sensory to pin in the upper and lower extremities
Tandem walking	Motor of the upper and lower extremities
Romberg's position	Muscle stretch reflexes of the upper and lower extremities
	Plantar response
	Rapid alternating movements
	Heel-to-shin movements
	Finger-to-nose movements
	Pronator drift

Pain Provocation Examination

It will be discussed in the next chapter that seeking the answer to diagnostic question #2 ("Where is the pain coming from?") involves a detailed examination attempting to *reproduce the patient's pain*. If the pain is not reproduced during this examination, concern should be raised for the possibility of a non-musculoskeletal cause of the pain. This is particularly a concern if one or more of the other factors discussed in this chapter are present.

Abdominal Examination

In patients whose history suggests the possibility of gastrointestinal disease as a contributor to their LBD, abdominal examination should be carried out.

For the purpose of examining the LBD patient the most important aspects of the abdominal examination are inspection and palpation. With the patient supine the practitioner can observe the contour and symmetry of the abdomen and look for visible masses. The practitioner then performs superficial and deep palpation and notes any muscular resistance, superficial or deep masses and pain or tenderness. In some cases the practitioner may want to palpate the kidneys with one hand on the posterior aspect of the trunk to lift the kidney and the opposite hand palpating deeply in the abdomen.

Peripheral pulses

In a patient with lower extremity symptoms or who is over the age of 50, the lower extremity peripheral pulses should be palpated. This should include the posterior tibial and/or dorsalis pedis pulses (the dorsalis pedis pulse may be congenitally absent in some individuals). For the posterior tibial pulse, the index and middle fingers are placed just posterior to the medial malleolus. For the dorsalis pedis pulse the index and middle fingers are placed on the dorsum of the foot just lateral to the tendon of the extensor hallucis longus muscle. If the pulse is diminished or absent on one or both sides, the popliteal and femoral pulses can be palpated in an attempt to localize the site of arterial occlusion.

Palpation and auscultation of the abdominal aorta

The spine practitioner may choose to include palpation and auscultation of the abdominal aorta as a routine part of the examination of the LBD patient who is over the age of 50, particularly if there is suspicion of abdominal aortic aneurism. The palpating hands or stethoscope should be placed in the upper abdomen, just to the left of midline.

Percussion

If fracture, infection or localized spine malignancy is suspected based on the history, percussion of the spinous processes may reveal severe pain at the effected level. The reflex hammer can be used to tap lightly over each spinous process and the patient asked if any particular level is painful. Mild or moderate tenderness in one or more spinous processes may be normal but severe pain at a single level may suggest fracture, infection or malignancy.

Special Tests

The vast majority of patients with LBDs do not require any special tests. In those who do, there are specific factors derived from the history and/ or examination that determine the most useful test to order.

Plain film radiographs

Plain film radiographs are indicated when there is suspicion of bony pathology, i.e., the history and/ or examination suggest the presence of fracture, bone infection or benign or malignant bone tumor. Flexion-extension studies are often useful in patients with clinical signs and/or symptoms specifically suggesting passive instability, particularly in patients with degenerative spondylolisthesis.

Computed Tomography

There are some patients in whom bony pathology is strongly suspected and plain film radiographs are inconclusive. In these cases computed tomography (CT) can be useful for more detailed examination of bone. In many cases CT can also identify problems in certain soft tissues, such as disc herniation, although MRI is far more useful than CT for this purpose. However in patients for whom MRI is indicated but who cannot have MRI, such as patients with a pacemaker, severe claustrophobia or metallic implant such as a surgical device, CT is the imaging modality of choice.

CT myelography is considered by many spine surgeons to be a useful tool in evaluating spinal stenosis or disc herniation but has little if any utility for the primary spine practitioner.

Magnetic Resonance Imaging

Magnetic resonance Imaging (MRI) is currently the Gold Standard for identifying anatomical abnormalities in the spine. As it is expensive, time-consuming and has a high false-positive rate, it should only be used in the presence of specific indications. MRI is only indicated on the initial visit in cases in which there is significant suspicion of serious disease such as cancer, spine infection, cauda equina syndrome or space occupying lesion other than disc herniation or spinal stenosis. In patients who have clear signs of radiculopathy but do not have signs or symptoms suggestive of disease other than disc herniation or spinal stenosis, MRI is not immediately necessary as it will not alter the management strategy. However, after at least 4-6 weeks of non-surgical management without improvement or in cases of progressive neurologic deficit, MRI should be considered. In addition, in a patient with radiculopathy who develops signs or symptoms suggestive of cauda equina syndrome, MRI should be ordered.

Recent evidence (see Albert, et al in Recommended Reading list) suggests that some patients with chronic LBDs may have infection within the disc, resulting in inflammation of the adjacent vertebral bodies due to cytokine and propionic acid production. The most common organism implicated in this infection is *Propionibacterium acnes*. It is thought that this anaerobic bacterium may find the avascular disc to be an ideal place to breed. The vertebral body inflammation can be visualized on MRI as Modic type 1 change (Fig. 4-1) in which decreased signal on T1 images and increased signal on T2 images is seen within the vertebral bodies. It is speculated that this inflammation can lead to pain.

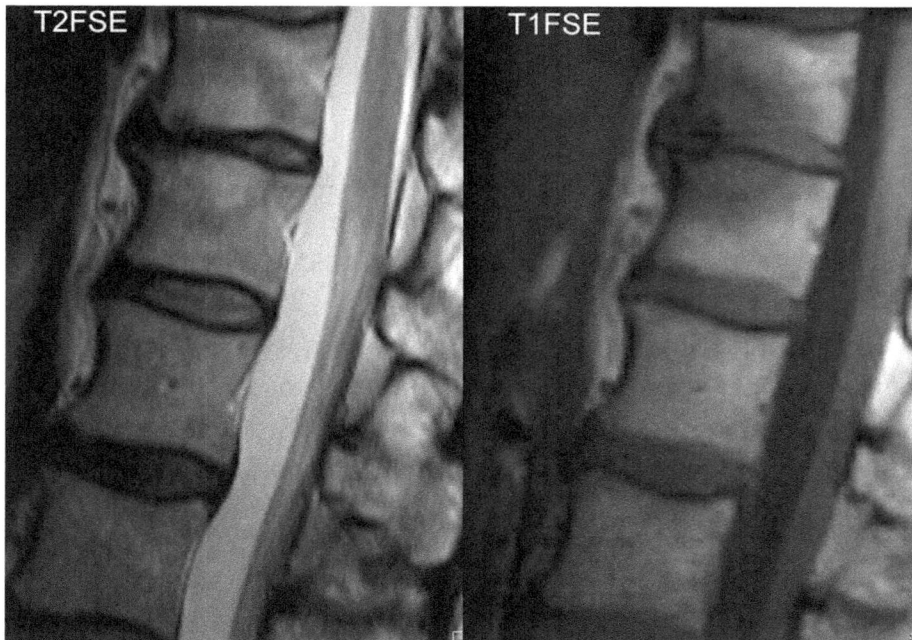

Figure 4-1. Modic type 1 change seen on a T2 weighted MRI image (left) and T1 weighted image (right). Image courtesy of Bill Hsu, DC, DACBR.

How commonly *P. acnes* infection may cause low back pain is unknown as Modic type 1 change is frequently found in asymptomatic individuals. Future work can be expected to shine light on whether this is a major factor in the etiology of LBDs.

Blood tests

As with the other special tests discussed here, blood tests are uncommonly necessary but when they are indicated they can be quite useful. Blood tests are indicated in cases in which an inflammatory process is suspected such as polymyalgia rheumatica or seronegative spondyloarthropathy. In these cases, the most important tests for the spine practitioner are erythrocyte sedimentation rate (Sed rate) and C-reactive protein (CRP).

Sed rate and CRP, as well as white blood cell count, may be indicated in patients with suspected infection although if epidural abscess is suspected, emergency referral is indicated rather than further testing.

Other tests such as thyroid function tests, complete blood count and blood chemistry screen may be warranted depending on the specifics of any individual case. Urine specimen may be indicated in some cases, particularly if multiple myeloma is suspected.

Bone scan

Bone scan can be useful in isolated circumstances in which cancer, infection or fracture is suspected and other imaging studies are not definitive. It may sometimes also be useful in cases of a pediatric patient with spondylolysis to determine the degree of metabolic activity at the site of fracture.

It should be expected that only approximately 1-3% of patients with LBDs will have significant findings suggestive of visceral disease or potentially serious illness. Therefore, it is important that the spine practitioner remain alert to these uncommon conditions. Once the practitioner is reasonably certain of a "no" answer to the first question of diagnosis, consideration of questions #2 and 3 can be made. These will be the topics of the next 2 chapters.

Recommended Reading:

Albert HB, Lambert P, Rollason J, Sorensen JS, Worthington T, Pedersen MB, et al. Does nuclear tissue infected with bacteria following disc herniations lead to Modic changes in the adjacent vertebrae? Eur Spine J. 2013 Feb 10.

Blumenfeld H. Neuroanatomy Through Clinical Cases. 2nd ed. Sunderland, MA: Sinaouer Associates, 2010.

Gardner A, Gardner E, Morley T. Cauda equina syndrome: a review of the current clinical and medico-legal position. Eur Spine J 2011;20(5):690-7.

Goldberg S. The 4-Minute Neurologic Exam. Miami FL: MedMaster, Inc, 1999

Joines JD, McNutt RA, Carey TS, Deyo RA, Rouhani R. Finding cancer in primary care outpatients with low back pain: A comparison of diagnostic strategies. J Gen Intern Med 2001;16(1):14-23.

Klineberg E, Mazanec D, Orr D, Demicco R, Bell G, McLain R. Masquerade: medical causes of back pain. Cleve Clin J Med 2007;74(12):905-13.

Papagoras C, Drosos AA. Seronegative Spondyloarthropathies: Evolving Concepts Regarding Diagnosis and Treatment. J Spine 2011;1(1).

Pateder DB, Brems J, Lieberman I, Bell GR, McLain RF. Masquerade: Nonspinal musculoskeletal disorders that mimic spinal conditions. Cleveland Clinic J Medicine 2008;75(1).

Siemionow K, Steinmetz M, Bell G, Ilaslan H, McLain RF. Identifying serious causes of back pain: cancer, infection, fracture. Cleve Clin J Med 2008;75(8):557-66.

· CHAPTER 5 ·

Diagnostic Question #2: Where is the pain coming from?

Another way of asking this question is "Are there characteristics of the pain generating tissue or tissues that can be identified and that allow treatment decisions to be made?" In the majority of patients with low back disorders (LBDs) there is no way to identify the pain generating tissue objectively and with 100% certainty. But history and examination can at least provide clues regarding the painful tissue. Treatment decisions can be made based on these clues and the practitioner can monitor the patient's response to treatment. It is not necessary to be absolutely certain of the pain generator to make treatment decisions. In addition, the patient can be provided with an evidence-based explanation as to the most likely cause of the pain.

In the context of Clinical Reasoning in Spine Pain™ (the CRISP™ protocols) there are four diagnostic entities that are investigated with diagnostic question #2:

1. Disc derangement: Diagnosed through historical factors and the end range loading examination.

2. Joint dysfunction: Diagnosed through historical factors and pain provocation maneuvers that are designed to identify pain from the lumbar facet joints or the sacroiliac joint.

3. Radiculopathy: Diagnosed through historical factors, neurologic examination and pain provocation maneuvers designed to identify nerve root pain.

4. Myofascial pain: Diagnosed through historical factors and pain provocation maneuvers designed to identify myofascial trigger points

The investigation of diagnostic question #2 involves asking the patient about movements, positions and activities that provoke or relieve the symptoms, along with a detailed examination. The examination involves applying specific maneuvers in an attempt to *reproduce the symptoms* (and, in the case of disc derangement, centralize and/or reduce the symptoms). The general principles of history taking were presented in Chapter 3 and details regarding each pain generator will be discussed in this chapter.

The examination for diagnostic question #2 involves the application of pain provocation tests; with each test the practitioner asks the patient whether the maneuver is painful and, more important, whether each maneuver *reproduces the pain for which the patient is seeking help*. The more definitively these examination procedures reproduce concordant pain, the more confident the practitioner can be in the diagnosis.

It is important during the process of applying pain provocation tests to help the patient *objectively observe* the sensation that is created by the maneuver. That is, to ask the patient "What do you feel when I perform this maneuver", "where do you feel it" and, ultimately, "does this reproduce the pain for which you are seeking my help?" In some cases a patient may become upset and begin talking about how he or she *feels about* the pain that is produced by the examination procedure, rather than simply reporting the presence or absence of concordant pain. When this occurs it gives the practitioner clues as to the patient's beliefs, judgments and cognitions about the pain - important information in seeking the answer to diagnostic question #3 (see Chapter 6). But for the purpose of seeking the answer to diagnostic question #2, it is important for the practitioner to acknowledge the patient's feelings and then to gently direct the patient to simply observe the actual sensation itself, identify its location, and determine whether the sensation reproduces the pain for which he or she is seeking help. This not only allows the practitioner to gain accurate information about the pain generator, it also begins the process of teaching *mindfulness*, i.e. teaching the patient to become an objective observer of the pain. This is a very powerful method of helping patients overcome fear and catastrophizing. Mindfulness will be discussed in more detail in Chapters 8, 9 and 11.

For a review of the evidence upon which the assessment of diagnostic question #2 is based, the reader is directed to the papers by Murphy and Hurwitz in the Recommended Reading list.

Disc Derangement

Historical factors that are associated with suspected lumbar disc pain include:

- Patients often present with antalgia or have a history of antalgia (kyphotic, lordotic or lateral shift). In some cases transient antalgia may be experienced upon arising from bed in the morning or arising from sitting.

- Pain and impairment tend to be worse in the morning, attributed to imbibition of fluid by the unloaded nucleus of the intervertebral disc when in bed, resulting in greater intradiscal pressure in the morning.

- The pain commonly increases pain with flexion: Flexion increases intradiscal pressure and thus often provokes disc pain. However increased pain with flexion is not universal in patients with disc derangements and, as will be seen, other patterns exist as well. There are some patients with disc derangements who prefer the flexed position.

- The pain is increased with sitting: As with flexion, sitting increases intradiscal pressure. However it is important to note that some patients with disc derangement feel comfortable sitting and do not experience pain until they stand up.

- The pain is increased with standing from a sitting position: Patients will often not only report pain on standing from a sitting position but also great difficulty extending the lumbar spine as they try to reach an upright position. It typically takes time to gradually reach the upright position, after which the pain is often somewhat better.

- The pain is worse in the morning: The intervertebral discs imbibe water during sleep, thus the discs are typically "swollen" in the morning.

- Antalgic posture: This will be discussed in detail later.

Essential to the identification of disc derangement is the end range loading (ERL) exam. With the ERL exam the spine is moved to end-range in multiple directions to detect a movement direction that has no pain during the arc but reveals a painful obstruction at the end of range. That direction is then explored with repeated movements or sustained positioning for beneficial symptomatic responses (diminution or "centralization" of pain) and beneficial mechanical responses (improved ROM).

The End Range Loading Examination to Identify Disc Derangement – by Gary Jacob, DC, LAc, MPH, DipMDT and Steven Heffner, DC, DipMDT

This section is an introduction to the diagnosis and treatment of "derangement syndrome" as first described by Robin A. McKenzie (see Recommended Reading list) as *part of* a system known as the

McKenzie Method or Mechanical Diagnosis & Therapy (MDT). The reader is encouraged to take advantage of the texts authored by Robin A. McKenzie and the educational program of the McKenzie Institute International for a more complete understanding of the diagnosis and treatment of disc derangement as well as other aspects of the McKenzie Method. See the Recommended Reading list for specifics.

Lumbar Disc Derangements as Antalgias and "Shades of Antalgia"

As discussed above, one common characteristic of disc derangement is antalgia. That is, antalgic posture is common in patients with disc derangement, particularly in the acute stage. However, antalgia is not seen universally with disc derangement; the majority of patients with this diagnosis will not exhibit antalgia. But an understanding of the identification and treatment of derangements that exhibit antalgia helps the practitioner understand the identification and treatment of derangements that do not exhibit antalgia.

Antalgia involves the spine being "fixed," "stuck," or "crooked" in a certain direction, with inability to move enough in the opposite direction to achieve neutral positioning. This inability is due to the perception of pain or mechanical obstruction. The types of antalgia commonly seen in patients with disc derangement are *kyphotic* (Fig. 5-1), *lateral shift* (Fig. 5-2) and *lordotic* (Fig. 5-3). In the lexicon of the McKenzie Method, the three antalgias are described in terms of the theorized direction of intradiscal displacement:

- Kyphotic Antalgia (Posterior Derangement): The kyphotic antalgia is fixed in flexion and leans away from the back pain.

- Lateral Shift Antalgia (Posterolateral Derangement): Lateral shift antalgia is fixed in lateral shift (the torso is translated lateral to the pelvis) and is typically associated with unilateral pain. A lean away from the side of pain (contralateral lateral shift antalgia) is more common than a lean towards the side of pain (ipsilateral lateral shift antalgia).

- Lordotic Antalgia (Anterior Derangement): The lordotic antalgia is fixed in extension and leans toward the back pain.

There is a specific treatment protocol for each of the three antalgias. Derangements presenting without visible antalgia are diagnosed and treated based on the findings of the ERL examination. If one understands the way frank antalgias behave mechanically and symptomatically, one can then understand how to identify and treat derangements that do not exhibit antalgia. If there is a presenting antalgia

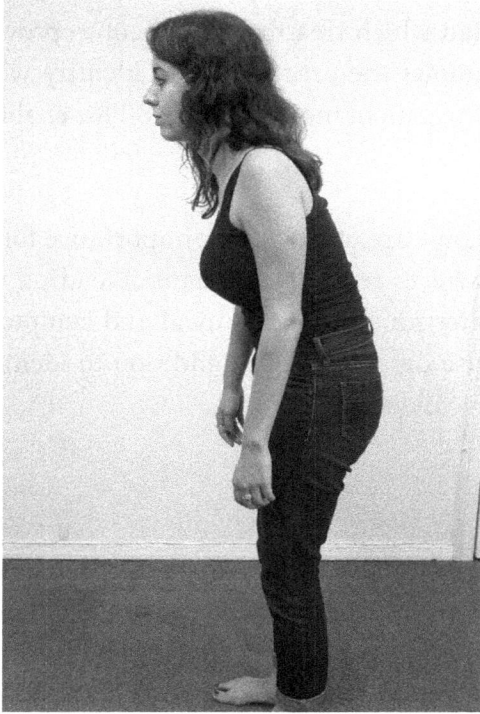

Figure 5-1. Kyphotic antalgia.

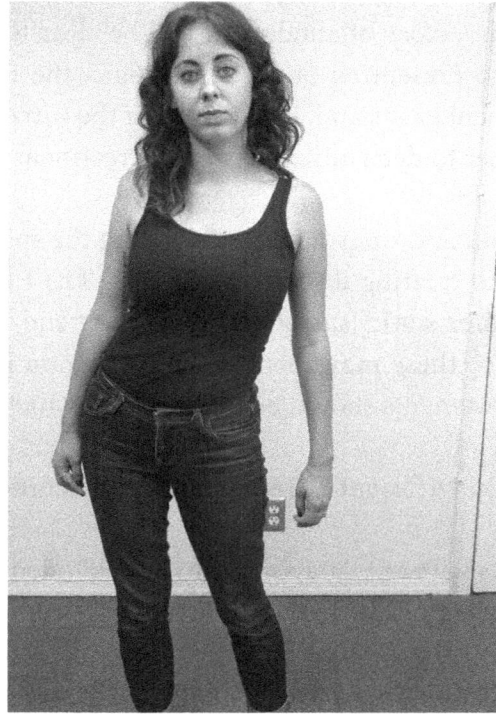

Figure 5-2. Lateral shift antalgia. Presented here is a left lateral shift antalgia. The antalgia is named according to the direction the trunk has deviated relative to the pelvis.

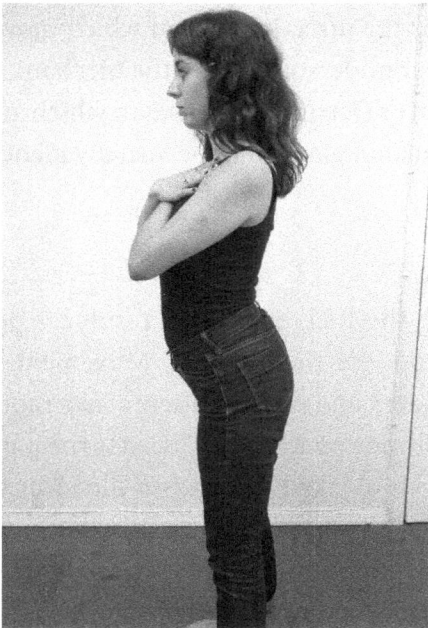

Figure 5-3. Lordotic antalgia.

or a *recent history* of antalgia, it will be clear to the clinician which treatment protocol to provide. If there is no presenting or recent antalgia, the ERL exam allows the practitioner to identify whether derangement exists and, if so, which of the three antalgias the patient most resembles. This enables the practitioner to determine the correct treatment protocol.

The pursuit and/or avoidance of loading the spine at end range are of particular importance for diagnosing and treating disc derangements. The ERL exam involves repetitive (dynamic) loading *to* end range and/or static (sustained) loading *at* end range to determine the mechanical and symptomatic response to these movements. The ERL exam identifies disc derangement in addition to identifying which movements should be pursued and which should be avoided. .

Loading in Different Directions Has Different Effects

In patients with antalgia, the trunk is held fixed in one direction due to a painful obstruction to movement in the opposite direction. Treatment protocols involve avoiding movement and positioning in the direction of the antalgia (the direction that is detrimental) and pursuing movement and positioning in the direction opposite the antalgia (the direction that is beneficial). Symptoms and mechanics are monitored to judge the appropriateness of the strategy.

The direction of the antalgia is the direction within which movement results in negative outcomes, i.e., the *Direction of Detriment*. The direction opposite the antalgia is the direction within which movement results in positive outcomes, i.e., the *Direction of Benefit*. A deeper understanding of the mechanical and symptomatic profiles of the Direction of Benefit and the Direction of Detriment in cases in which antalgia is present will increase the ability to identify derangements when antalgia cannot be visually identified.

Direction of Benefit: Mechanical and Symptomatic Profile

The Direction of Benefit is the direction of movement during the ERL exam that produces positive mechanical and symptomatic outcomes. It is the direction opposite the antalgia. Movement in the Direction of Benefit is typically restricted by a painfully obstructed end range. Patients may report the perception of an obstruction, rather than pain, as the reason for motion loss (i.e., "it's not the pain that is stopping me, it just doesn't go any farther; that's the end; it feels blocked"). Repetitive loading to end range in the Direction of Benefit results in positive mechanical and symptomatic responses including reduction of the obstruction to movement (i.e., improved range of motion) in that direction and favorable changes in symptoms (i.e., reduction and/ or centralization of pain when moving in that direction). The Direction of Benefit has been referred to by others as the "Directional Preference."

Favorable changes in derangement-related symptoms include diminution of symptom frequency or intensity as well as a unique pattern of favorable changes that McKenzie described as "centralization phenomena."

Centralization Phenomena: Retreat of Distal Symptoms

Centralization phenomena are patterns of symptomatic responses to loading, wherein there is a *retreat of distal symptoms*, i.e., reduction in the distance that symptoms extend away from the spine. There are various patterns of change that can represent centralization. Some examples are:

- Symptoms radiating from the back to the foot change to symptoms radiating only as far as the knee.

- Lower extremity pain without back pain changes to back pain without lower extremity pain.

- A localized area of back pain becomes smaller in size

The association of centralization phenomena with the McKenzie Method should not be interpreted to mean that centralization is the only favorable symptomatic change that occurs during the ERL exam. There are many cases of derangement in which the distance the symptoms extend does not change, but the symptoms simply reduce in intensity as a result of repetitive movement or sustained positioning.

Increase of Proximal Symptoms: A Centralization-Associated Response

It is important to note that during the ERL exam, when a Direction of Benefit is identified it is very likely that proximal symptoms will increase, at least initially. That is, if centralization occurs, in which the peripheral symptoms retreat proximally as a result of repetitive or sustained movement, the proximal symptoms will likely become more intense. This increase of proximal symptoms is a "favorable" response as long as centralization (retreat of distal symptoms) occurs.

Antalgias typically exhibit centralization (retreat of distal symptoms) and increase of proximal symptoms when movement occurs in the direction opposite the antalgia. In fact, *the reason the antalgic position is assumed is to avoid the increase of proximal symptoms experienced with movements in the opposite direction of antalgia.* However, in most cases that is the very movement that is required to correct the problem. Thus, it is important for the practitioner to help the patient navigate through the increase of proximal symptoms so that mechanical correction and centralization may occur. Also, it is important for the practitioner to carefully monitor the mechanical and symptomatic response to movement to be sure that a beneficial response (i.e., centralization or reduction of symptoms with improved freedom of movement) occurs rather than a detrimental response (i.e., peripheralization of symptoms).

Direction of Detriment: Mechanical and Symptomatic Profile

The Direction of Detriment is the direction of movement during the ERL exam in which loading during the arc of motion and/or at the end range of motion has negative mechanical and symptomatic effects. In patients with antalgia, the Direction of Detriment is *into* the direction of the antalgia. It was stated earlier that ERL in the Direction of Benefit is met by a painful obstruction at some point during the range. In the Direction of Detriment there can be pain during the arc of motion as well at end range. In addition, movement is not obstructed; in fact, there may be excessive movement. When voluntary motion is limited it is the perception of pain and a feeling of instability as opposed to the perception of a mechanical obstruction that is reported as prohibiting further movement (i.e., "I *could* go farther but it would hurt me too much").

Loading in the Direction of Detriment results in negative mechanical and symptomatic responses. These may include excessive range of motion or aberrant movement (e.g., a painful "catch") in that direction, the creation of a painfully obstructed end range in one or more *other* directions of movement, increased symptom intensity or frequency and *peripheralization phenomena.*

Peripheralization phenomena are symptomatic responses to repetitive or sustained loading in which there is *advance* of distal symptoms; it is the opposite of centralization in that symptoms radiate farther from the spine. In addition, in the Direction of Detriment there typically occurs a *decrease of proximal symptoms.* This is in contrast to the *increase of proximal symptoms* that is associated with the centralization response that occurs with the Direction of Benefit.

The "McKenzie Reflex": Directions of Benefit and Detriment Affect Each Other

The responses to loading in the Direction of Detriment can result in a mechanical obstruction to movement in the Direction of Benefit. Subsequent loading in the Direction of Benefit will then diminish the mechanical obstruction. Stated another way, *loading in a direction that promotes peripheralization or increase of peripheral symptoms can lead to mechanical obstruction to movement in another direction. Conversely, loading in a direction that diminishes the mechanical obstruction to movement diminishes the adverse effects of loading in the direction that promoted peripheralization.*

As was discussed in Chapter 2, it is not known for certain what causes disc pain. However, the working model is one of "derangement" in which a part of the nucleus pulposis migrates into a radial tear in the annulus.

While further research is needed to explore the derangement mechanism, this theoretical model can help the practitioner conceptualize the effects of the ERL exam as well as the treatment that arises from this exam.

Conceptual explanations based on the derangement theory of disc pain are as follows:

- Loading in the Direction of Detriment causes further displacement of intradiscal material during the arc of motion and at the end of range, thus causing peripheralization of symptoms. Loading in the Direction of Detriment promotes intradiscal displacement to a more distal location, reflected by peripheralization phenomena (advance of distal symptoms) and, at times, decrease of proximal symptoms. Range of motion may be excessive, as the displaced intradiscal material does not offer resistance to movement in the Direction of Detriment; the displacement encourages movement in that direction. As the derangement worsens, movement into the direction in which the nuclear material became displaced (anterior, posterior or posterolateral) is increasingly obstructed until antalgia develops.

- The Direction of Benefit is movement in the direction obstructed by the displacement of nuclear material. In the Direction of Benefit, there is no pain until end range, at which point the displaced nuclear material offers resistance to motion, resulting in a painfully obstructed end range. Loading at the painfully obstructed end range in the Direction of Benefit returns the displaced intradiscal material to a more central location, reflected by the symptomatic phenomena of centralization (retreat of distal symptoms). Proximal increase of symptoms associated with centralization represents the "pressure pain" of returning the nuclear material to "a smaller container." Reduction of the derangement diminishes the chances and severity of the adverse effects that result from loading in the Direction of Detriment.

Antalgia Spectrum Phases

As antalgia resolves, derangement features are increasingly subtracted from the clinical picture (conversely, as antalgia develops, derangement features are added). An idealized day-to-day scenario of the order in which derangement features are subtracted from the clinical picture as antalgia resolves is considered below; the opposite order would represent antalgia development. In the treatment of disc derangement with antalgia, loading in the Direction of Benefit results in progressive improvement, typically (though certainly not universally) in the following order:

Day 1: Increase of proximal symptoms associated with centralization and recovery of movement in the obstructed direction in order to achieve neutral posture

Day 2: Increase of proximal symptoms no longer occurs as centralization continues

Day 3: Symptoms and mechanical aberrations during the arc of motion in the Direction of Detriment resolve; centralization continues.

Day 4: Symptoms at the end range of motion in the Direction of Detriment resolve; centralization continues

Day 5: The painful obstructed end range in the Direction of Benefit resolve; centralization continues

Day 6: No complaints; no findings during motion or at end range in any direction

It should be noted that *the most basic mechanical and symptomatic pattern of disc derangement is the painfully obstructed end range in a movement plane direction that is unremarkable during the arc of movement.* This mechanical feature is more important than the topography of the symptoms that the patient describes during history taking.

Antalgia Treatment-Based Protocols:

For each type of antalgia the classic McKenzie Derangement nomenclature is provided in parentheses. Then the Direction of Benefit and the Direction of Detriment are identified. A detailed description of the skills required to reduce derangements and to maintain their reduction is considered at length for the antalgias, which represent the most severe manifestation of disc derangement. In cases in which there is no antalgia it is the practitioner's task, through the ERL exam, to determine which antalgia the patient most resembles and then to use that antalgia treatment protocol to correct the derangement.

The majority of patients respond to the treatment protocols for kyphotic antalgia (except those who present with lateral shift or lordotic antalgia), independent of where the presenting symptoms are located. So in the patient who does not have antalgia it is best to explore sagittal plane movements first (this will be discussed later).

Kyphotic AntalgiaTreatment Protocols (Posterior Derangement Protocols)

- Direction of Benefit: Extension

- Direction of Detriment: Flexion

For patients with a frank kyphotic antalgia, symptoms are typically central or symmetrical and do not radiate into the lower extremities. However, the majority of patients with asymmetrical lumbosacral symptoms radiating down the lower extremity (a Posterolateral Derangement) but who do not have a lateral shift antalgia, respond to Kyphotic Antalgia Treatment Protocols (i.e., the ERL examination reveals centralization with extension movements, as will be discussed later). In those cases, the obstruction offered by the posterior component of the nuclear displacement is more relevant to loading than the lateral component; it is thought that the reduction of the posterior component takes the lateral component "along for the ride," i.e. is able to draw the lateral component forward and to the center as well.

The patient presenting with kyphotic antalgia (Fig. 5-1), cannot tolerate the increase of proximal symptoms associated with centralization in the Direction of Benefit (i.e., extension) in the standing position. Therefore treatment is initiated from the prone position and the patient is asked to report on centralization and peripheralization phenomena each step of the way. The progression is as follows:

- The patient lies prone, preserving the kyphosis (Fig. 5-4): The patient is made comfortable with a roll placed under the abdomen to "accommodate" the antalgia.

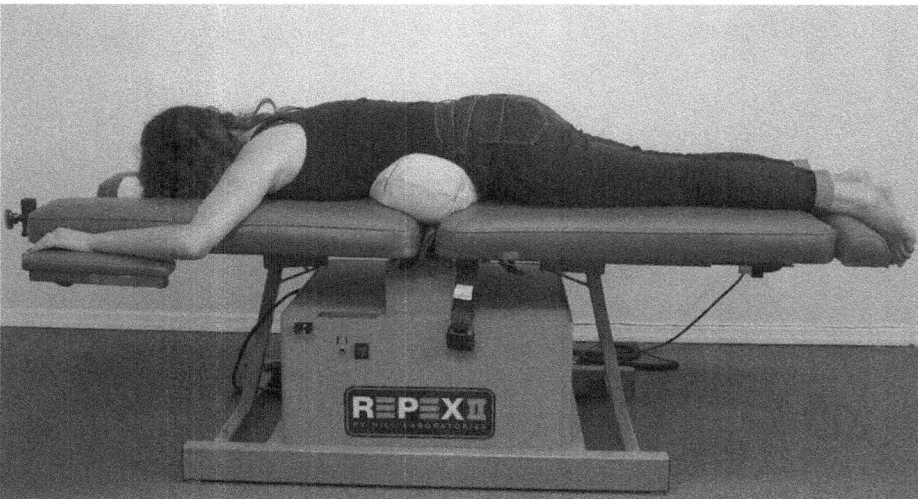

Figure 5-4. Prone lying with a roll to accommodate the kyphosis.

- Prone Lying (Fig. 5-5): After the patient relaxes, the roll is removed so the patient lies flat on the support surface, thus diminishing the kyphosis and perhaps introducing slight lordosis.

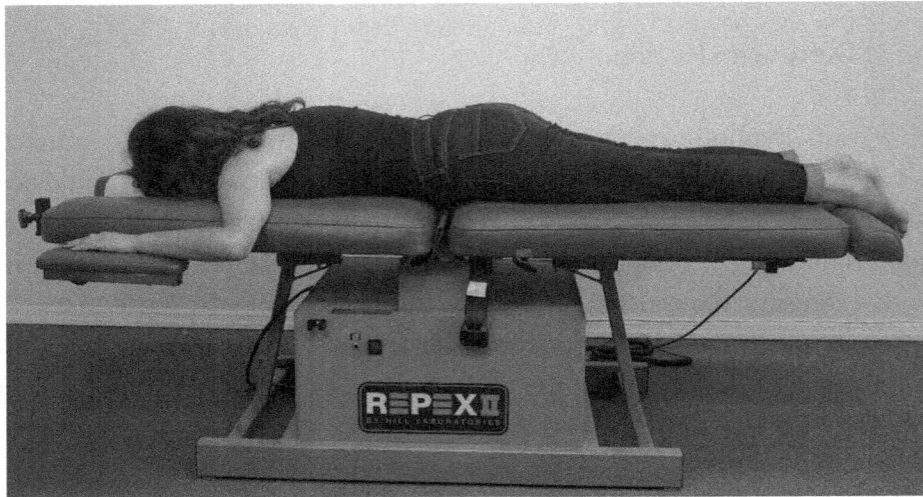

Figure 5-5. Prone lying without support.

- Reclining on Elbows (Fig. 5-6): The patient is asked to raise the trunk up to rest on bent elbows and forearms. The patient lets the abdomen sag, thus introducing lordosis.

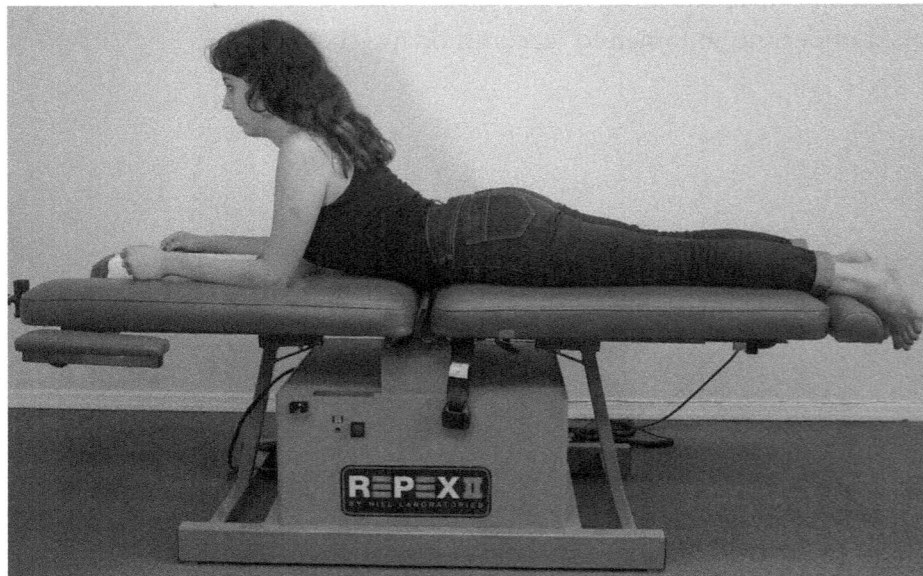

Figure 5-6. Reclining on elbows.

- Prone extension (Fig. 5-7): From the prone position, the hands are placed between the level of the ears and the shoulders and the elbows are extended to passively extend the trunk. The patient lets the abdomen and pelvis "sag down." It is important to avoid contraction of the gluteal muscles as this limits lumbar extension. Gluteal contraction can be prevented by placing the lower extremities in a pigeon-toed (hip internal rotation) position. Prone extension is performed as far as possible to end-range, with instructions to hold the end range of extension for a second or two. The patient then returns to the prone position, completely relaxes for a moment, and then repeats the "press-up" for up to 10 repetitions, attempting to extend further each time. The recovery of extension in the prone position translates into resolution of the kyphotic antalgia in the standing position.

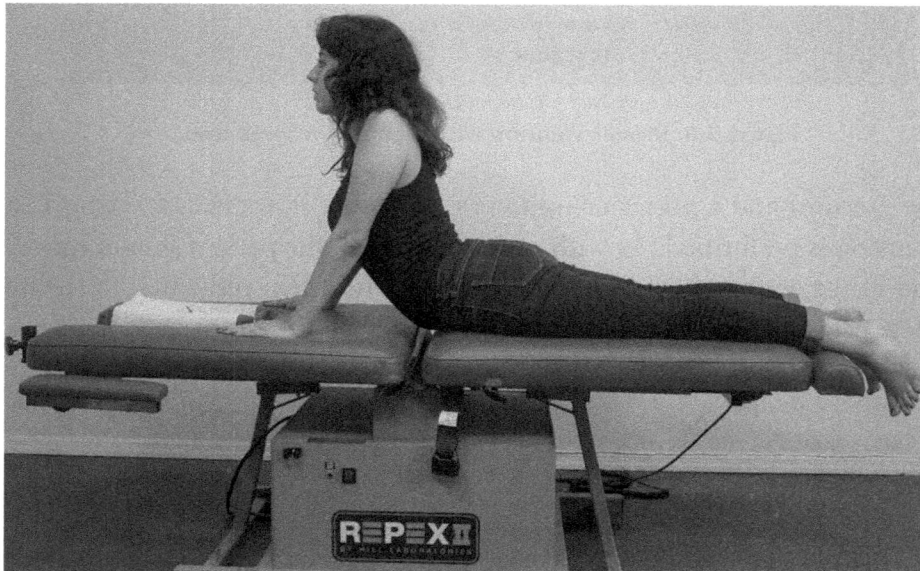

Figure 5-7. Prone extension.

- Prone extension with manual overpressure (Fig. 5-8): When performing prone extensions, manual overpressure (mobilization with patient generated movement) may be applied to help promote end range extension and centralization.

- Standing extension (Fig. 5-9): As the derangement improves (typically by the second visit), extension exercises in the standing position are introduced as an alternative to prone extension; these are useful in circumstances (such as at work) when exercising in the prone position is not possible. The patient's hands are placed on both sides of the lumbosacral spine (typically the

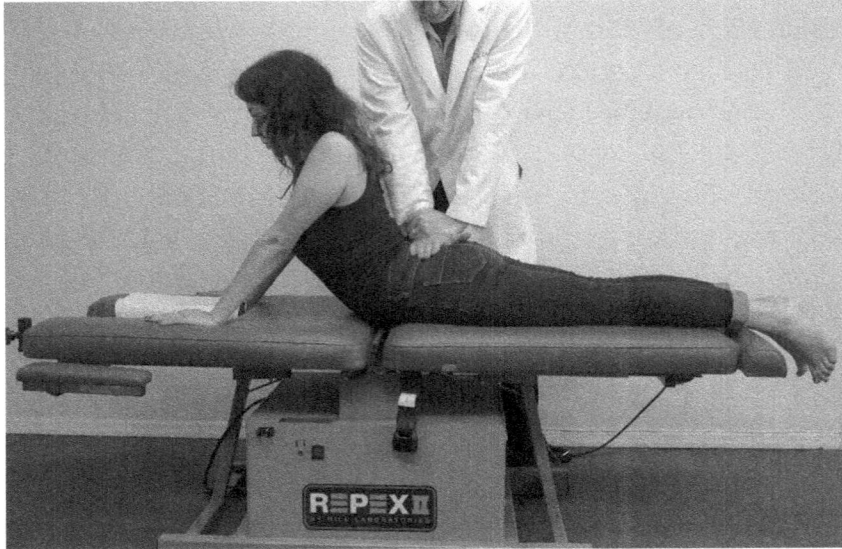

Figure 5-8. Prone extension with manual overpressure.

base of the sacrum) and a posterior-to-anterior pressure is applied, creating a fulcrum about which extension is performed. As with prone extension, the patient should move as far as possible to end-range, with a pause both at end-range and when returning to the neutral staring position between repetitions. The exercise is repeated 10 times. Prone extensions are typically

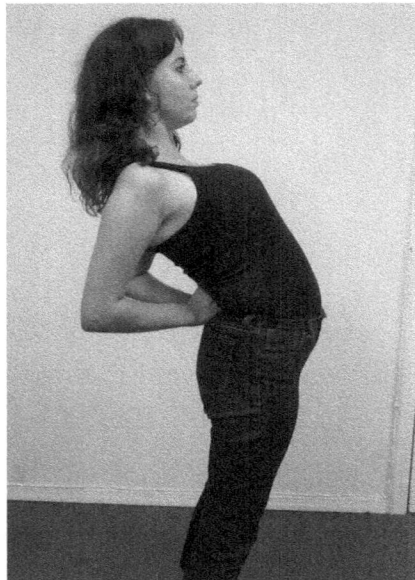

Figure 5-9. Standing extension.

more effective than standing extensions but in certain circumstances it might not be convenient for the patient to perform prone extensions. In these circumstances, standing extensions are usually an adequate substitute. However the patient should be instructed to perform the extension exercises in the prone position whenever possible.

Avoiding Loading in the Direction of Detriment (Flexion)

The kyphotic antalgia patient is advised to avoid any exercises, movements or positions that flex the lumbar spine, i.e., anything that brings the chest and knees closer together. Education is provided regarding the maintenance of lumbar lordosis (slight extension) when sitting, lifting, performing manual handling tasks, making transitions between postures, etc (see Chapter 9 for additional recommendations).

If lordotic sitting posture results in centralization and flexed, slouched sitting posture results in peripheralization, those reactions can be used as educational and motivational tools. However, it must be remembered that increase of proximal symptoms associated with centralization is common in patients with disc derangement. In these cases, the practitioner must provide appropriate guidance. But even in cases where there is obvious benefit from "sitting up", patients may not comply because they feel they "look weird" when doing so. This psychosocial obstacle to assuming a lordotic sitting posture can be overcome with various simple educational techniques.

Two effective approaches to teaching how to achieve lumbar lordotic sitting and how to help overcome the psychosocial barriers to lordotic sitting are McKenzie's "Slouch-Overcorrect-Relax 10%" and the senior author's (GJ) "Stand Alert-Sit Alert-Stand Alert" and "Sit Slouched-Stand Slouched" exercises.

Slouch-Overcorrect-Relax 10%

Step 1: Slouched sitting posture (Fig. 5-10) - The patient is asked to assume a slouched sitting posture, i.e., to load the lumbosacral spine at the end range of flexion. Adverse symptoms are noted.

Step 2: Over-corrected sitting posture (Fig. 5-11) - The patient simultaneously rolls the pelvis forward to increase lumbar lordosis, rotates the chest upward and retracts the head and neck backward, all to end-range. The shoulders should not be thrown back in a "military" posture but should relax "down." Essentially, body parts are moved to the end of range in the direction opposite the slouched positioning.

Step 3: "Let go 10%" (Fig. 5-12) - From the overcorrected position, the patient is asked to let go ~10% to find correct lordotic sitting posture

For those who "feel weird" when "sitting up," the overcorrected posture feels even weirder. The result of this is that the normal lordotic sitting posture does not feel so weird after all.

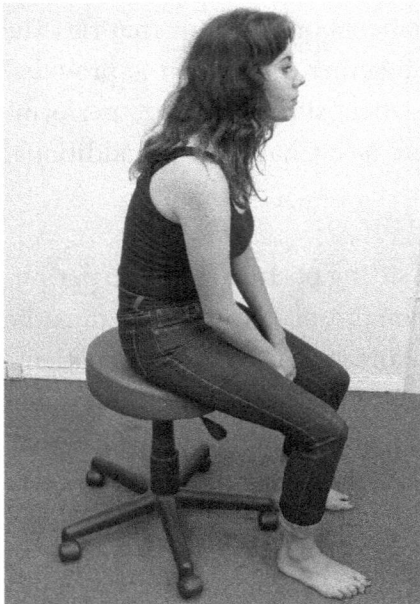

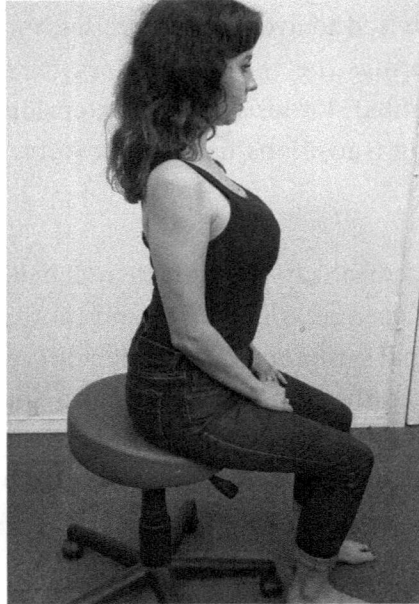

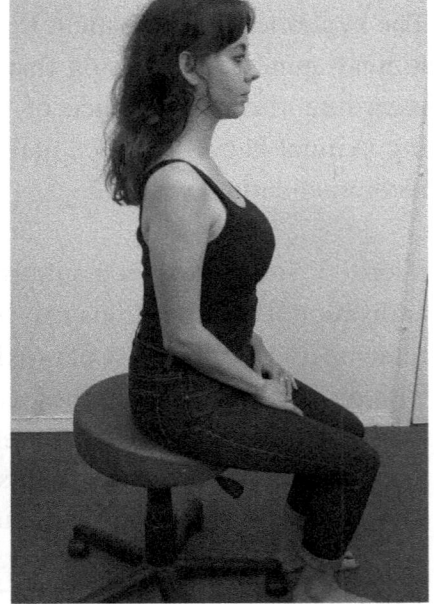

Figure 5-10. Slouched sitting posture. Figure 5-11. Over-corrected sitting posture. Figure 5-12. Letting go 10% to attain the correct lordotic sitting posture.

Stand Alert-Sit Alert-Stand Alert

This trains lordotic sitting by maintaining the lordosis of standing.

Step 1: Stand alert - The patient is asked to stand with alert (not military) posture.

Step 2: Standing to sitting maintaining alert upper body posture (Fig. 5-13) - From alert standing, the patient is guided into a seated position while maintaining the lumbar lordosis of standing. The practitioner's hands may be strategically placed on the sternum (to prevent flexion) and on the low back (to preserve lordosis) during the transition. The patient is asked to imagine having a glass on his or her head that is filled to the brim. Some patients may have to "stick the buttocks out backwards" a bit in order to ensure lordosis is maintained during the transition.

Step 3: Sitting to standing maintaining lumbar lordosis - From the lordotic sitting posture, the patient is transitioned from sitting to standing, maintaining lumbar lordosis. Again the practitioner's hands may be applied to ensure the maintenance of the lordosis

With this exercise the patient realizes that sitting up does not look weird because, from the waist up, he or she looks the same as when standing.

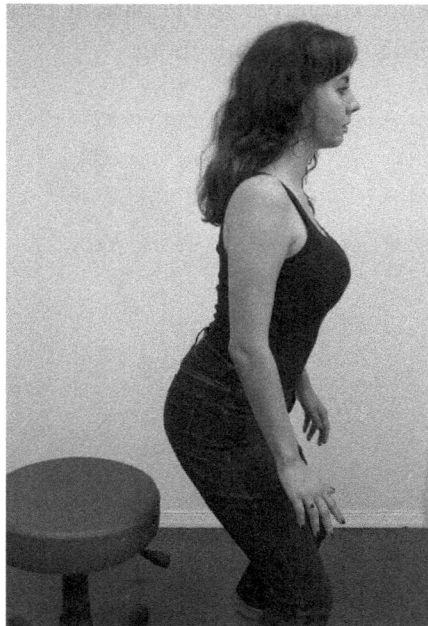

Figure 5-13. Standing to sitting maintaining alert upper body posture

Sit Slouched-Stand Slouched

This exercise, employed subsequent to the Stand Alert-Sit Alert-Stand Alert Exercise, is merely a psychosocial ploy to help the patient better appreciate the how the slouched sitting posture that feels "normal" is not advantageous, whether the concern is about appearance or health.

Step 1: Sit slouched (Fig. 5-10) - The patient is asked to sit in a relaxed, slouched position.

Step 2: Sitting to standing maintaining upper body slouched posture (Fig. 5-14) - The slouched (flexed) position of the trunk is maintained as the patient is transitioned to standing. The practitioner's hands may be strategically placed on the upper back and abdomen to maintain the slouched posture. Once standing, the practitioner removes the hands and the patient is left to contemplate the disadvantages of maintained flexion of the lumbar spine.

With this exercise the patient immediately understands that it looks strange and would be unduly stressful to stand and walk with the lumbar spine in the flexed, slouched position that is so often assumed when sitting. The patient can then easily generalize these principles to the sitting position. Neutral lordotic sitting becomes more attractive as the patient realizes it resembles the way he or she prefers to look and feel when standing and walking about.

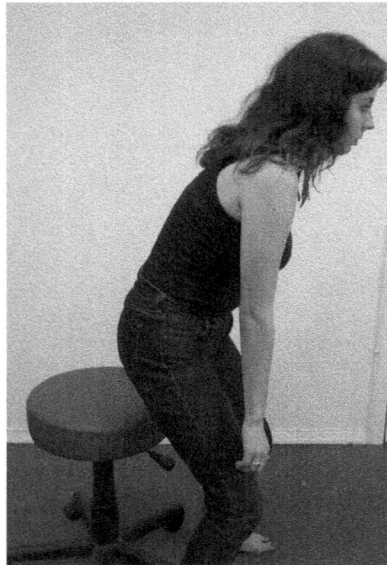

Figure 5-14. Sitting to standing maintaining upper body slouched posture.

Kyphotic Antalgia Treatment Protocols for Patients with Postero-lateral Derangements

The Kyphotic Antalgia Treatment Protocols are the ones most patients initially respond to. It was noted earlier that kyphotic antalgia correlates to the "posterior derangement" in the McKenzie lexicon. However, the Kyphotic Antalgia Treatment Protocols are also the most common method to treat posterolateral derangements when there is no lateral shift antalgia. In those cases, the posterior component of the derangement is more relevant to the loading strategy than the lateral component. The lateral component is not significant; obstruction to movement in the coronal plane may be slight or non-existent. The nuclear displacement theory would indicate that the extension forces that are employed manage to reduce both the posterior component and the lateral component of the derangement. The lateral component of the nuclear migration is reduced by direct effect or by being "brought along" by the posterior component.

In cases in which the size of the lateral component is sufficient to significantly obstruct movement in the coronal plane, the Lateral Shift Antalgia Treatment Protocols are required. Those cases are identified as having a "relevant lateral component," meaning the lateral component is relevant to the loading strategy; the loading strategy should be *lateral* and not in the sagittal plane. In these cases, the lateral component of the derangement is more relevant to the loading strategy than the posterior component. Even in cases of frank lateral shift antalgia, once the lateral component is sufficiently reduced (with resolution of antalgia and other signs and symptoms), the Kyphotic Antalgia Treatment Protocols are required for complete resolution.

Lateral Shift Treatment Protocols (Postero-Lateral Derangement Protocols)

- Direction of Benefit: Side gliding in the opposite direction of antalgia

- Direction of Detriment: Side gliding into the antalgia, extension, flexion

Lateral shift antalgia (Fig. 5-2) involves an obstruction to movement in two movement-plane directions. The obvious one is in the coronal direction opposite the antalgia (the lateral component of the posterolateral derangement). The less obvious obstruction to movement is in extension (the posterior component of the posterolateral derangement).

Recovery of motion in the coronal direction is required before recovery of extension motion can be achieved. After recovery of movement in the direction opposite the antalgia, extension changes from a Direction of Detriment to a Direction of Benefit. At that point treatment continues according to Kyphotic Antalgia Treatment Protocols.

The explanation according to nuclear displacement theory for extension being detrimental and then becoming beneficial after coronal plane loading is as follows:

If the lateral component is significant, extension cannot sufficiently drive the lateral component of the displaced intradiscal material to the center and instead "squeezes" the material more laterally.

However, after coronal loading *sufficiently* reduces the lateral component, extension is then not only effective in reducing the posterior component of the derangement but is also able to drive the remaining lateral component of the derangement to the center as well.

Lateral shift antalgia represents the *fixed position* in which the torso is translated to the right or left in relation to the pelvis. *Side gliding* is the *translation movement* employed to correct the lateral shift antalgia. Both the lateral shift position and the side gliding movement are named "right" or "left" according to the direction the torso is positioned or moves relative to the pelvis.

The reader should recall that treatment of the kyphotic antalgia has to be initiated in the prone position (because the proximal increase of symptoms cannot be tolerated standing), and then progressed to standing. Treatment of the lateral shift antalgia is initiated in the standing position, with prone procedures added later. Described here are exercise progressions for a patient presenting with a *left lateral shift antalgia* (Fig. 5-2).

Wall Side Gliding

There are three variations of Wall Side Gliding, each involving different degrees of extension. These are Flexion Side Gliding, Neutral Side Gliding and Extension at Side Gliding End Range (i.e. extension from a lateral shift position).

Flexion Side Gliding is required for a minority of patients who cannot tolerate Neutral Side Gliding due to proximal increase of symptoms or who peripheralize during Neutral Side Gliding. Once Flexion Side Gliding is tolerated and is of benefit, the patient can be progressed to Neutral Side Gliding. Once Neutral Side Gliding is tolerated and is of benefit, the patient can be progressed to Extension at Side Gliding End Range (i.e. from a lateral shift position).

Neutral Trunk Wall Side Gliding (Fig. 5-15): The exercise description will be of a patient with a left lateral shift antalgia. The patient is asked to flex the elbow to 90° and to "lean" against the wall so the entire lateral aspect of the left arm presses firmly against the wall without the left shoulder "hunching up" or becoming unleveled. The axillary line of the patient's trunk leans into the medial epicondyle. The feet are placed away from the wall. The right hand is placed just below the right iliac crest and applies pressure to translate the pelvis leftward, toward the wall (right side gliding). The pelvis is translated left towards the wall until the obstructed end range prevents further movement. This position is maintained for a moment and then the pelvis is slowly backed away from the wall just enough to decrease the pain. The exercise is performed up to 10 repetitions, the patient attempting to translate the pelvis farther towards the wall with each repetition. Unlike prone extensions, in which the patient returns to the starting position with each repetition, side gliding is more of a ratchet-like pattern of recovering motion, i.e., backing off a little, recovering more motion, backing off a little, etc., without returning to the starting point for each cycle. After the exercise is completed it is important for the patient to slowly and carefully move back into the upright position so as to not recreate the antalgia.

Flexed Trunk Side Gliding (Fig. 5-16): In a minority of patients, slide gliding in the neutral position produces proximal increase of symptoms that is intolerable, or peripheralization occurs with this movement. In these cases the exercise is modified to be performed from a slightly flexed trunk position.

Extension at the End Range of Side Gliding (Fig. 5-17): When slide gliding in the neutral position is tolerated with benefit, the degree of extension is ramped up by the patient performing extension at the point of maximum side gliding, i.e. from a lateral shift position opposite that of the antalgia. After achieving the lateral shift position, the patient extends the trunk by sliding the lateral aspect of the arm against the wall, as if the patient were cleaning the wall.

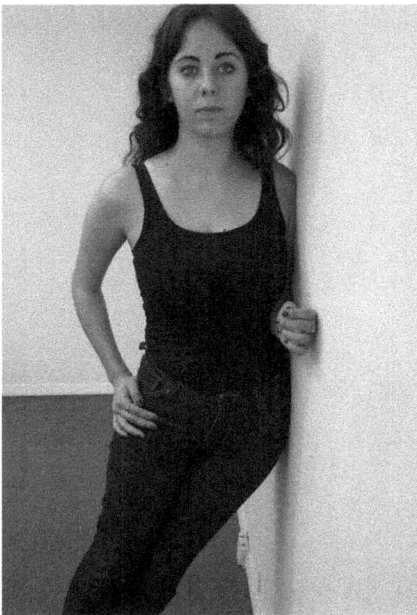

Figure 5-15. Neutral trunk wall side gliding.

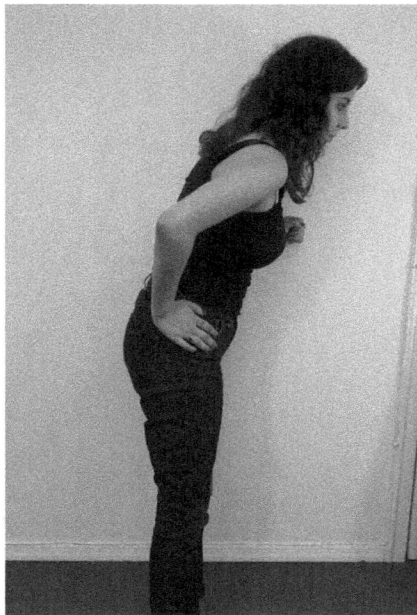

Figure 5-16. Flexed trunk wall side gliding.

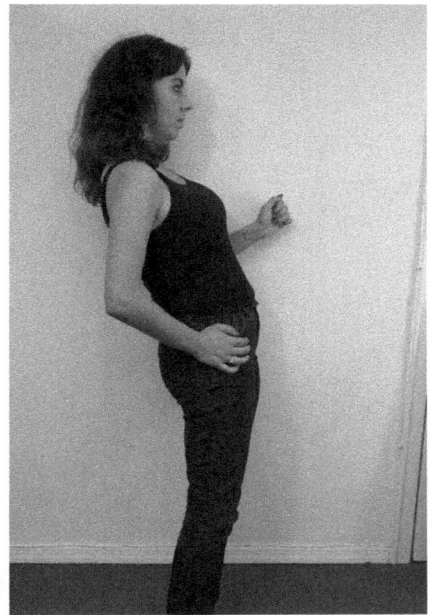

Figure 5-17. Extension at the end range of side gliding.

Practitioner-Assisted Side Gliding (Fig. 5-18): If the patient is unable to adequately conduct the Wall Side Gliding exercise to end range, practitioner assistance is required.

The patient stands with the feet shoulder width apart. The medial epicondyle of the left elbow is placed against the axillary line. The practitioner approaches the patient from the left, oriented in the coronal plane and places the forward foot behind the patient and the rear foot perpendicular to the forward foot. The practitioner's left upper trapezius contacts the patient's left arm just above left elbow. The practitioner reaches around the patient, interlacing the fingers just below the crest of the right ilium. The practitioner's hands pull the pelvis while at the same time the practitioner's shoulder pushes the trunk away. Practitioner-assisted side gliding employs the same variations as wall side gliding. For Extension at the End Range of Side Gliding, there is no wall to brush against; the patient obtains stability by holding/leaning on to the practitioner's wrist (Fig. 5-19).

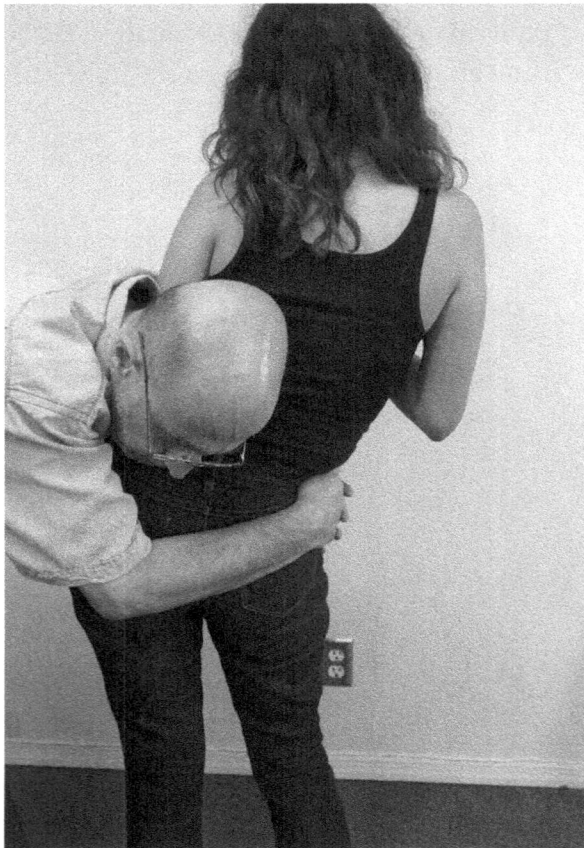

Figure 5-18. Practitioner-assisted side gliding.

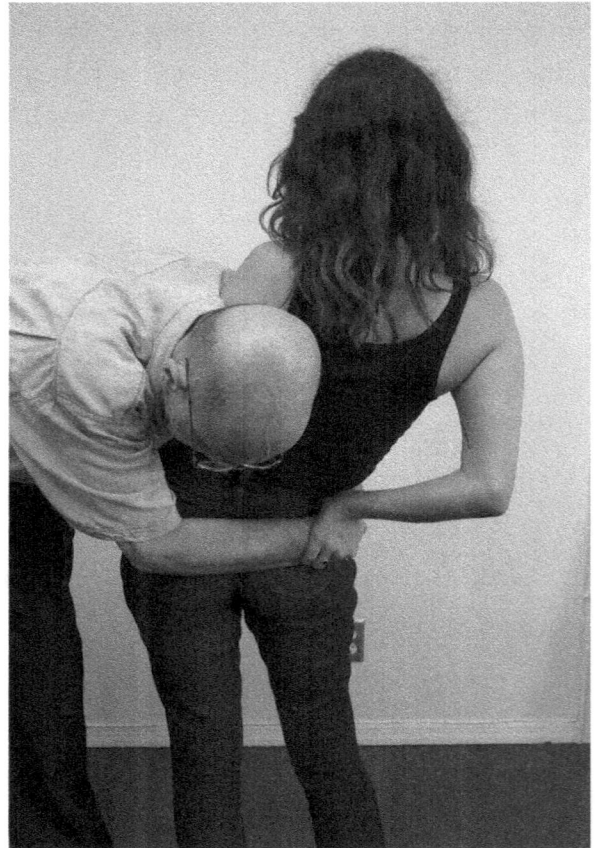

Figure 5-19. Practitioner-assisted extension at the end range of side gliding.

Prone Extension from a Lateral Shift Position (Fig. 5-20): If Extension at the End Range of Right Side Gliding is beneficial, the patient is progressed to the same exercise performed in the prone position.

The prone patient is asked to translate the pelvis in the direction opposite that of the presenting antalgia. For the patient with left lateral shift antalgia the pelvis is moved to the left, creating a right lateral shift. Prone extensions are then performed from the right lateral shift position up to 10 times in the manner described for the kyphotic antalgia, the only difference being the laterally shifted starting position. With each repetition of the exercise, further extension is attempted.

Once Prone Extensions from a Lateral Shift position are tolerated and are of benefit, the patient is progressed to the Kyphotic Antalgia Treatment Protocols, i.e. prone extensions (Fig. 5-7).

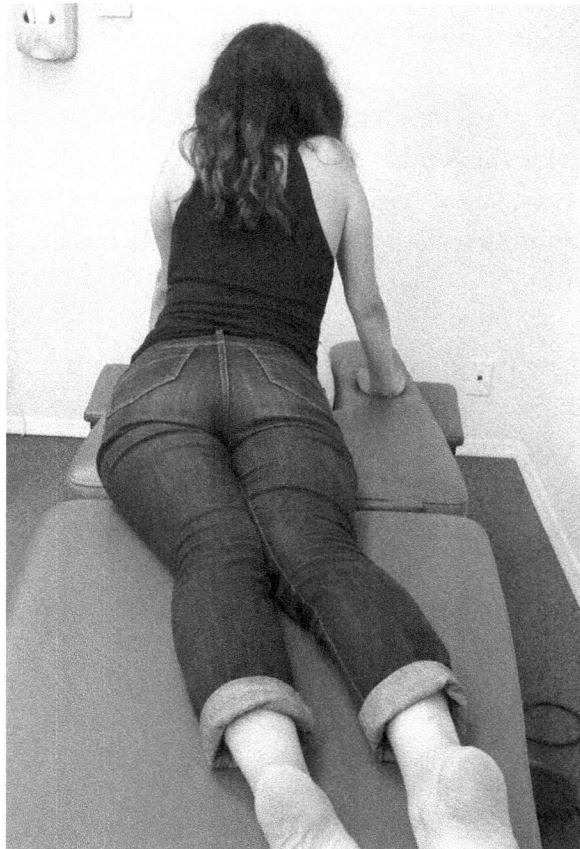

Figure 5-20. Prone extension from a lateral shift position.

An example of five-visit treatment progression for lateral shift antalgia is as follows. It is noted that each progression increases the degree of extension.

Day 1: Flexion Side Gliding (if necessary) (Fig. 5-16).

Day 2: Neutral Side Gliding (Fig. 5-15).

Day 3: Extension at the End Range of Side Gliding (Fig. 5-17).

Day 4: Prone Extension from a Lateral Shift Position (Fig. 5-20).

Day 5: Prone Extensions (Fig. 5-7)

Avoiding Mid- or End-Range Loading in Flexion Direction of Detriment

As with the kyphotic antalgia patient, the lateral shift antalgia patient is advised to avoid any exercises, movements or positions that flex the lumbar spine. As with the kyphotic antalgia patient, the lateral shift antalgia patient receives education regarding the maintenance of lumbar lordosis when sitting, lifting, performing manual handling tasks, making transitions between postures, etc (see Chapter 9 for additional recommendations).

The difference between the lateral shift antalgia and the kyphotic antalgia is that while flexion is a Direction of Detriment for both, extension is initially a Direction of Detriment for the lateral shift antalgia but is the Direction of Benefit for the kyphotic antalgia. While it is important for the lateral shift antalgia patient to avoid flexion by maintaining some lordosis in the lumbar spine, the degree of lordosis that is tolerated may be limited until the lateral component is reduced.

Lordotic Antalgia Treatment Protocols (Anterior Derangement Protocols)

- Direction of Benefit: Flexion

- Direction of Detriment: Extension

The treatment protocols for lordotic antalgia (Fig. 5-3) are the opposite of those for the kyphotic antalgia. Flexion end range loading exercises are advised. Extension is avoided. Patients are encouraged to slouch when sitting. Flexion may be performed from the supine, sitting or standing position (Fig. 5-21).

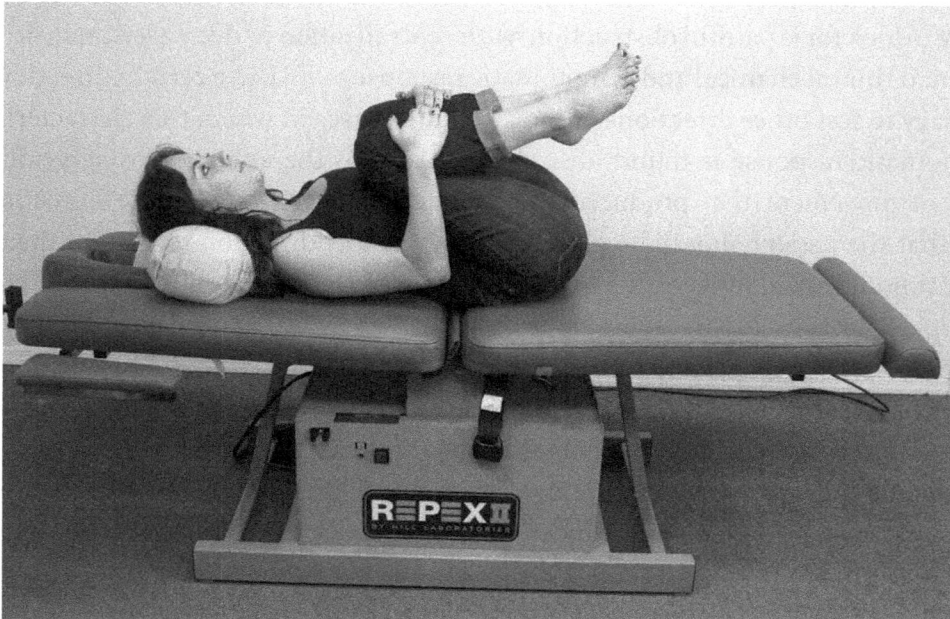

Figure 5-21. Flexion exercises in the supine position.

Anterior disc derangements typically do not radiate beyond the knee and pain often refers to the groin or anterior thigh.

The End Range Loading Exam for Detecting Derangement in the Absence of Antalgia

As discussed earlier, the majority of patients with disc derangement do not exhibit antalgia. But the treatment protocols for the different antalgias can help the practitioner conceptualize how to determine whether a patient who does not exhibit antalgia has disc derangement.

Disc derangements are identified based on their characteristic response to the ERL exam, i.e., moving the spine to end-range in the various directions presented here. The characteristic response is:

- Movement in one direction results in painful obstruction. Repetitive movement in this direction causes proximal increase in symptoms, centralization or reduction of peripheral symptoms and gradual easing of the painful obstruction.

- Movement in another direction results in normal or excessive range of motion and peripheralization of symptoms with repetition.

The key feature to look for is painful obstruction, with centralization or decreased intensity of symptoms upon repetition. If this mechanical and symptomatic response to ERL in a certain direction is identified, it is not necessary to test other directions of movement. In cases in which this characteristic mechanical and symptomatic response is found, disc derangement is the answer to diagnostic question #2. The direction of movement that produced this characteristic response is the Direction of Benefit, which means that the patient should be given exercises in this direction to correct the derangement. And the patient should avoid movements in the Direction of Detriment, at least until the derangement is corrected.

The Directions of Benefit discussed with regard to the treatment of the antalgias are the directions that are pursued in the ERL exam in patients without antalgia. Consistent with the fact that the most common antalgia is the kyphotic type, the most common Direction of Benefit in patients with disc derangement is extension. Therefore, it is most sensible to check this direction of movement first during the ERL exam.

Extension ERL

To perform ERL in extension, the same process used for the Kyphotic Antalgia Treatment Protocols is followed, however in most cases the practitioner can start with Step 4, the prone extension maneuver (Fig. 5-7). The patient presses up until the painful obstruction is engaged, relaxes in that position for a moment, and then returns to the starting position. The practitioner observes the range of motion and asks the patient to report any symptoms. If there is a painful obstruction, particularly if the patient's presenting pain is reproduced, the patient is then asked to perform this maneuver repetitively and to observe and report to the practitioner what "happens" to the pain as well as to the obstruction. Typically, up to 10 repetitions may be necessary to fully evaluate the mechanical and symptomatic response to this repetitive movement. Again, a characteristic response of disc derangement would be for the pain to gradually centralize or decrease in intensity and the mechanical obstruction to ease as the movement is repeated.

It is important for the practitioner to remember that increase in proximal symptoms is common in patients with disc derangement. Because of this, the patient may report that the pain is "worsening." Therefore the practitioner should always ask the patient to report on the location of the pain as well as the nature of the obstruction, rather than using judgmental terms such as "getting better" or "getting worse." This helps the practitioner gain accurate information regarding the response to the ERL movement but also trains the patient to objectively observe the pain without judgment or evaluation. Objectively observing the pain is an important skill that will be discussed further in Chapters 8, 9 and 11.

Side Gliding ERL

Assessing side gliding is done in the same manner as was used for the Lateral Shift Treatment Protocols. It is done in the neutral position and either the patient-generated wall side gliding method (Fig. 5-15) or the practitioner-assisted method (Fig. 5-18) can be used. As with the assessment of extension, the mechanical and symptomatic response to repetitive movements is explored. The spine is moved to end-range until the painful obstruction is engaged. The patient relaxes in that position for a moment, and then returns to the starting position. The practitioner observes the range of motion and asks the patient to report any symptoms. If there is a painful obstruction, particularly if the patient's presenting pain is reproduced, this maneuver is repeated up to 10 times. While the repetitions are being performed, any changes in the mechanics and/or symptoms are noted.

In some patients, rather than moving back to the neutral position after moving to end-range, it is helpful to move the spine to end-range, then just away from that point with the movement repeated in a ratchet-like pattern, each repetition involving the patient moving to the point of obstruction, then away, etc., without returning to the starting point for each cycle.

In other patients, when assessing side gliding, sustained positioning can be helpful. With sustained positioning the spine is moved to the point at which the painful obstruction is engaged. The patient then stays at that point for an extended period of time (as short as 20 seconds, as long as 60 seconds). The patient moves away from the painful obstruction, and then moves back to that point again. The patient observes and reports on the mechanical and symptomatic response to returning to end-range after sustained positioning.

Side gliding is often the Direction of Benefit in patients with unilateral pain (although, as was stated earlier, most patients with unilateral pain respond positively to extension). Either direction of side gliding (i.e., left or right) can conceivably be the Direction of Benefit however it is more common for side gliding toward the side of pain to be the Direction of Benefit then side gliding away from the side of pain (recall that the direction of side gliding is named by the direction the torso moves). So in a patient with unilateral pain, if centralization or improvement of symptoms is not found with extension, side gliding toward the side of pain should be explored. If centralization or improvement is not found with this, side gliding away from the side of pain should be explored.

Flexion ERL

Flexion is uncommonly the Direction of Benefit and should only be explored if centralization or improvement is not found with extension or with side gliding to both sides. The flexion ERL examination is performed in the same manner as described earlier for the Lordotic Antalgia Treatment Protocols. The assessment is best done in the supine position (Fig. 5-21). As with side gliding, repetitive movements or sustained positioning can be explored.

Additional Tips for Detecting Derangement in the Absence of Antalgia

When a patient presents with antalgia, disc derangement is strongly suspected and the treatment protocol is to reverse the antalgia and monitor for centralization or improvement of symptoms. Therefore, in patients with antalgia a meticulous evaluation of mechanical and symptomatic responses to determine the Direction of Benefit and the Direction of Detriment is typically not required, although *monitoring* the mechanical and symptomatic responses to treatment is always necessary. When patients do not present with an antalgia, but derangement is suspected (based on historical factors related to disc pain), detective work is required to confirm whether derangement exists and, if so, which antalgia treatment protocol is the best fit (i.e., what is the Direction of Benefit). In addition to the ERL exam as described above, the following derangement detection and correction tips are helpful.

Recent History of Antalgia: When a patient presents without antalgia, disc derangement (and the type of derangement) may be determined by obtaining a history of recent antalgia. Even if patients deny recently "being crooked," it is important to specifically ask if they have difficulty standing erect upon awakening in the morning or after prolonged sitting. If that is the case, further inquiry should be made as to whether they are "stuck" forward (kyphotic antalgia) or to the side (lateral shift antalgia).

Pain Worse on Awakening: Awakening with back pain or pain that is significantly worse in the morning is typical of disc derangement. This is thought to be due to imbibition of fluid into the disc, resulting in increased intradiscal pressure.

Relative Effects of Sitting Compared to Standing or Walking: For many patients with disc derangement, history will uncover that one offers more relief than the other. Relaxed sitting results in flexion of the lumbosacral spine. Standing and walking extend the lumbar spine as compared to sitting. Many practitioners assume that if a patient reports being "worse" when sitting and "better" when standing or walking that the Direction of Detriment is flexion and the Direction of Benefit is extension, and vice versa. That assumption may not be correct and should be corroborated with what the patient experiences and displays during the ERL exam.

When there is significant intradiscal displacement resulting in significant range of motion loss (as with the antalgias), there may initially be greater pain perceived in the Direction of Benefit due to proximal increase of symptoms. As a result, the Direction of Detriment may actually be preferred by the patient. As improvement occurs, the Direction of Benefit begins to feel better than the Direction of Detriment.

For any of the antalgias, the relative effects of sitting and standing can change, depending on the phase of recovery. Using the kyphotic antalgia as an example, it is recalled that the kyphotic antalgia occurs as the body's attempt to avoid the proximal increase of symptoms that is precipitated by extension. It is also recalled that the likelihood and degree of the proximal increase of symptoms is proportional to the loss of motion in the Direction of Benefit. The kyphotic antalgia patient may feel "worse" when standing because extension precipitates a proximal increase of symptoms that is so distressing that flexion (the Direction of Detriment) is chosen instead, and is perceived to be "better." As the kyphotic antalgia resolves and extension is recovered, the proximal increase of symptoms no longer occurs and the Direction of Detriment (sitting flexed) then feels "worse" than the Direction of Benefit.

Alternate Methods for Diagnosing Disc Pain

Discogram is sometimes used to identify disc pain. This is an expensive and invasive test that requires meticulous identification of psychological distress as well as injection of control disc levels to allow for reliable findings. Discogram is rarely, if ever, necessary, particularly at the primary spine care level. In addition, it is not necessary to know with absolute certainty that the disc is the pain generating tissue, or which particular disc is involved, in order to make decisions based on the findings of the ERL examination.

Discoblock shows promise as a confirmatory test of suspected disc pain. This is a procedure in which anesthetic is injected into a suspected painful disc to determine whether decrease in pain results. Further research is needed to determine the clinical utility and potential side effects of this procedure.

Joint Dysfunction

Joint dysfunction can either involve the lumbar facet joints or the sacroiliac (SI) joints. This condition has been labeled by various professions as joint dysfunction, joint fixation, joint blockage, osteopathic lesion, somatic dysfunction, chiropractic subluxation, as well as other names.

Lumbar Facet Pain

Lumbar facet pain is identified through the criteria adapted from the work of Laslett, et al and Young, et al (see Recommended Reading list). These criteria include:

- Age≥50.

- The pain is best when the patient is walking and/or;

- The pain is best when the patient is sitting.

- The primary focus of the pain is paraspinal.

- There is no pain on standing from a sitting position.

- The extension/rotation test is positive.

- Disc derangement has been ruled out.

From these criteria it can be seen that before drawing conclusions about the presence of suspected facet pain the ERL examination must be carried out to rule out disc derangement.

Extension-Rotation Test

1. With the patient in the standing position the practitioner asks what, if any, symptoms he or she has.

2. The patient places both hands at the lumbosacral junction and bends backward as far as possible (Fig. 5-22). The practitioner asks if this provokes pain.

3. The patient returns to the starting position. The patient extends again and then rotates to either side from the extended position (Fig. 5-23).

4. The practitioner asks the patient if this provokes pain. If it does, the practitioner asks if it *reproduces the chief complaint.*

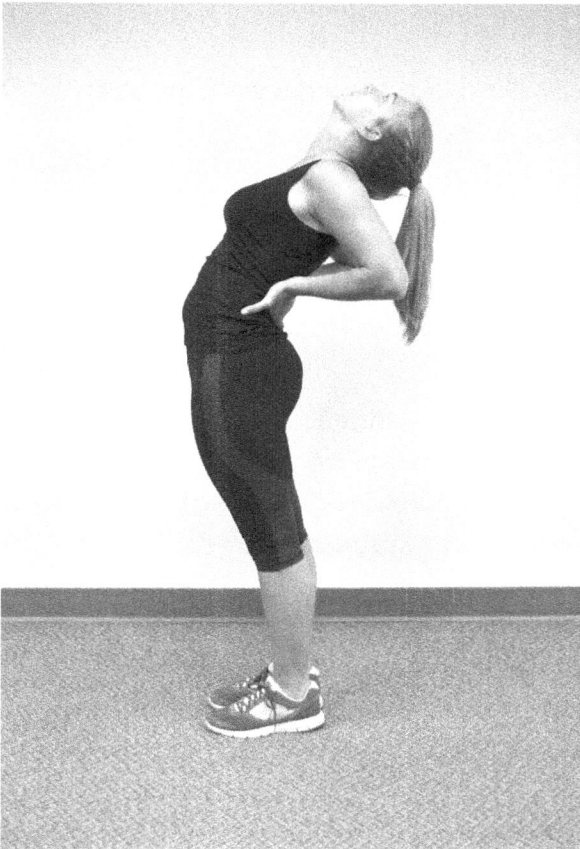

Figure 5-22. Extension phase of the extension-rotation test

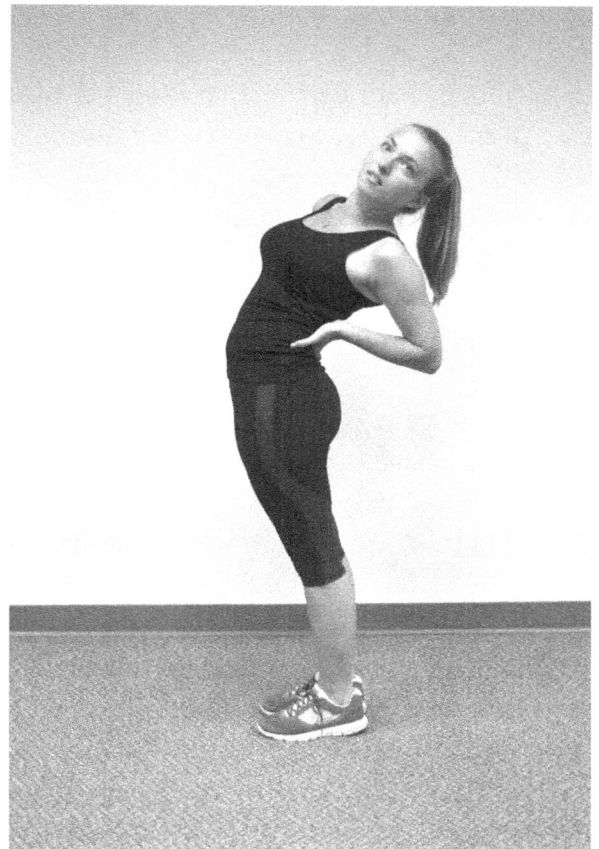

Figure 5-23. Rotation phase of the extension-rotation test. The pati nt rotates to both sides.

If the patient's pain is reproduced by the addition of rotation, the test is positive. If pain is provoked by extension but not rotation, or if no pain is provoked at any point in the test, the test is negative. It is important to distinguish reproduction of the patient's pain from "strain pain" resulting from an unfamiliar movement. Also, if the patient's pain is unilateral, it is important to check rotation to both sides because the pain may be provoked by rotation toward the side of pain or away from the side of pain.

The extension-rotation test is very sensitive. So if this test is negative, it is doubtful that the patient has facet joint dysfunction. However the test is not very specific so if it is positive, this does not "rule in" facet joint dysfunction. The test has to be combined with the other criteria provided here to make the diagnosis. It is also important to note that patients with facet pain do not necessarily fit all the criteria. Clinical reasoning is necessary, in light of the entire clinical picture, to make the diagnosis.

Sacroiliac Pain

Pain from SI joint dysfunction is identified though criteria developed from the work of Laslett, et al and Young, et al (see Recommended Reading list). Historical factors associated with SI pain are:

- The pain is located entirely below the lumbosacral junction (i.e., SI joint pain is rarely perceived at L5 or above).

- The pain is unilateral and is not found in the midline.

- The pain is worse when the patient stands from a sitting position – this will typically be expressed differently by the SI joint patient than by the disc derangement patient. The patient with SI pain will describe this as pain while moving from the seated to the standing position but will not typically describe the painful obstruction and difficulty with straightening up described by the patient with disc derangement.

Examination for suspected SI pain is carried out through SI provocation tests. There are five such tests that have been found to be most useful. The strict criterion is that if three out of these five tests are positive, the diagnosis of SI joint dysfunction is established. However, not all patients will have three unequivocally positive tests so clinical reasoning in light of the entire clinical picture is necessary. Additionally, it is important to note that, as is the case with facet pain, the diagnostic accuracy of the examination for SI pain is greatly improved when disc derangement is ruled out first. Therefore, the ERL exam should be carried out prior to considering SI pain.

The five SI provocation tests are:

1. Distraction Test: The patient lies supine and the practitioner applies anterior to posterior pressure on the anterior superior iliac spines bilaterally in an attempt to distract the SI joint (Fig. 5-24).

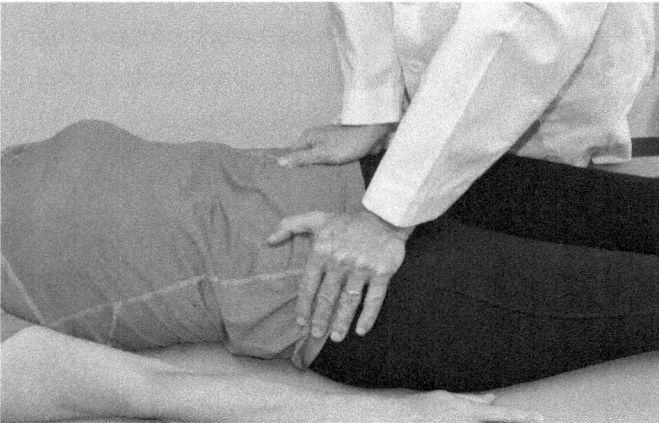

Figure 5-24. The Distraction Test.

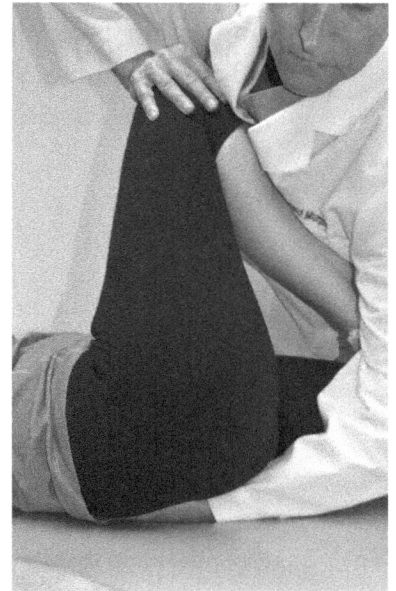

Figure 5-25. The Thigh Thrust Test.

2. Thigh Thrust Test: The patient lies supine and the practitioner flexes the involved hip to 90 degrees. The practitioner then places one hand on the sacrum to stabilize it and applies downward pressure along the long axis of the thigh in an attempt to shear the SI joint (Fig. 5-25).

3. Gaenslen's Test: The patient lies supine with one leg hanging off the table and the other hip fully flexed. The practitioner places downward pressure on the extended leg to move it further into extension while placing pressure on the flexed leg to move it further into flexion. The attempt is to rotate one innominate posteriorly and the other anteriorly (Fig. 5-26). If the test is negative with one leg off the table the test is repeated with the other leg off the table, as reproduction of pain can occur on either side.

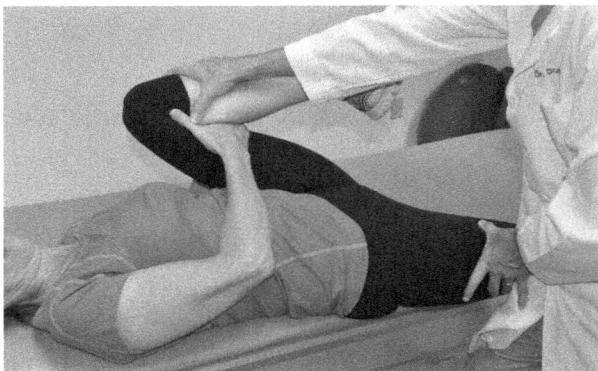

Figure 5-26. Gaenslen's Test.

4. Compression Test: With the patient in the side lying position the practitioner presses downward on the ilium in a lateral-to-medial direction in an attempt to apply a compression force to both SI joints (Fig. 5-27).

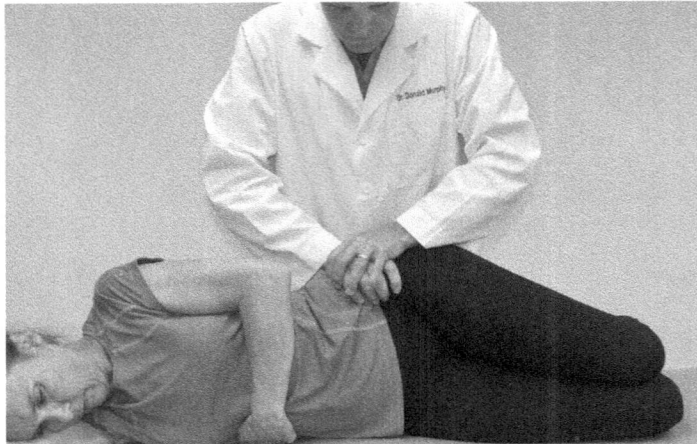

Figure 5-27. Compression Test.

5. Sacral Thrust Test: The patient lies prone and the practitioner applies pressure in a posterior to anterior direction on the apex of the curve of the sacrum in an attempt to shear the SI joints (Fig. 5-28).

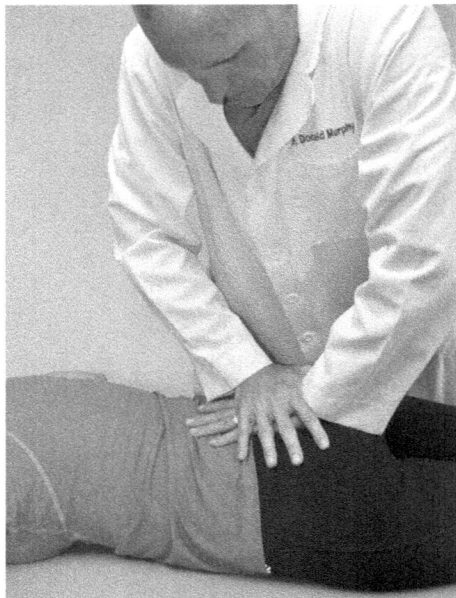

Figure 5-28. The Sacral Thrust Test

The purpose of the tests described here is to identify pain from the SI joint itself, i.e., intra-articular or capsular SI joint pain. There are some patients who will present with pain in the SI area but who will not have intra-articular pain, and thus the pain-provocation maneuvers shown here may not reproduce the pain. In these patients the pain is often arising from the long dorsal SI ligament and the pain can be reproduced by palpating that ligament.

With the patient lying prone, the long dorsal SI ligament can be located by palpating just inferior to the posterior superior iliac spine. The ligament often feels like a hard ridge. Reproduction of the patient's pain on palpation of the ligament suggests the dorsal SI ligament as the primary pain generator.

Alternate Methods for Diagnosing Joint Pain

Anesthetic joint injections (joint blocks) are occasionally used in an attempt to identify pain arising from the facet or SI joints. However, as was discussed earlier with regard to discogram, joint blocks are invasive and expensive and require a meticulous approach to blinding and confirmation in order to produce reasonably reliable findings. Most important, however, is that in most cases it is not necessary to know with *absolute certainly* the precise tissue origin of pain in order to make treatment decisions based on the historical and examination findings presented here. Therefore, injections for diagnostic purposes are uncommonly necessary, particularly at the primary spine care level. Nevertheless, they are an option in cases in which diagnostic clarity is lacking, and a more precise tissue diagnosis is considered to be clinically important. Substantial temporary relief ("substantial" being defined as a minimum of 80% improvement in pain intensity that is measured prior to and following the injection) strongly suggests that the joint that was injected is the primary pain generator.

Another invasive diagnostic test for joint pain is the medial branch block (MBB). The medial branch of the spinal nerve innervates the facet joints. MBB is an injection technique in which the medial branch is anesthetized temporarily. As with joint blocks, if significant pain relief occurs shortly after the procedure, based on pre- and post-injection pain measures, the facet joint at that level is implicated. This test is only recommended if radiofrequency neurotomy is being considered (see Chapters 10 and 12).

Joint injections and MBBs should be performed under fluoroscopic guidance and are typically performed by an anesthesiologist or a physiatrist.

Radiculopathy

Pain of neural origin occurs with radiculopathy, although it is also found with piriformis syndrome (see below). For the purpose of this book, the diagnostic term radiculopathy is used for any disorder involving a nerve root. This can involve nerve root pain in isolation, symptoms of neurologic dysfunction (such as paresthesia, sensory loss or motor loss) in isolation, or both pain and neurologic dysfunction. The most common causes of radiculopathy are spinal stenosis and disc herniation. Younger patients with radiculopathy are more likely to have disc herniation and older patients are more likely to have spinal stenosis. Historical factors associated with radiculopathy are:

- Lower extremity pain that typically extends below the knee (in the case of L5 or S1 radiculopathy).

- The lower extremity pain typically is more intense than the back pain.

- Neurologic symptoms such as paresthesia, dysesthesia, sensory loss or motor loss.

- Neurogenic claudication, in patients whose radicular pain is secondary to spinal stenosis. With neurogenic claudication the pain begins during walking and progressively worsens as the patient continues walking. Sitting or bending into flexion typically provides relief.

- Severe low back pain, particularly in patients whose radicular pain is secondary to disc herniation (though a patient with a sequestrated fragment may have lower extremity pain without low back pain).

- In patients whose radicular pain is secondary to disc herniation, the pain is often worse with flexion whereas in those whose radicular pain is secondary to spinal stenosis, the pain is often improved with flexion.

Examination for radicular pain is done through the neurodynamic exam, using what are commonly called "nerve root tension tests." During the neurodynamic exam the practitioner utilizes maneuvers that apply tension to the nerve root, looking for reproduction of the patient's pain. Maneuvers are then applied that slacken the nerve root to see if this reduces or eliminates the pain. The neurodynamic exam actually applies tension and slackening not only to the nerve roots but to the entire neural tract that the nerve roots are a part of. So, strictly speaking, the neurodynamic exam is designed to identify pain that is arising from a neural source anywhere along the neural tract to which the movement is being applied. The history and the remainder of the examination can then provide clues as to the likelihood that the source of pain is the nerve root itself (although, as will be seen, there are aspects of the neurodynamic exam that can help in this localization). Because patients with nerve root pain may have other manifestations of radiculopathy, namely neurologic deficit, a careful neurologic exam should be performed (see Chapter 4).

There are three principles that are useful in maximizing the understanding of the neurodynamic exam:

1. All neural structures are part of anatomical continuum: As mentioned earlier, the nerve root is anatomically just one aspect of a continuous neural tract that extends from the brain, along the spinal cord to the nerve root and plexus and ending at the distal end of the peripheral nerve. Tension applied to one end of the tract, if it is of sufficient magnitude, can ultimately be transmitted along the entire tract. This tension results from movement of the parts of the body through which that neural tract extends. For example, if a person were to sit upright and move the head and spine into flexion, this would apply tension to the spinal cord. If the person were then to extend the knee, this would apply tension to the sciatic nerve, thus increasing the tension on the entire neural tract that extends from the brain to the distal end of the sciatic nerve. Dorsiflexion of the ankle would then increase this tension even further. Clinical application of this group of movements will be seen later when the Slump Test is presented.

2. Tension is applied first and to a greatest extent at the point closest to which movement is initiated: In the above example, the movement started with flexion of the cervical spine. Thus, the initial tension occurs in the cervical spinal cord, and then spreads as the other body parts are moved. This is helpful in conducting the neurodynamic exam because starting the examination procedure close to the suspected pain source (i.e. the nerve root) may be helpful in maximizing tension on the nerve root, which increases the likelihood that nerve root pain will be reproduced.

3. Structural differentiation: The movements that produce tension on neural structures also produce tension on certain musculoskeletal structures. Therefore, pain with movement does not necessarily implicate the neural structure as the pain source. Maneuvers that *slacken* the neural structure, without changing the tension on the musculoskeletal structures, will help to differentiate the pain source. If pain that is elicited on the initial maneuver is lessened or eliminated with the structural differentiation (i.e., neural slackening) maneuver, it is likely that the pain is of neural origin. However if the structural differentiation maneuver fails to reduce or eliminate the pain (particularly if more than one structural differentiation maneuver fails to do this) it is unlikely that the pain is of neural origin.

The usefulness of these principles will become clear as the neurodynamic exam is further explored.

The Straight Leg Raise Test

The Straight Leg Raise is the basic neurodynamic test for pain arising from the sciatic nerve, the lumbosacral plexus, and the nerve roots that contribute to this neural complex (primarily L5, S1 and, in some cases, L4). This test is very sensitive for the presence of nerve root pain but it is not very specific. That is, if a patient has radiculopathy involving one or more of the nerve roots that make up the sciatic nerve, it is very likely that the Straight Leg Raise will be painful. However, there are many patients in whom the Straight Leg Raise will be painful but who do not have lumbosacral radiculopathy. Therefore tests of structural differentiation will have to be applied to increase the specificity of making the diagnosis of nerve root pain involving these nerve roots.

The Straight Leg Raise is most commonly performed with the patient in the supine position. The lower extremity on the side of pain is raised such that the hip is flexed while the knee remains extended (Fig. 5-29). The patient is asked to indicate the point at which he or she feels pain and whether this pain reproduces the chief complaint. Again, because of the high sensitivity of this basic test, if this maneuver is non-painful, this argues against the presence of radicular pain (but does not rule it out, especially in patients with spinal stenosis). However, because of the low specificity of this basic test, reproduction of the patient's pain does not allow the practitioner to be confident in the diagnosis of radicular pain. Further testing is necessary to establish the diagnosis.

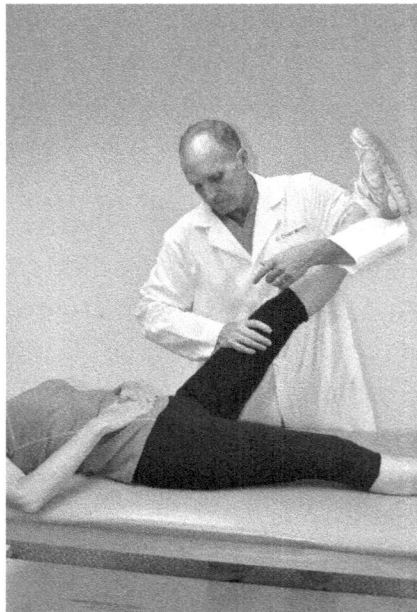

Figure 5-29. The basic Straight Leg Raise.

The simplest way to confirm the presence of radicular pain is to assess the effect that ankle dorsiflexion and ankle plantar flexion has on the pain. The easiest way to do this is to initially dorsiflex the ankle prior to raising the leg. Then while ankle dorsiflexion is maintained, the lower extremity is raised such that the hip is flexed while the knee remains extended as with the basic Straight Leg Raise test (Fig. 5-30). The patient is asked to indicate the point at which he or she feels pain and whether this reproduces the chief complaint. While the leg is maintained in this position the foot is then plantar flexed (Fig. 5-31). The patient is asked whether this maneuver has any effect on the pain. If this maneuver lessens or eliminates the pain, this suggests the presence of neural pain involving the sciatic nerve complex - the history and the remainder of the examination will help the practitioner determine whether this pain is likely from radiculopathy. If ankle plantar flexion has no effect on the pain, this argues against the presence of radicular pain.

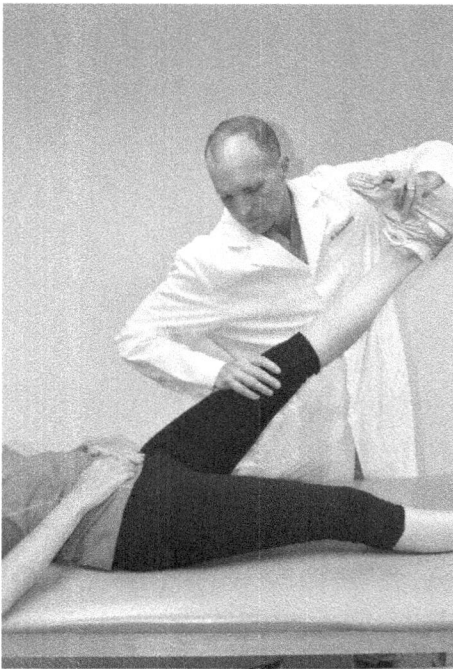

Figure 5-30. Applying ankle dorsiflexion during the Straight Leg Raise.

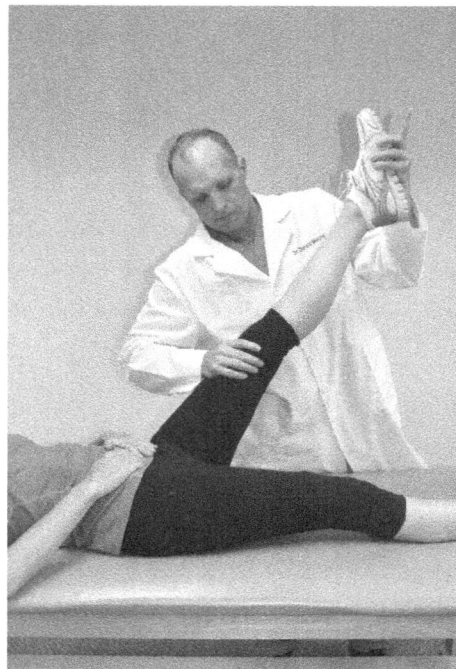

Figure 5-31. Applying ankle plantar flexion with the leg in the raised position.

There are cases in which the Straight Leg Raise, even with ankle dorsiflexion, does not place enough tension on the nervous system to provoke symptoms. A simple way to increase this tension is to add medial hip rotation and adduction to the test. With the patient in the supine position the ankle is dorsiflexed and the hip medially rotated. Then as the Straight Leg Raise is being performed, the lower extremity is

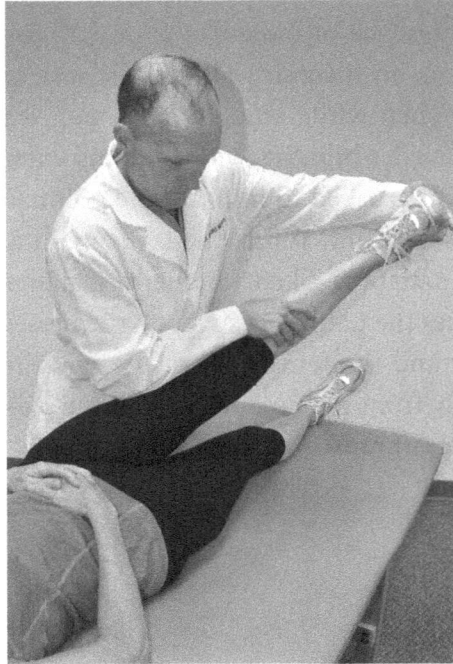

Figure 5-32. Straight Leg Raise with ankle dorsiflexion, medial hip rotation and hip adduction.

moved into adduction as well (Fig. 5-32). The leg is raised to the point at which the patient's symptoms are elicited. Structural differentiation can then be sought by moving the ankle into plantar flexion.

In patients with radicular pain that is primarily proximal, i.e. in the buttock, proximal thigh or lower back, there are some cases in which the standard neurodynamic exam will not elicit symptoms. In these cases it is often useful to start the process of applying tension to the nervous system proximally rather than distally. To do this, begin with flexion of the hip to approximately 90 degrees. Follow this with knee extension, then ankle dorsiflexion.

In some cases a greater degree of tension on the nerve root is required to reproduce the patient's symptoms. This is common in patients whose radiculopathy is caused by spinal stenosis as opposed to those whose radiculopathy is caused by disc herniation. In these cases the Slump Test is useful.

The Slump Test

This is carried out with the patient seated. To begin the process of elongating the central nervous system as well as the involved nerve roots the patient moves the head, neck and trunk into a flexed position. The patient is asked if this is painful and, if so, if it reproduces the chief complaint. Then the practitioner dorsiflexes the ankle and extends the knee while head, neck and trunk flexion are maintained (Fig. 5-33). The patient is again asked if this is painful and, if so, if it reproduces the chief complaint.

If this maneuver reproduces the patient's chief complaint, structural differentiation of a neural source of this pain is sought via maneuvers that take tension off the nervous system. The patient is asked to extend the head and neck while the lower extremity position is maintained (Fig. 5-34). If this reduces or eliminates the pain, this suggests a neural source of pain. This can be further confirmed by having the patient move the head and neck back into a flexed position to the point at which pain is again produced and then plantar flexing the ankle to see if this reduces or eliminates the pain (Fig. 5-35).

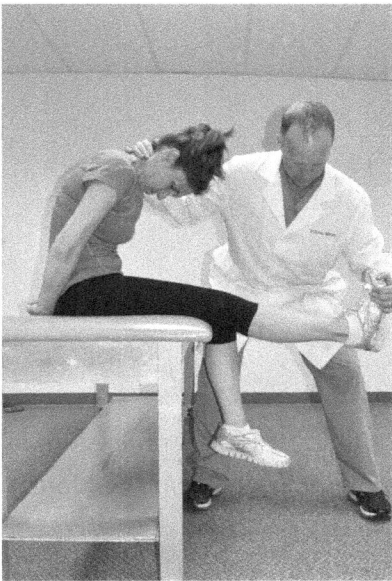

Figure 5-33. The slump position.

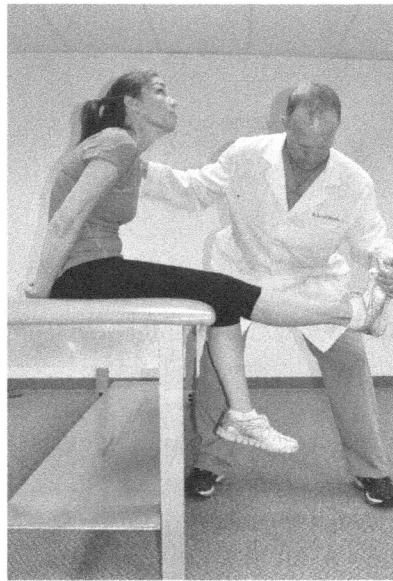

Figure 5-34. Extending the head and neck from the slump position.

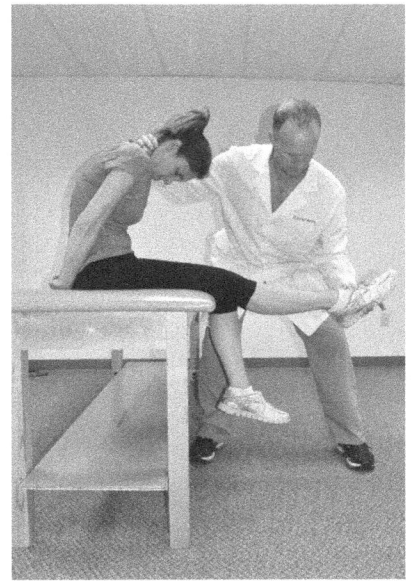

Figure 5-35. Plantar flexing the ankle while maintain the slump position.

A variant of the Slump Test that can be useful is performed with the patient in the long sitting position on the examining table so that both hips are flexed and both knees extended. The patient is asked if this is painful and, if so, if it reproduces the chief complaint. In patients with radicular pain, this will often reproduce the pain in the involved leg with little or no pain on the uninvolved side. The patient is moved into the slump position by flexion of the head, neck and trunk. Again the patient is asked about symptom reproduction. If the initial position reproduced the patient's pain, increased pain in the second position suggests a neural origin of the pain. Further tension on neural structures can then be produced by having the patient dorsiflex the ankle on the involved side (Fig. 5-36). If reproduction of pain is not produced until this fully slumped position is established, structural differentiation can be sought either with extension of the head or plantar flexion of the ankle on the involved side. In a patient with radiculopathy these maneuvers will be expected to reduce or eliminate the pain.

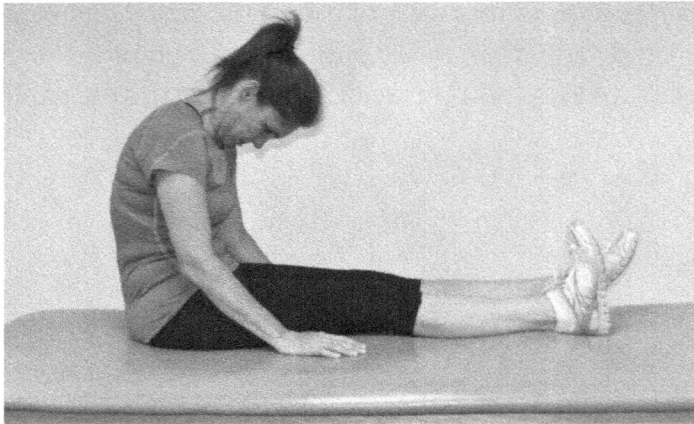

Figure 5-36. Slumping with ankle dorsiflexion in the long sitting position.

In patients with radiculopathy involving the L2through L4 levels the Straight Leg Raise and its derivatives presented here will not be expected to reproduce the pain. As these nerve roots form the lumbar plexus and, ultimately, the femoral nerve, the Femoral Nerve Stretch Test, along with its derivatives, is the procedure of choice.

The Femoral Nerve Stretch Test

With the patient in the prone position the practitioner stabilizes the pelvis with one hand, and then flexes the knee with the other (Fig. 5-37). The patient is asked to indicate the point at which he or she feels pain and whether this pain reproduces the chief complaint.

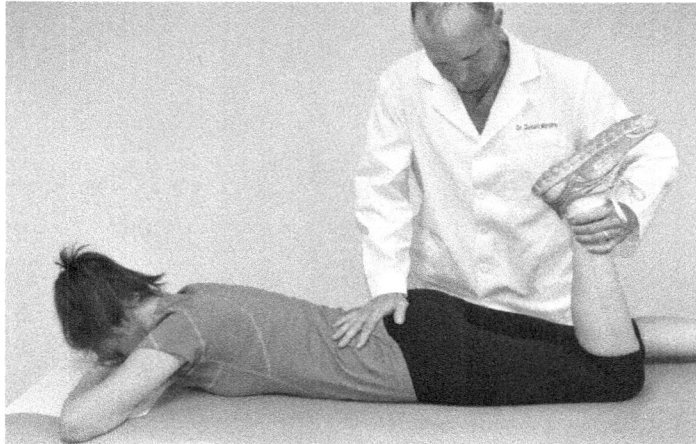

Figure 5-37. The Femoral Nerve Stretch Test.

As with the Straight Leg Raise, this test is very sensitive for the presence of radicular pain but is not very specific. Therefore, structural differentiation is required to increase the specificity of the examination.

One simple addition to the Femoral Nerve Stretch Test is to perform the test with the patient lying prone on the examining table with the head off the edge of the table and the cervical spine flexed. The Femoral Nerve Stretch Test is performed to the point at which pain is elicited (Fig. 5-38). The patient is then asked to look up as far as possible, extending the cervical spine (Fig. 5-39). The patient is asked if this changes the pain. In most patients extension of the spine will decrease tension on the nerve root and thus reduce or eliminate the pain. However there will be some patients for whom this maneuver will increase the pain. Either way, the change in symptoms with movement of the head suggests the presence of neural pain.

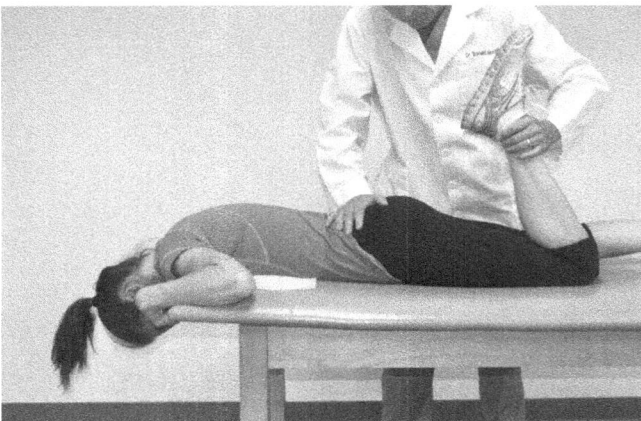

Figure 5-38. The Femoral Nerve Stretch Test with the cervical spine fully flexed.

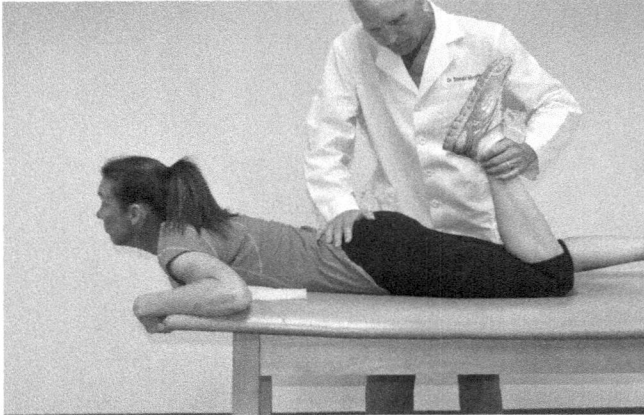

Figure 5-39. The Femoral Nerve Stretch Test with the cervical spine fully extended.

The Femoral Nerve Slump Test

This is a more definitive test for radicular pain involving L2 through L4. With this test the patient is side-lying. The involved leg can be on the up side or the down side. The test will be presented here with the involved leg on the up side. The patient is placed in a fully slumped position and pulls the knee of the uninvolved side toward the chest. The involved leg is moved into a position of knee flexion and hip extension (Fig. 5-40) and the patient is asked to indicate the point at which he or she feels pain and whether this pain reproduces the chief complaint. The patient is then asked to move out of the slumped position and to extend the head, neck and trunk (Fig. 5-41). The patient is asked if this changes the symptoms. In most patients with radiculopathy involving the L2-L4 levels extension will decrease or eliminate the pain. However there will be some patients in whom this movement increases the pain. Either way, the change in symptoms with movement out of the slumped position suggests the presence of neural pain.

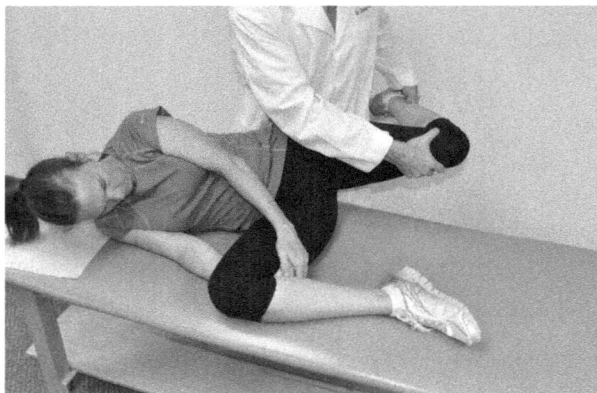

Figure 5-40. The Femoral Nerve Slump Test.

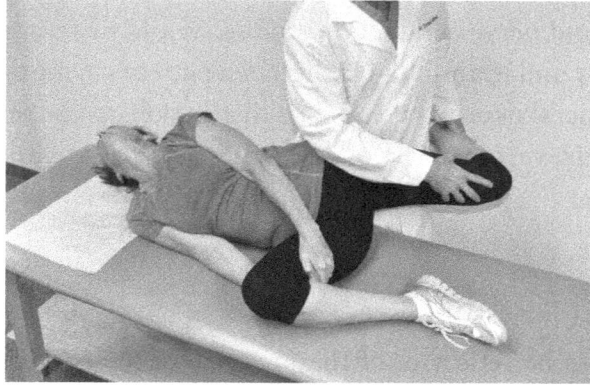

Figure 5-41. The Femoral Nerve Slump Test with extension of the head, neck and trunk for structural differentiation.

As was stated earlier the neurodynamic examination does not, in itself, localize the pain to a nerve root. This examination process identifies pain that is of neural origin and theoretically the pain can be arising from any part of the nervous system to which tension is being applied. So the portion of the neurodynamic examination discussed in this chapter relative to patients with L5 or S1 radicular pain may be positive in patients with piriformis syndrome in addition to those with lumbosacral radiculopathy. Likewise, the portion of the neurodynamic examination relative to patients with L2-L4 radicular pain may also be positive in patients with femoral neuropathy. Thus, the findings of the neurodynamic examination, as with all examination procedures discussed in this book, must be considered in light of the findings from the remainder of the patient assessment.

Alternate Methods for Diagnosing Radicular Pain

Epidural steroid injection or nerve root block (in which the nerve root is injected with anesthetic) can be useful to confirm radicular pain. As with other diagnostic injection procedures, they are typically provided by an anesthesiologist or a physiatrist. Also, as with other diagnostic injection procedures, the presence of nerve root pain can usually be determined quite well through history and examination. Therefore it is very uncommon that the primary spine practitioner would need to order injections for diagnostic purposes.

There are some patients in whom electromyography and nerve conduction studies are a useful tool in assessing radiculopathy. These are electrophysiological tests of the function of the nerve root (more specifically, the motor branch of the nerve root) and the peripheral nerves. These studies do not evaluate pain and thus cannot be used to identify the nerve root or peripheral neural structures as pain sources. Electromyography and nerve conduction studies should be reserved for those cases in which it is not clear based on history and examination whether a patient's symptoms are arising from radiculopathy, plexopathy or peripheral neuropathy. As this distinction can be made on the basis of a careful history and examination in the vast majority of cases, these studies are uncommonly necessary.

Myofascial pain

Myofascial pain is thought to be reflective of the presence of myofascial trigger points (TrPs). TrPs are very common in patients with LBDs but they typically form in response to one of the other pain generators discussed in this chapter and it is relatively uncommon for TrPs to be the primary source of pain. In most patients, when the pain from the primary source (disc derangement, joint dysfunction, radiculopathy) is resolved, any TrP pain that may be present will resolve on its own. However, there are a significant number of patients in whom residual TrP pain remains after resolution of the primary pain generator. In these patients, it is important to identify and treat the TrPs.

TrPs are primarily identified through palpation. In deciding which muscles to examine it is helpful to be familiar with the typical referred pain patterns of the various muscles that can contribute to LBDs. There are good sources of trigger point pain referral maps, the best of which is the book by Simons, Travell and Simons entitled Myofascial Pain and Dysfunction: The Trigger Point Manual (see Recommended Reading list). Knowing the typical referred pain patterns of various muscles and getting a clear description from the patient of the pain location allows the practitioner to narrow the likely potential muscular pain sources.

With the presence of a TrP, there is usually a taut band within the muscle that can be identified through skilled palpation. This taut band will be tender to palpation but may not reproduce the patient's pain. By moving along the taut band the practitioner will typically find the TrP, which will feel like a nodular formation. The TrP will be painful upon palpation and, if it is involved in the generation of the patient's pain, will reproduce the pain.

The muscles that are most commonly involved in patient with LBDs are:

Lumbar erector spinae

The erector spinae muscles are primarily located in the thoracic and thoracolumbar spine with most of the lumbar spine covered by the tendons of these muscles. TrPs in this group of muscles can cause localized pain as well as pain that can extend into the sacroiliac and buttock areas. With the patient lying prone, the bulk of the muscle should be palpated in the thoracolumbar area (Fig. 5-42).

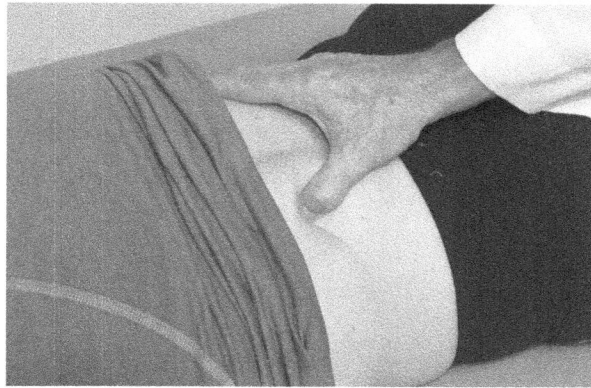

Figure 5-42. Palpation of the lumbar erector spinae muscles.

Lumbosacral multifidis

The multifidis muscles make up the bulk of the musculature in the lumbosacral junction and are a common cause of localized lumbosacral pain. To examine these muscles the patient lies prone and palpation is applied at the lumbosacral junction just lateral to the spine (Fig. 5-43).

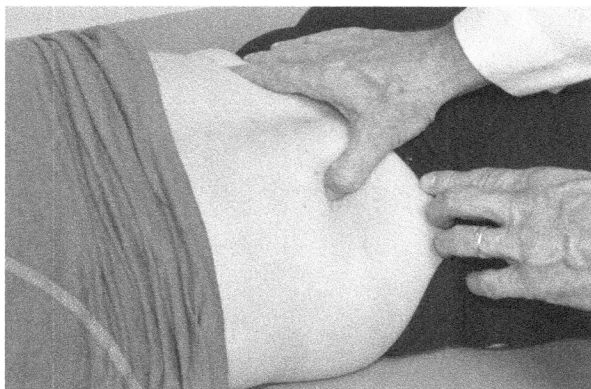

Figure 5-43. Palpation of the lumbosacral multifidis

Quadratus lumborum

TrPs in the quadratus lumborum can cause pain in the flank area as well as in the sacroiliac and buttock areas. They can sometimes mimic sacroiliac pain. They are palpated with the patient lying on his or her side. It is best to peak the table or to place a roll on the underside of the patient to laterally flex the spine away from the side being examined (Fig. 5-44). The lower extremity on the side being examined should be placed behind the other and the upper extremity on the side being examined should be placed over-head to further laterally flex the spine. The muscle is palpated between the 12th rib and the iliac crest.

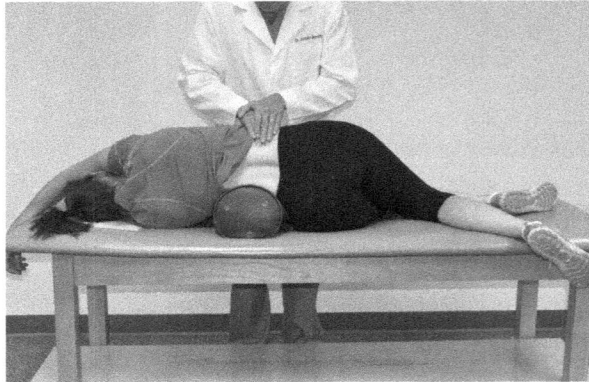

Figure 5-44. Palpation of the quadratus lumborum.

Gluteus maximus

The gluteus maximus can cause localized buttock pain. It can be palpated with the patient lying prone. The most common area for trigger points is near the medial attachment of the muscle (Fig. 5-45).

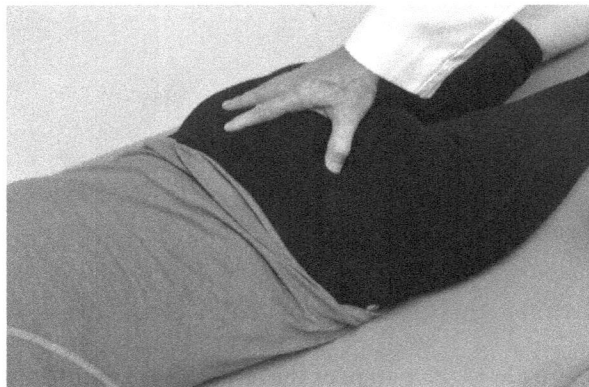

Figure 5-45. Palpation of the gluteus maximus.

Piriformis

Trigger points in the piriformis muscle can cause localized buttock pain. In addition, tightness in the piriformis muscle can cause piriformis syndrome, in which the muscle entraps the sciatic nerve. In most people, the sciatic nerve passes inferior to the piriformis as it descends down the posterior aspect of the lower extremity. However, in some people the sciatic nerve pierces through the piriformis as it descends. In these patients, tightness in the muscle, which may or may not be accompanied by TrPs, can lead to irritation of the sciatic nerve, resulting in neural pain. The pain will typically be identified with the neurodynamic examination (see above).

There often is no way to definitively distinguish piriformis syndrome from radiculopathy, however, patients with piriformis syndrome will typically have buttock and posterior lower extremity pain but no low back pain. Patients with radiculopathy secondary to spinal stenosis or disc herniation will typically, but certainly not always, have low back pain in addition to lower extremity pain. Also, patients with radiculopathy will be more likely to have substantial neurologic deficit than patients with piriformis syndrome however, many patients with radiculopathy will not exhibit neurologic deficit.

Many patients with piriformis syndrome will have pain with sitting that results from pressure on the entrapment site. When asked, these patients will often say that if they lean away from the side of involvement while sitting, the pain is reduced. Patients with radiculopathy secondary to disc herniation will often report pain with sitting, but it is the *position* of sitting that provokes the pain in these patients, rather than the pressure on the buttock of the involved side. So it is important to ask whether it is the position of sitting or the pressure on the buttock that causes pain and if leaning away from the side of involvement provides relief. Of course, patients with radiculopathy secondary to spinal stenosis typically report relief of pain when sitting.

MRI is useful to rule in or out the presence of disc herniation or spinal stenosis but one has to recall that these findings on MRI can occur asymptomatically. Distinguishing between lumbar radiculopathy and piriformis syndrome can usually be made on the basis of history and examination, so MRI is not usually necessary for this purpose. Often a trial of treatment is required before a determination can be made as to which disorder is present.

The piriformis muscle can be palpated with the patient prone (Fig. 5-46). The muscle is palpated toward the center of the buttock but just lateral to the sciatic nerve to distinguish TrPs in the muscle from tenderness of the sciatic nerve. In normal circumstances it will be difficult or impossible to distinguish the piriformis muscle from the remainder of the buttock muscles. If the piriformis is tight, it will be clearly distinguishable as a taut cord extending from the sacrum to the greater trochanter. The piriformis can also be palpated with the patient side-lying with the involved side up.

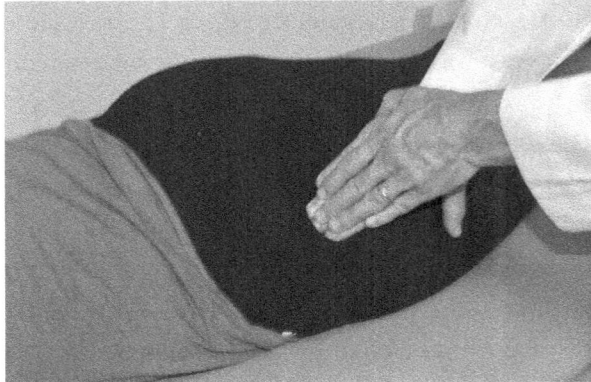

Figure 5-46. Palpation of the piriformis with the patient prone.

While patients certainly are allowed to have more than one of these pain generators, typically they do not. The exception is myofascial pain which commonly coexists with one of the other pain sources and is usually secondary.

Answering diagnostic question #2 is only one part of the overall diagnostic process, particularly in patients whose LBD is in the subacute or chronic stage. To complete the diagnostic picture, answering diagnostic question #3 is necessary. That will be the topic of the next chapter.

Recommended reading:

Butler DS, Moseley GL. Explain Pain. Adelaide, Australia: Noigroup Publications; 2003.

Butler DS. The Sensitive Nervous System. Adelaide, Australia: Noigroup Publications; 2000.

Clare HA, Adams R, Maher CG. A systematic review of efficacy of McKenzie therapy for spinal pain. Aust J Physiother 2004;50:209-16.

Clare HA, Adams R, Maher CG. Reliability of McKenzie classification of patients with cervical or lumbar pain. J Manipulative Physiol Ther 2005;28(2):122-7.

Hancock MJ, Maher CG, Latimer J, Spindler MF, McAuley JH, Laslett M, et al. Systematic review of tests to identify the disc, SIJ or facet joint as the source of low back pain. Eur Spine J 2007;16(10):1539-50.

Laslett M, Aprill CN, McDonald B, Oberg B. Clinical predictors of lumbar provocation discography: a study of clinical predictors of lumbar provocation discography. Eur Spine J 2006;15(10):1473-84.

Laslett M, Aprill CN, McDonald B, Young SB. Diagnosis of sacroiliac joint pain: validity of individual provocation tests and composites of tests. Man Ther 2005;10:207-18.

Laslett M, Birgitta O, Aprill CN, McDonald B. Centralization as a predictor of provocation discography results in chronic low back pain, and the influence of disability and distress on diagnostic power. Spine J 2005;5(4):370-80.

Laslett M, McDonald B, Aprill CN, Tropp H, Oberg B. Clinical predictors of screening lumbar zygopophyseal joint blocks: development of clinical prediction rules. Spine J 2006;6(4):370-9.

Laslett M, McDonald B, Tropp H, April CN, Oberg B. Agreement between diagnoses reached by clinical examination and available reference standards: a prospective study of 216 patients with lumbopelvic pain. BMC Musculoskel Disord 2005;6:28.

Laslett M, Oberg B, April CN, McDonald B. Zygapophysial joint blocks in chronic low back pain: a test of Revel's model as a screening test. BMC Musculoskel Disord 2004;5:43.

Laslett M, Williams M. The reliability of selected pain provocation tests for sacroiliac joint pathology. Spine 1994;19(11):1243-9.

Laslett M, Young SB, Aprill CN, McDonald B. Diagnosing painful sacroiliac joints: A validity study of a McKenzie evaluation and sacroiliac provocation tests. Aus J Physiother 2003;49:89-97.

Long A, Donelson R, Fung T. Does it matter which exercise? A randomized control trial of exercise for low back pain. Spine 2004;29(23):2593-602.

May S, Donelson R. Evidence-informed management of chronic low back pain with the McKenzie method. Spine J 2008;8(1):134-41.

McKenzie Institute International http://www.mckenziemdt.org/ [accessed 26 July 2012]

McKenzie RA, May S. The Lumbar Spine: Mechanical Diagnosis and Therapy. 2nd ed. Waikenae, NZ: Spinal Publications; 2003.

Murphy DR, Hurwitz EL, Nelson CF. A diagnosis-based clinical decision rule for patients with spinal pain. Part 2: Review of the literature. *Chiropractic & Osteopathy* 2008;16:8

Murphy DR, Hurwitz EL. A theoretical model for the development of a diagnosis-based clinical decision rule for the management of patients with spinal pain. BMC Musculoskeletal Disorders 2007;8:75.

Murphy DR, Hurwitz EL. Application of a Diagnosis-Based Clinical Decision Guide in Patients with Low Back Pain. Chiropr Man Therap 2011;19(1):26.

Murphy DR, Hurwitz EL: Application of a Diagnosis-Based Clinical Decision Guide in Patients with Neck Pain. Chiropr Man Therap 2011, 19(1):19.

Shacklock M. Clinical Neurodynamics. A New System of Musculoskeletal Treatment. Edinburgh: Elsevier; 2005.

Simons DG, Travell JG, Simons LS. Myofascial Pain and Dysfunction: The Trigger Point Manual. Volume 1. Baltimore: Williams and Wilkens; 1999.

Young S, Aprill C, Laslett M. Correlation of clinical examination characteristics with three sources of chronic low back pain. Spine J 2003;3(6):460-5.

· CHAPTER 6 ·

Diagnostic question #3: What has happened with this person as a whole that would cause the pain experience to develop and persist?

Another way of asking this question is, "what factors are present that are perpetuating the ongoing pain, disability and suffering experience or are causing recurrent episodes?" There are several factors that can contribute to the perpetuation of low back disorders (LBDs). It should be noted that diagnostic question #3 (in addition to diagnostic questions #1 and 2) is important in the subacute or chronic patient; in the acute patient, diagnostic questions #1 and 2 are most critical. Diagnostic question #3 is also important in the patient who initially presents in the acute stage but does not fully recover (or does not improve at all) from the acute episode.

The perpetuating factors that are considered with diagnostic question #3 are presented in Table 6-1:

Table 6-1. **Perpetuating factors to be considered in diagnostic question #3.**

Somatic/ Neurophysiological factors	Psychological factors
Dynamic Instability	Fear
Passive Instability	Catastrophizing
Nociceptive system sensitization	Passive coping
	Poor self-efficacy
	Depression
	Perceived injustice
	Hypervigilance for symptoms
	Cognitive fusion
	Anxiety

Dynamic Instability

Dynamic instability is believed to result from impairment of the motor control system (see Chapter 2).

Historical factors that are consistent with dynamic instability include:

- Recurrent episodes of pain.

- Pain aggravated by quick movements.

- Feeling of "giving way" in the back.

- Frequent self-manipulation for relief.

- Frequent painful "catching" during movements.

- Pain when turning in bed.

In addition, dynamic instability occurs more commonly in younger people, i.e., those under 40 years old.

The following tests can be useful in examining for the presence of dynamic instability:

1. Hip Extension Test: The patient lies prone and is asked to raise one leg from the table by extending at the hip, maintaining an extended knee (Fig. 6-1). The weight of the leg causes perturbation to the spine, requiring a protective response from the motor control system. Normally it should be expected that the lumbar spine will maintain its neutral position in response to raising the leg. Lateral shift, rotation or hyperextension of the lumbar spine suggests the presence of dynamic instability.

2. Prone Instability Test: In the standard application of this test the patient lies prone with the upper body (from the waist up) on the table and the lower body hanging off the table. The feet are resting on the floor so the trunk muscles can be relaxed (Fig. 6-2). The examiner applies posterior-to-anterior pressure to the spinous processes of each segment in the lumbar spine. If the patient reports pain when pressure is applied to one or more segments the patient is asked to raise the feet off the floor, activating the lumbar extensors (Fig. 6-3).

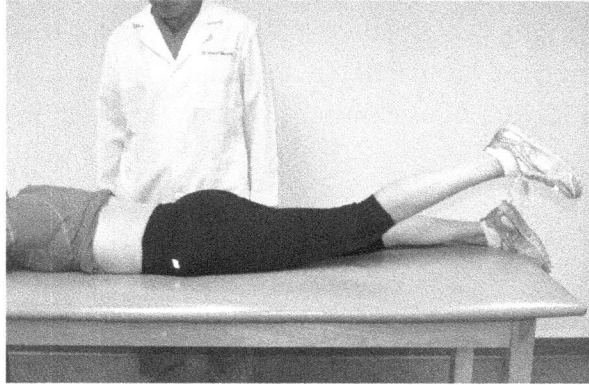

Figure 6-1. The Hip Extension Test.

Posterior-to-anterior pressure is again applied to the segment(s) that were painful at rest and the patient is asked if this is still painful. If pain that was reported at rest is reduced or eliminated when the muscles are activated, the test is positive, suggesting the presence of dynamic instability.

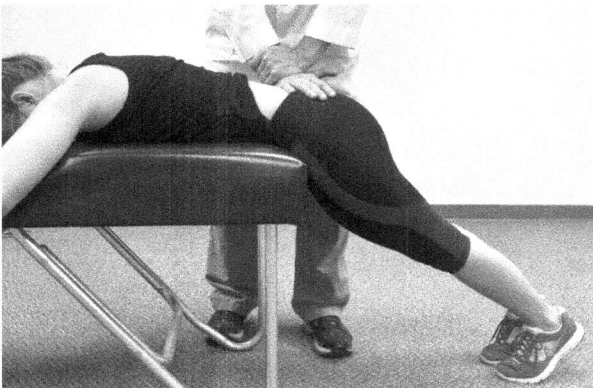

Figure 6-2. Starting position for the standard application of the Prone Instability Test.

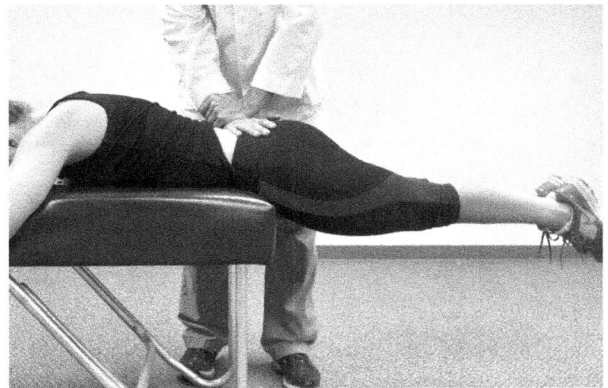

Figure 6-3. Re-application of pressure with the feet off the floor during the standard application of the Prone Instability Test.

Many patients will have difficulty with the standard application of this test. An alternative method that is more universally applicable than the standard procedure is to have the patient lie prone on the table (Fig. 6-4). As with the standard application of the test, pressure is applied to each segment of the lumbar spine and the patient is asked if this produces pain at any segment.

If pain is elicited at a segment the patient is asked to raise the head, shoulders and arms off the table without extending the lumbar spine. Pressure is again applied at the painful segment(s) (Fig. 6-5). If the pain is reduced or eliminated, dynamic instability is suspected.

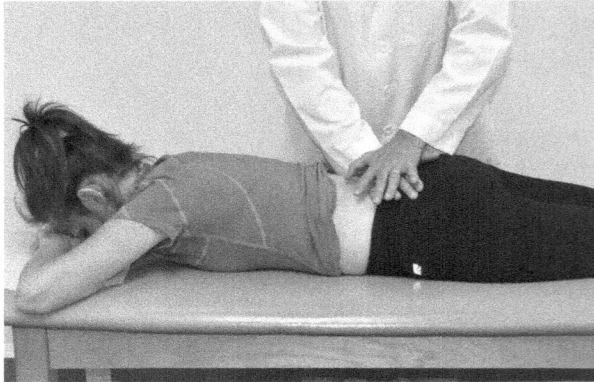

Figure 6-4. Starting position for the alternate application of the Prone Instability Test.

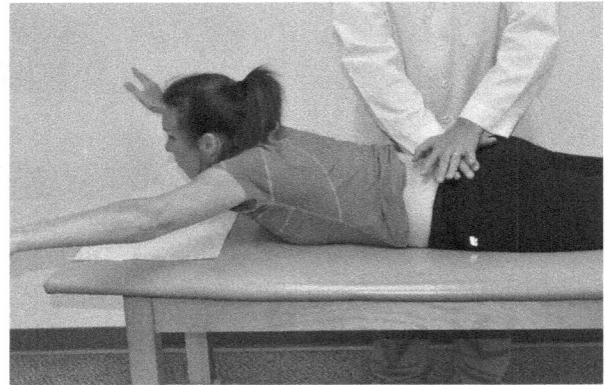

Figure 6-5. Re-application of pressure with the head, shoulders and arms elevated during the alternative application of the Prone Instability Test.

3. Active Straight Leg Raise Test: The patient lies supine and is asked to raise one leg approximately 5 cm from the table (Fig. 6-6). The patient is asked if this causes pain or discomfort. If it does, overpressure is applied in a lateral to medial direction on the posterior aspect of the pelvis, theoretically mimicking the action of the multifidis muscles. The patient is then asked

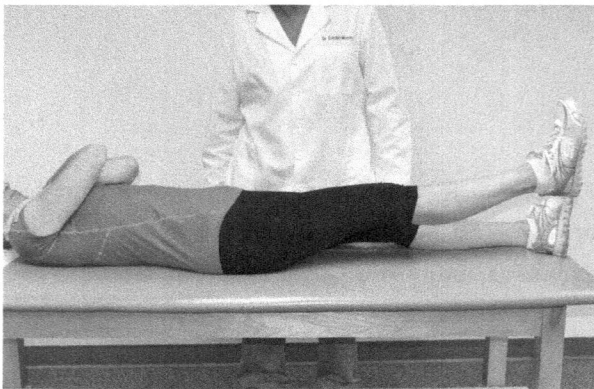

Figure 6-6. Active Straight Leg Raise.

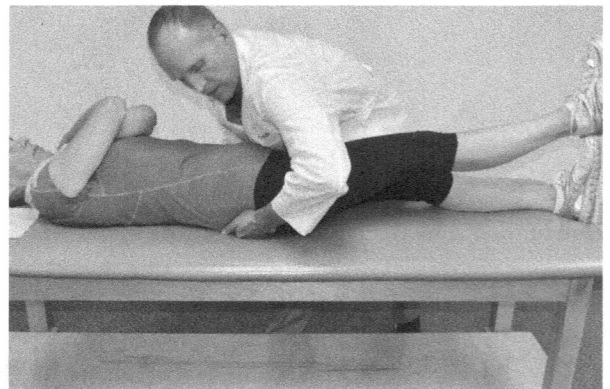

Figure 6-7. Lateral-to-medial overpressure in the posterior portion of the pelvis.

140

to raise the leg again (Fig. 6-7). If the pain is reduced or eliminated with the application of overpressure, dynamic instability is suspected. If the application of overpressure in this position does not eliminate or reduce the pain, the examiner applies overpressure in a lateral to medial direction in the anterior aspect of the pelvis, theoretically mimicking the action of the transverse abdominis muscle (Fig. 6-8). The patient is again asked to raise the leg. Again, if the pain is reduced or eliminated dynamic instability is suspected. The procedure is repeated with the other leg.

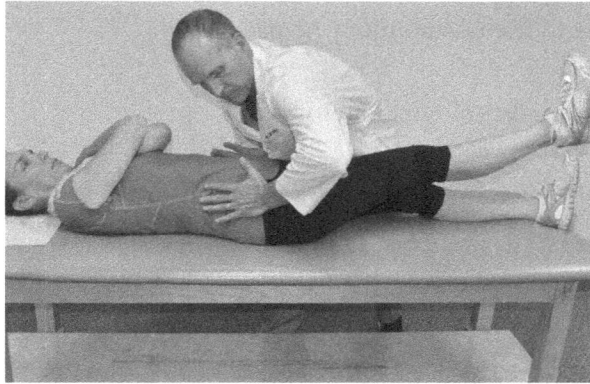

Figure 6-8. Lateral-to-medial overpressure in the anterior portion of the pelvis.

Passive Instability

Passive instability should be suspected in patients who have had trauma severe enough to cause ligamentous disruption or who have degenerative spondylolisthesis. Passive instability can occur in other circumstances but this is very uncommon. If there are clear reasons to suspect passive instability, flexion-extension radiographs are the preferred means of diagnosis. The standard criteria for determining segmental instability on flexion-extension radiographs are that of White and Panjabi (see Recommended Reading list) although more research is needed to investigate the clinical utility of these criteria. The criteria consider both translation of the segment and flexion or extension of the segment.

Anterior or posterior translation greater than 4.5 mm or greater than 15% of the vertebral body width is considered excessive translation. Flexion or extension of the segment greater than 15 degrees at L1-2, L2-3 or L3-4, greater than 20 degrees at L4-5 or greater than 25 degrees at L5-S1 is considered excessive movement.

Nociceptive System Sensitization

NSS should be suspected in any patient whose reported pain intensity is out of proportion to the clinical findings. Further investigation can then be carried out to support or refute the initial impression.

Smart, et al (see Recommended Reading list) developed the following criteria for the identification of NSS through a Delphi process and found good discriminative validity:

- Pain disproportionate to the tissue injury or pathology.

- Strong association with psychological factors.

- Disproportionate, non-mechanical and unpredictable exacerbating and remitting factors in the history.

- Diffuse, nonanatomic areas of pain/ tenderness.

The utilization of these criteria forms a good basis for screening for the presence of NSS. In most patients, no further investigation is necessary.

Waddell's nonorganic signs are likely in part reflective of the presence of NSS although it would appear that nonorganic signs indicate a more complex picture. As has been discussed throughout this book, NSS is part of a larger clinical picture of chronic LBD in which several somatic, neurophysiologic and psychological factors contribute to the overall pain, disability and suffering experienced by the patient. It appears that the presence of nonorganic signs is reflective of an intense interaction between NSS and at least some of the psychological factors that contribute to the LBD experience.

Waddell's nonorganic signs involve 5 categories of findings, each of which is given one point. The categories are:

1. Tenderness
   a. Superficial palpation: Widespread sensitivity to light touch of superficial soft tissues over the lumbar spine.
   b. Nonanatomic: Deep tenderness is felt over a wide area, is not localized to one structure and often extends to the thoracic spine, sacrum or pelvis.

2. Simulation
   a. Axial loading: Increased low back symptoms in response to light pressure to the top of the head of the standing patient (Fig. 6-9)
   b. Rotation: Back pain is reported when the shoulders and pelvis are passively rotated in the same plane as the patient stands relaxed with the feet together (Fig. 6-10).

3. Distraction: Marked difference in the report of pain when a Straight Leg Raise test is performed in the supine position as part of the pain provocation examination and when the same maneuver is performed in the seated position in a different part of the exam, such as during the neurologic exam while testing the plantar response.

4. Regional Disturbances
   a. Motor: "Breakaway" weakness identified during the neurologic examination in which the patient demonstrates full strength (5/5) initially but then "breaks away", losing the ability to provide resistance as a result of what the patients deems as "weakness."

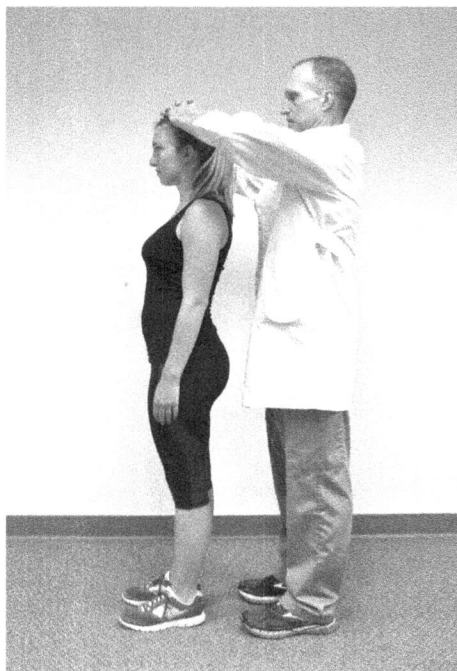

Figure 6-9. Axial loading during simulation assessment.

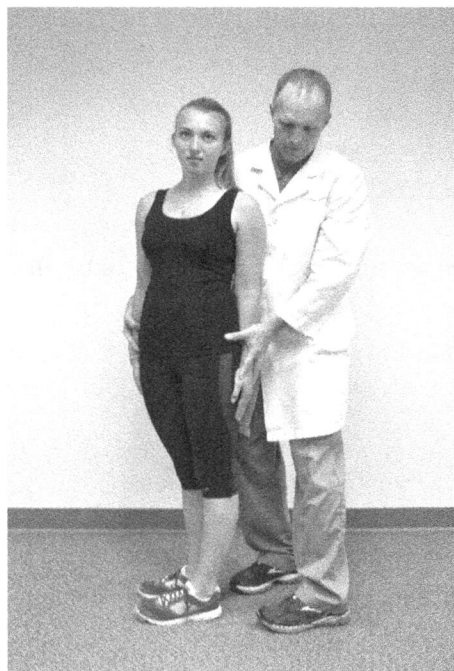

Figure 6-10. Rotation during simulation assessment.

b. Sensory: Regional sensory disturbance unexplained on a neurological basis. The most common manifestation of this is stocking distribution hypoesthesia, in which the patient's foot is examined with a pin and he or she reports an inability to feel the pinprick in any part of the foot. Of course, lower extremity peripheral polyneuropathy would have to be ruled out in this situation, which can usually be done through history (diabetes, family history of congenital neuropathy, exposure to toxic metals, etc.) and examination (vibration sense, joint position sense).

5. Overreaction: Excessive guarding, bracing, rubbing, grimacing, sighing or limping that is out of proportion to the severity or acuteness of the injury.

A positive finding in any category is given 1 point. In categories 1, 2 and 4, which have more than one potential finding, if *any* of the listed findings are present, one point is applied to that category. It is generally considered that a score of 3 or more out of a possible 5 is clinically meaningful for the presence of nonorganic pain behavior that likely arises in part from NSS.

The approach from Smart, et al discussed above is the most clinically useful means of suspecting NSS. It is less time-consuming and probably more sensitive than examination for Waddell's nonorganic signs.

Psychological Factors

Psychological factors that can perpetuate an ongoing pain, disability and suffering experience are sometimes referred to as "Yellow Flags." As was discussed in Chapter 2, the "Big 5" psychological factors in LBD patients are:

1. Fear

2. Catastrophizing

3. Passive coping

4. Poor self-efficacy

5. Depression

In addition, other factors such as perceived injustice, cognitive fusion, hypervigilance for symptoms and anxiety are important. See Chapter 2 for a complete discussion of these psychological processes.

The astute and experienced spine practitioner can probably get a good sense of the presence of many of these psychological factors simply by interacting with the patient; indeed, it is in establishing a relationship with the patient that allows the spine practitioner to gather the most important insights. Simply by asking questions like "are there certain activities that you would normally be engaging in but are avoiding because of the pain? If so, why are you avoiding them?" will often open the door for an understanding of the patient's beliefs, cognitions and assumptions about the pain.

There are also a variety of questionnaires available that are useful in detecting clinically meaningful psychological factors that may potentially contribute to the perpetuation of the pain, disability and suffering experience. While it is probably important to measure more than one of the important psychological factors in LBDs, it is not necessary to obtain a detailed quantitative assessment of all these factors. This would be burdensome to the patient and impractical in a busy practice environment. Described here are some of the more useful questionnaires. This is certainly not an exhaustive list, but the questionnaires discussed are ones that the busy spine practitioner may fund useful in practice.

Keele STarT Back 9-item Screening Tool

This is perhaps the most useful tool in identifying psychological factors that may be perpetuating the LBD. There are three different STarT Back questionnaires applicable to the LBD patient – a 6-item screening tool, a 9-item screening tool and a 9-item clinical tool. The most important for the spine practitioner in identifying problematic psychological factors is the 9-item screening tool (the 9-item clinical tool may also be useful as an outcome measure, as will be discussed in Chapter 7). This questionnaire can also be used as a general measure of risk for chronicity.

Questions 5 through 9 on the STarT Back 9 item questionnaire are useful for detecting psychological factors. These items assess fear (item 5), anxiety (item 6), catastrophizing (item 7), depression (item 8) and overall "bothersomeness" (item 9). A total score of 3 or less on the complete questionnaire indicates that the patient is at low risk of chronicity. In those patients with a total score above 4 on the entire questionnaire, a combined score of 3 or less on items 5-9 places the patient at medium risk of chronicity. A combined score of 4 or more places the patient at high risk of chronicity. Thus it is reasonable to extrapolate from this that a combined score on items 5-9 of 3 or more suggests the presence of clinically

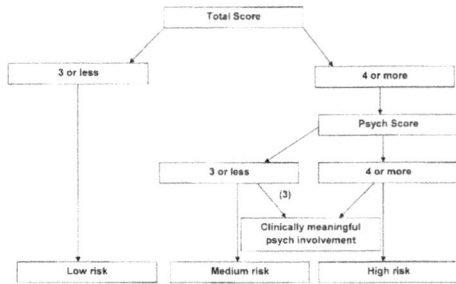

Figure 6-11. Interpreting the scores on the STarT Back Questionnaire (adapted from http://www.keele.ac.uk/sbst/usingscoringthesbst/ [accessed 29 July 2013])

meaningful psychological factors that have the potential to perpetuate the LBD. This is represented schematically in Fig. 6-11.

All STarT Back tools can be found at:

http://www.keele.ac.uk/sbst/downloadthetool/ [accessed 29 July 2013]

The Tampa Scale for Kinesiophobia

This questionnaire is designed to evaluate and measure fear beliefs. The original questionnaire contained 17 items however an 11-item version has been developed and validated that is easier for patients as well as clinic staff. These questions focus on the patient's beliefs about the pain with regard to its overall meaning and its relationship with movement and activity. In addition, the instrument contains a question about the patient's perception of how seriously people are taking the pain. The questionnaire is scored by totaling the responses to each question, with the score being expressed out of a total of 44 (e.g. 29/44). In general, a score of 27 or higher should be considered the threshold for clinically meaningful fear beliefs. So if a patient's score on this questionnaire is at or above this threshold, the practitioner should be concerned that fear beliefs are an important component to the 3rd question of diagnosis.

The full 11-item Tampa scale can be obtained at:

http://www.lni.wa.gov/ClaimsIns/Files/OMD/IICAC/FunctionalScales.pdf [accessed 29 July 2013].

The Fear Avoidance Beliefs Questionnaire

The Fear Avoidance Beliefs Questionnaire (FABQ) also measures fear beliefs although it does so in a slightly different manner than the Tampa Scale. There are two subscales of the FABQ – the Activity Subscale (the first 5 questions) and the Work Subscale (questions 6 through 16). The Activity subscale is appropriate for use in all LBD patients and the Work Subscale is specific to patients in whom the onset of the LBD has been attributed to work. Therefore, the best use of the FABQ is for all patients to complete the Activity subscale and for patients with work related LBD to complete both subscales. As with the Tampa scale, the questionnaire is scored by adding the scores for each individual question, although with the FABQ not all the items are included in the total score. For the Activity subscale, only items 2-5 are scored while for the Work subscale items 6, 7, 9, 10, 11, 12, 15 are scored. This is expressed as the score out of a total of 24 for the Activity subscale and 42 for the Work subscale. The threshold for clinically meaningful fear beliefs using the FABQ is a score of 15 or higher on the activity subscale.

The FABQ can be obtained at:

http://www.qcomp.com.au/media/29364/fear--avoidance-beliefs-questionnaire%5B1%5D.pdf [accessed 29 July 2013]

The Two-Question Coping Screen

This consists of two questions taken from the larger Coping Strategies Questionnaire. The questions address the patient's perception regarding the effectiveness of his or her coping strategies. The score of the two questions is totaled. A score below eight is considered the threshold for clinically meaningful coping difficulties. The questions are:

Based on all the things you do to cope, or deal with, your back pain, on an average day, how much control do you feel you have over it? Please circle the appropriate number. Remember, you can circle only one number along the scale.

No control   Some   Complete Control

0   1   2   3   4   5   6

Based on all the things you do to cope, or deal with, your back pain, on an average day, how much are you able to decrease it? Please circle the appropriate number. Remember, you can circle only one number along the scale.

Can't	Can decrease	Can decrease
Decrease	it somewhat	it completely
it at all		

0   1   2   3   4   5   6

A score less than 4 on the combined scales should be considered the threshold for clinically meaningful coping difficulties.

The Bournemouth Disability Questionnaire

This is a seven-item questionnaire that is primarily designed as a functional outcome measurement tool (see Chapter 7). However one of the items relates to depression and another relates to anxiety. So observation of the scores on these two items can give the practitioner an idea as to the degree to which depression and/ or anxiety are contributing to the patient's pain, disability and suffering experience. There is no established threshold for clinical significance using these scales.

The Bournemouth Disability Questionnaire can be obtained at:

http://www.aecc.ac.uk/system/site/uploads/content/docs/Research/BQ%20ONLY%20%28BACK%29.pdf [accessed 29 July 2013]

Self-efficacy

The Chronic Pain Self-Efficacy scale can be used to assess this important construct however this is a 22-item questionnaire that is not conducive to use in a busy clinical environment. The spine practitioner can informally assess a patient's self-efficacy by simply asking:

How confident are you in your ability to overcome your problem?

Total confidence										No confidence
0	1	2	3	4	5	6	7	8	9	10

The preceding questionnaires are probably the most useful scales currently available for use in the clinic. There are other tools that a practitioner may find useful, such as the Pain Catastrophizing Scale, the Beck Depression Questionnaire and the Beck Anxiety Questionnaire.

A great deal of information regarding psychological factors can be obtained with the Keele STarT Back screening tool, the two-question coping screen and the single self-efficacy question. This is the best general approach that is applicable to the vast majority of patients.

It is important to note that while these scales are very useful in measuring several important psychological factors that can contribute to patients' pain, disability and suffering experience, they do not replace good one-on-one communication between practitioner and patient. A great understanding can be gained through mindful observation of the way in which the patient talks about his or her LBD and the patient's pain behavior. Developing skills in this area is at least as important as developing skills in all other areas of evaluation and management discussed in this book.

Answering the third question of diagnosis allows the spine practitioner to complete the process of obtaining quality information regarding the biopsychosocial factors that are contributing to each patient's pain, disability and suffering experience. The remaining chapters will discuss how to put this information together into a working diagnosis and form a management strategy designed to address each contributing factor.

Recommended Reading

Bolton JE, Breen AC. The Bournemouth Questionnaire. A short-form comprehensive outcome measure I: Psychometric properties in back pain patients. J Manipulative Physiol Ther. 1999;22(8):503-10.

Cook C, Brismee JM, Sizer PS. Subjective and objective descriptors of clinical lumbar spine instability: A delphi study. Man Ther 2006;11:11-21.

Fishbain DA, Cole B, Cutler RB, Lewis J, Rosomoff HL, Rosomoff RS. A structured evidence-based review on the meaning of nonorganic physical signs (Waddell Signs). Pain Med 2003;4(2):141-81.

Hill JC, Dunn KM, Lewis M, Mullis R, Main CJ, Foster NE, et al. A primary care back pain screening tool: identifying patient subgroups for initial treatment. Arthritis and Rheumatism 2008;59(5):632-41.

Kendall NAS, Burton AK, Main CJ, Watson PJ, on behalf of the Flags Think-Tank. Tackling musculoskeletal problems: a guide for the clinic and workplace - identifying obstacles using the psychosocial flags framework. London, The Stationery Office, 2009. www.tsoshop.co.uk/flags [accessed 29 July 2013]

Leeuw M, Goossens ME, Linton SJ, Crombez G, Boersma K, Vlaeyen JW. The fear-avoidance model of musculoskeletal pain: current state of scientific evidence. J Behav Med 2007;30(1):77-94.

Linton SJ, Shaw WS. Impact of psychological factors in the experience of pain. Phys Ther 2011;91(5):700-11.

Main CJ, Buchbinder R, Porcheret M, Foster N. Addressing patient beliefs and expectations in the consultation. Best Pract Res Clin Rheumatol 2010;24(2):219-25.

Main CJ, Foster N, Buchbinder R. How important are back pain beliefs and expectations for satisfactory recovery from back pain? Best Pract Res Clin Rheumatol 2010;24(2):205-17.

McGill S. Low Back Disorders. Evidence-Based Prevention and Rehabilitation. Champaign, IL: Human Kinetics; 2002.

Miles CL, Pincus T, Carnes D, Taylor SJ, Underwood M. Measuring pain self-efficacy. Clinical J Pain 2011; 27(5):461-70.

Murphy DR, Hurwitz EL. The Usefulness of Clinical Measures of Psychologic Factors in Patients with Spinal Pain. J Manipulative Physiol Ther 2011;34:609-13.

Robinson ME, Riley JL, Myers CD, Sadler IJ, Kvaal SA, Geisser ME, et al. The Coping Strategies Questionnaire: a large sample, item level factor analysis. Clin J Pain 1997;13:43–9.

Smart KM, Blake C, Staines A, Doody C. Clinical indicators of 'nociceptive', 'peripheral neuropathic' and 'central' mechanisms of musculoskeletal pain. A Delphi survey of expert practitioners. Man Ther 2010;15(1):80-7.

Smart KM, Blake C, Staines A, Doody C. The Discriminative Validity of "Nociceptive," "Peripheral Neuropathic," and "Central Sensitization" as Mechanisms-based Classifications of Musculoskeletal Pain. Clin J Pain 2011;27(8):655-63.

Waddell G, Newton M, Henderson I, Sommerville D, Main CJ. A fear-avoidance beliefs questionnaire (FABQ) - the role of fear-avoidance beliefs in chronic low back pain and disability. Pain 1993; 52:157-168.

Waddell G. The Back Pain Revolution. 2nd ed. Edinburgh: Churchill Livingstone; 2004.

White AA, Panjabi MM. Clinical Biomechanics of the Spine. 2nd ed. Philadelphia: Lippincott, 1990.

Woby SR, Roach NK, Urmston M, Watson PJ. Psychometric properties of the TSK-11: a shortened version of the Tampa Scale for Kinesiophobia. Pain 2005;117(1-2):137-44.

· CHAPTER 7 ·

Establishing a Diagnosis, Clinical Decision Making and Outcome Measurement

Multidimensional Working Diagnosis

Clinical Reasoning in Spine Pain™ (the CRISP™ protocols) involves the practitioner seeking the answers to the three questions of diagnosis. This allows for the establishment of a working diagnosis. The term "working diagnosis" is used here because for most of the factors that contribute to the low back disorder (LBD) experience there is no way to definitively prove their existence. Thus, using the CRISP™ protocols the spine practitioner develops *the most accurate impression* as to what diagnostic factors are contributing to each patient's pain, disability and suffering experience. From this, the practitioner can decide on the combination of treatments that are most appropriate. In so doing, the practitioner tests the diagnosis with a trial of treatment, carefully monitoring the patient's response.

In many patients the diagnosis is multidimensional, including one or more pain sources and one or more perpetuating factors (on the primary spine care level, at the initial visit only about 1-3% of patients should be expected to have significant findings in response to diagnostic question #1). Some possible diagnoses might be:

- Lumbar disc derangement with dynamic instability, need to rule out infection. This diagnosis would be made in a patient who may have a history of fever or elevated temperature on examination, whose pain centralizes with end range loading examination and who has one or more stability test that is positive.

- Sacroiliac joint dysfunction with elevated fear beliefs. This diagnosis would be made in a patient whose pain does not centralize on end range loading examination, whose pain is reproduced with sacroiliac provocation maneuvers, and who has an elevated score on a questionnaire related to fear beliefs, such as the STarT Back questionnaire, Fear-Avoidance Beliefs Questionnaire or Tampa Scale for Kinesiophobia.

- Radiculopathy with nociceptive system sensitization and dynamic instability. This diagnosis would be made in a patient in who has historical factors suggestive of radiculopathy and whose pain is reproduced with the neurodynamic examination. The patient may or may not have neurologic signs or symptoms. The patient would also have signs and symptoms suggestive of elevated pain perception as well as positive tests for dynamic instability.

These are just a few examples of possible working diagnoses. Any combination of the potential answers to the three questions of diagnosis can serve as the working diagnosis in any given patient.

Outcome Assessment

It is important to measure, using reliable and valid tools, whether the patient is improving as a result of care. Most importantly, these measures must be *clinically relevant*. That is, the outcome assessment tool must measure factors that are of importance to the patient. In the past, range of motion (ROM) has been a popular measure used by practitioners of all kinds. This popularity stemmed in part from the fact that ROM is easy to measure and intuitively it would appear that ROM would be an important determiner of spine function, and thus of the patient's clinical status. However we now know that ROM does not correlate well with an individual's functional abilities (see Nattrass, et al and Parks, et al in the Recommended Reading list). That is, an individual's ability to conduct and enjoy life does not generally depend on precise ROM measures.

This gets to the crux of the measurement of treatment outcome. The most relevant question one can ask a LBD patient is, *"what is the extent to which this problem is interfering with your ability to conduct and enjoy your life?"* This is the question that a good outcome assessment tool asks, in a detailed and psychometrically valid manner. The measurement of functional outcome is best done by one or more simple questionnaires. There are a variety of such questionnaires that are specific to the LBD patient and that require only a few minutes for the patient to complete and even less time for clinic staff to score. A number of LBD-specific questionnaires are available. Presented here are the best known and most clinically useful.

The purpose of these outcome assessment instruments is to determine the perceived functional ability of the patient at baseline (prior to starting treatment) then to determine the perceived functional ability again after an initial trial of treatment, as well as at each re-examination thereafter. This allows the practitioner to determine whether the management strategy being employed is making a relevant difference for the patient in terms of his or her ability to conduct and enjoy life. The patient completes the questionnaire on the first visit, prior to seeing the practitioner. The patient then completes the questionnaire at each re-examination, again prior to seeing the practitioner. The score of the instrument at re-examination is compared with that from the initial visit to see if a *clinically meaningful* improvement has taken place. *Clinically meaningful* improvement is the change in score from baseline to re-examination (or from one re-examination to the next) that correlates with a perceptible change in functional abilities that is meaningful to the patient. For man outcome assessment tools the threshold for minimal clinically meaningful change has been established. In order for a change in score to be considered clinically meaningful, it must exceed that threshold.

STarT Back 9-item Clinical Tool

The STarT Back 9-item *Screening* Tool was discussed in Chapter 6 with regard to its use in assessing risk of chronicity and detecting psychological factors that may contribute to the perpetuation of chronic LBD. The STarT Back 9-item *Clinical* Tool is designed to be used as an outcome measure instrument. It includes the same questions as the screening tool, except the patient responds to the questions according to scales numbered 0-4 or 0-10. The questions relate to the "bothersomeness" of the patient's symptoms, the effect of the LBD on the patient's ability to dress and walk, and the intensity of fear, anxiety, catastrophizing and depression the patient is experiencing.

This instrument can be found at:

http://www.keele.ac.uk/sbst/downloadthetool/ [accessed 29 July 2013]

The Bournemouth Disability Questionnaire

This is a 7-item questionnaire with a 0-10 scale for each question. The questionnaire covers pain intensity, interference with daily activities, interference with recreational, social and family activities, anxiety, depression, interference with work activities and control of symptoms. The score for each scale is added to calculate the total score for the questionnaire. The threshold for clinically meaningful change using this instrument is 13 points or 35% change.

The Bournemouth Disability Questionnaire can be obtained at:

http://www.aecc.ac.uk/system/site/uploads/content/docs/Research/BQ%20ONLY%20%28BACK%29. pdf [accessed 29 July 2013]

The Oswestry Low Back Pain Disability Questionnaire

This is a 10-item questionnaire that obtains information regarding pain intensity, the pattern of improvement or worsening of the pain and interference with personal care, lifting, walking, sitting, standing, sleeping, socializing and traveling. The response to each item is scored from 0 to 5 and the total number of points from each item is added. This number is then doubled and expressed as a percentage.

The Oswestry Low Back Pain Disability Questionnaire can be obtained at:

http://www.workcover.com/workcover/search?q=oswestry *[accessed* 29 July 2013*]*

The Roland-Morris Low Back Pain and Disability Questionnaire

This is a 24-item questionnaire that asks various questions about the effects of the LBD on the patient's behavior and ability to perform activities. Each item that is checked is worth 1 point and the total number of items checked represents the total score on the instrument.

The Roland-Morris Low Back Pain and Disability Questionnaire can be obtained at:

http://www.rmdq.org/ [accessed 29 July 2013]

The threshold for clinically meaning change using the StarT Back, Oswestry and Roland Morris instruments is a 30% change.

The Swiss Spinal Stenosis Questionnaire

As the name implies, this questionnaire is specific to patients diagnosed with spinal stenosis. It consists of 12 questions the patient answers at baseline and an additional 6 items the patient answers at re-examinations. The questionnaire includes items related to the severity of symptoms (questions 1–7), the effect of the symptoms on physical function (questions 8–12) and, for use at re-examinations, satisfaction with treatment (questions 13–18). Questions 1-7 are scored from 1-5 and the remaining questions are scored 1-4. The total score is expressed as a percentage of the highest score possible (55 for questions 1-12, 79 for the entire questionnaire, including the questions related to treatment outcome).

The Swiss Spinal Stenosis Questionnaire can be obtained at:

http://www.scientificspine.com/spine-scores/swiss-spinal-stenosis-questionnaire.html [accessed 29 July 2013]

Patient-Specific Functional Scale

The questionnaires discussed here are very useful for obtaining detailed quantifiable information regarding the patient's general perception of his or her functional abilities. However it is also important to ascertain the patient's perception regarding the ability to engage in *specific activities that are important to the patient*. Useful for this is a modification of the Patient-Specific Functional Scale (see Stratford, et al in Recommended Reading list). The patient provides two or more activities that he or she has difficulty with but would like to be able to participate in. The perceived ability to engage in each activity is rated on a numerical scale:

What are two important activities that you cannot do or are having trouble doing? (i.e., "I can't get dressed without help," "I can't play golf," "I can't go to work.")

Activity 1._____

Please rate activity

        0   1   2   3   4   5   6   7   8   9   10

   Unable to perform   *Able to perform at same level as before problem*

Activity 2._____

Please rate activity

        0   1   2   3   4   5   6   7   8   9   10

   Unable to perform   *Able to perform at same level as before problem*

The full Patient-Specific Functional Scale can be obtained here:

http://www.maic.qld.gov.au/forms-publications-stats/pdfs/the_patient_specific_functional_scale.pdf [accessed 29 July 2012]

Numeric Pain Rating Scale

The Numeric Pain Rating scale (NRS) is a simple 0-10 scale that allows the patient to indicate the intensity of the pain, with 0 representing "no pain" and 10 representing "the worst pain imaginable." Three- and four-level scales are sometimes used but it is adequate to use a single scale that measures the average pain intensity over the past week. An example of such a scale is:

Over the past week, on average how would you rate your back pain?

No pain   Worst possible pain

0   1   2   3   4   5   6   7   8   9   10

A reduction of 2 points is often used as the threshold for clinically meaningful change using the NRS. However using percentage change, rather than change in the raw score, likely more accurate reflects true meaningful improvement. Sloman, et al (see Recommended Reading list) found the following correlations between percentage change in pre- and post-operative NRS scores and the patients' actual experience of improvement:

35% reduction – "minimal" improvement

67% reduction – "moderate" improvement

70% reduction – "much" improvement

93% improvement – "complete" improvement

Establishing a Management Strategy Based on the CRISP™ Protocols

The three questions of diagnosis approach allows the practitioner to identify the key factors that are contributing to the patient's pain, disability and suffering experience and to develop a management strategy that is best able to address those key factors. This allows the practitioner to personalize the treatment approach to the needs of the patient.

A variety of treatment approaches have been shown to be useful in patients with LBD. However the vast majority of randomized, controlled trials regarding LBD treatments involve a single treatment being applied homogeneously to all patients who happen to be randomized to receive that treatment. Rarely can studies be found in which patients are evaluated through a meticulous history and examination process in an attempt to individualize a treatment plan for each patient. In addition, the focus of most studies is been to evaluate a particular *treatment procedure* or *modality* for a group of patients with LBD rather than evaluating a *thought process* that leads to a *management strategy* designed to help an individual patient overcome his or her particular LBD.

The CRISP™ protocols are designed to help the spine practitioner move beyond this limitation of the spine literature by utilizing an evidence-based thought process in making decisions as to how to best help each patient.

Decisions in response to diagnostic question #1

In a patient in whom visceral disease or potentially serious or life threatening illness is suspected, there are a number of potential actions steps that can be taken. These depend not only on the disorder suspected but also on the comfort level of the spine practitioner in pursuing further investigation. In some cases the practitioner may choose to refer the patient to the local emergency department (or, depending on the situation, have the patient transported by ambulance), to his or her primary care physician or to a specialist. In others the spine practitioner may choose to further evaluate the patient him- or herself. There are no well-defined rules in these cases.

Cancer

The important factors suggesting the possibility of cancer were discussed in chapter 4. They include:

- History of cancer (this is particularly important if the primary cancer was in a tissue that has predilection for metastasis to bone – see Chapter 4 and Table 4-2).

- Age over 50 years.

- Unexplained weight loss (defined as a 10-pound or greater weight loss over a period of 6 months or less).

- Smoking history.

- Failure to respond to a one-month trial of evidence-based care.

In addition, symptoms and signs of possible cancer should be considered, including:

- No position of relief

- Fever

- Chills

- Constitutional symptoms

- Pain in multiple sites

- Pain on percussion

- Pain is worse at night

The practitioner should consider the entire clinical picture in making decisions about further investigation. The combination of multiple factors favoring the diagnosis of cancer should be considered more strongly than any one individual factor.

With patients in whom further investigation is warranted, an approach based on the work of Joines, et al (see Recommended Reading list) is recommended. The practitioner should start with blood tests and plain film radiographs. The blood test must include erythrocyte sedimentation rate (Sed rate) and C-reactive protein (CRP). In addition, complete blood count with differential and chemistry screen should be included. If either the Sed rate or CRP is elevated (or both are elevated) or if the plain film radiographs are positive for potential pathology, MRI is indicated.

Infection

Spinal infection, such as epidural abscess or osteomyelitis, should be considered in a patient who reports recent fever, chills and/or rigors, particularly if these are detectable at the time of examination. There are several types of spine infection and epidural abscess is one of the most common. Because this is a rapidly progressive disorder, the febrile LBD patient, particularly if acute, should be strongly suspected of having an abscess. The imaging modality of choice is MRI. In a patient who appears acutely ill, accommodations should be made to have him or her brought to the nearest hospital emergency department. In those who are febrile but do not appear acutely ill, a stat (i.e., the same day) MRI should be obtained. If this is not possible, the patient should go to the nearest emergency department.

Benign Tumor

In a patient with suspected benign tumor (local severe pain, no position of relief, relief w/ NSAID, pain on percussion) MRI is the imaging modality of choice.

Fracture

Fracture should be suspected in patients who have had major trauma, or minor trauma if they are older or have other risk factors for bone density loss such as diagnosed osteopenia or osteoporosis or prolonged steroid use. Patients with spine fracture also will often have marked pain on percussion at the involved segment. In these patients, plain film radiographs should be ordered. If the radiographs are negative for fracture but the practitioner is still suspicious, bone scan or MRI is often useful.

Abdominal Aortic Aneurism (AAA)

In a patient who reports a feeling of pulsation in the abdomen, coldness or discoloration in the lower extremities or in whom auscultation and palpation raises the suspicion of aortic aneurism, abdominal ultrasound is the best screening tool. Generally, AAA of less than 5cm can be monitored. However, those of 6mm or more are at increased risk of dissection so more urgent action must be taken. Regardless, when the spine practitioner encounters a patient with AAA of any size the patient's primary care practitioner should be alerted.

Gastrointestinal (GI) and Genitourinary (GU) Disease

The diagnostic workup of the patient with suspected GI or GU is dependent on the particular disorder suspected. For the spine practitioner, the best course of action is to refer these patients to their primary care practitioner.

Cauda Equina Syndrome (CES)

In the patient with suspected CES, immediate surgical referral is necessary. However it is essential that the diagnosis first be confirmed by MRI. Because of the urgency of the situation, MRI should be obtained immediately. If it is not possible to order a stat MRI, or if immediate surgical referral is not possible, the patient should be transported to the nearest hospital emergency department. Particularly in patients with incomplete CES, the greatest likelihood for recovery of bowel and/or bladder function occurs when decompressive surgery is performed within 24 hours. With complete CES it is less clear as to whether recovery will occur even if decompression is done within 24 hours. Nonetheless, it is best for the primary spine practitioner to act immediately in suspected cases.

Spondyloarthropathy

In patients with suspected spondyloarthropathy, such as ankylosing spondylitis, reactive spondyloarthropathy, psoriatic spondyloarthropathy, spondyloarthropathy associated with inflammatory bowel disease or undifferentiated spondyloarthropathy, plain film radiography in the best screening imaging modality. In those cases in which further clarification is needed, MRI should be ordered. In addition, blood tests including Sed rate, CRP and HLA-B27 should be ordered.

It was discussed in Chapter 4 that concern should be raised in patients whose pain cannot be reproduced during the pain provocation examination. If this occurs in isolation, i.e., in the absence of other signs or symptoms suggesting a non-musculoskeletal cause of the pain, the patient can often be monitored and immediate investigation may not be necessary. However, it is best for the practitioner to have a low threshold for investigation in these cases.

Decisions in response to questions #2 and 3 are introduced here but will be discussed in great detail in Chapters 10 and 11.

Decisions in Response to Question #2

Diagnostic question #2 asks, "Where is the pain coming from?" As was discussed in Chapter 5, in most patients with LBD there is no way to determine with absolute certainly the precise tissue of origin. However, there are signs and symptoms that can give the practitioner an idea of where the pain is coming from and upon which the practitioner can make treatment decisions. The following clinical decisions are recommended for each of the findings under diagnostic question #2:

1. Disc derangement: End range loading maneuvers into the direction that centralized the pain. This is patterned after the work of McKenzie (see Recommended Reading list). In addition, distraction manipulation as discussed by Cox (see Recommended Reading list) has been shown to decrease intradiscal pressure. So this is likely a useful method in patients with suspected disc pain.

2. Joint dysfunction: Joint manipulation. There are a variety of techniques of manipulation and this treatment should not be attempted by someone with inadequate training. Joint manipulation has been found to have both mechanical and neurophysiological effects on the joints of the lumbar spine.

3. Radiculopathy: In the acute stage of radicular pain the clinical picture is dominated by nerve root inflammation. Therefore, anti-inflammatory measures should be the focus. This can be in the form of anti-inflammatory medications (most of which can be obtained over-the-counter), oral steroids (which must be obtained by prescription) or epidural steroid injection. In the chronic stage, i.e., in patients with chronic radicular pain secondary to disc herniation or spinal stenosis, peripheral inflammation is less prominent and the key aspect of the pathophysiology is congestion, fibrosis and sensitization of the nerve root. Neural mobilization is the treatment of choice in these patients.

4. Myofascial pain: In patients in whom myofascial pain is a prominent component of diagnostic question #2 a variety of myofascial methods are available, including lengthening techniques and direct manual techniques.

Decisions in Response to Question #3

Diagnostic question #3 asks, "What has happened with this person as a whole that would cause the pain experience to develop and persist?" That is, this question allows the spine practitioner to focus on factors that serve to perpetuate the ongoing pain, disability and suffering experience for which patients seek help. The following clinical decisions are recommended for each of the findings under diagnostic question #3:

1. Dynamic instability: Stabilization exercise. There are a variety of theories and methods of stabilization exercise. The purpose of this approach is to train the motor control system to function as effectively as possible. In most cases the exercises can be done at home or the health club with minimal equipment.

2. Nociceptive system sensitization (NSS): Education and graded exposure. The education of patients with NSS relates to the nature of pain and the physiologic mechanisms by which pain intensity becomes amplified. Once this understanding is clear, or at least the patient is open to it, the graded exposure process can be instituted. Graded exposure involves desensitization of the nociceptive system through the gradual introduction of movements, positions and activities that provoke the pain to a tolerable level.

3. Fear, catastrophizing, passive coping, poor self-efficacy, depression and other psychological factors: Education, counseling and guidance. The management of psychological factors in LBD patients is more contextual than it is literal. It occurs with each and every interaction between the spine practitioner and the patient.

Shared Decision Making

In most cases of LBDs, there are a variety of diagnostic and therapeutic options available. Shared decision making (SDM) is the process by which a discussion of these options takes place between the practitioner and the patient prior to decisions being made. SDM brings together the knowledge and skills of the practitioner with the values and desires of the patient. At times the process involves family members or other loved ones.

The content and depth of the discussion will vary depending on the clinical situation and the patient's values and desires. It is important for the practitioner and patient to discuss the patient's goals for recovery. Helpful in this regard is to encourage the patient to get in touch with his of her core values (see Chapter 8). In this way the patient can be clear about the goals of the practitioner-patient encounter.

Some patients will want to have a great deal of involvement in the decision making process while others will want far less. There is no "right" or "wrong" way to approach this, however it is essential for the practitioner to provide leadership (without dictating to the patient what he or she "must" do except in potentially life-threatening situations). Patient benefit should be the most important driver of the shared decision making process. It is not uncommon for patients to adopt an attitude of, "You're the doctor; I will do whatever you say." The patient certainly has the right to take that approach but in many cases this should raise concern that the patient may be too passive in the process.

Some decisions are straightforward and should be directed by the practitioner. For example in a case in which the practitioner strongly suspects cancer or infection, investigation is imperative and the practitioner should take charge of this process. However for most decisions there will be multiple options available – including the option to do nothing. Ultimately, the decision rests on the patient to decide on diagnostic and treatment options. But, again, the patient will look to the practitioner for leadership so it is incumbent upon the practitioner to provide the options as clearly and objectively as possible, being careful not to put his or her own desires above the welfare of the patient. The patient's deepest held values should be the ultimate deciding factor in most clinical decisions.

The SDM process involves several key aspects:

1. The practitioner should establish a partnership on the initial visit by soliciting from the patient his or her most important goals, and the values upon which the goals are based.

2. It should be made clear from the beginning that the practitioner and patient will be working together to help the patient achieve those goals.

3. During history and examination, the practitioner should explain what he or she is doing and why, thus keeping the patient engaged in the process of arriving at a diagnosis.

4. Patients are not ubiquitous when it comes to involvement in decision making. The practitioner should find out how much involvement the patient would like to have, as well as how much information the patient wishes to be provided.

5. It is important to encourage the patient to share ideas, perceptions, concerns and expectations about the problem and how best to overcome it.

6. Once a diagnosis is established, the practitioner should discuss this in detail with the patient along with the recommended management strategy.

7. Alternatives to the recommended management strategy should be provided to the patient, including the pros and cons (i.e., benefits and risks) of each. In most cases of LBDs, "doing nothing" is an option and this should be made clear to the patient. While most patients will not choose the "do nothing" option (or else they would not be seeking help in the first place), putting this option on the table establishes clear patient autonomy.

8. Conflicts between the practitioner's recommendation and the patient's desires should be rectified.

9. Finally, a course of action should be agreed upon, with full commitment of both parties.

More information about SDM can be found at:

http://patients.dartmouth-hitchcock.org/shared_decision_making.html [accessed 30 July 2013]

A Trial of Treatment

Once a working diagnosis is established a trial of treatment based on the diagnosis can begin. In most cases, two or more sessions will be required for the clinician to apply the treatment strategy, monitor the clinical response, determine whether the treatment is having a positive effect and plan for aftercare. Generally, some form of symptomatic or functional change should be seen within one to three treatment sessions, although this is highly variable. So the spine practitioner should expect to start thinking about whether the diagnosis is correct or the management strategy is effective within the first few visits. If a positive change in not seen in that time, the practitioner should begin to think about whether the diagnosis and/or treatment choices should be re-considered. At formal re-examination visits a more thorough assessment can be made. At the re-examination visits the patient should complete the outcome assessment questionnaires that were completed on the initial visit so the practitioner can determine quantitatively whether improvement in functional abilities and quality of life has occurred.

Re-examination

The duration of time between the initial examination and the first re-examination, and between each re-examination, is highly individual, but typically three weeks is a reasonable period of time to allow the management strategy to have its effect, and then to determine whether meaningful improvement is occurring.

If clinically meaningful improvement is occurring, the current management strategy should continue. It should be noted however that, as discussed previously, this does not necessarily mean that the same treatment approaches should continue. One must adhere to the principles or transition away from passive and practitioner-dependent care toward active and patient-directed self-care (see Chapter 8). However, clinically meaningful improvement indicates that the overall treatment plan is bringing about functional gains and should continue.

Clinical decision making in cases in which initial treatment has *not* resulted in clinically meaningful improvement will be discussed in Chapter 12.

The principles of management and general approaches that apply to all patients will be explored in the next two chapters. In Chapters 10 and 11 specific treatment approaches for the factors identified in diagnostic questions #2 and 3 will be presented in detail.

Recommended Reading

Comer CM, Conaghan PG, Tennant A. Internal construct validity of the Swiss Spinal Stenosis questionnaire: Rasch analysis of a disease-specific outcome measure for lumbar spinal stenosis. Spine (Phila Pa 1976) 2011;36(23):1969-76.

Cox, JM. Low Back Pain: Mechanism, Diagnosis, and Treatment, 7th edition, 2011, Lippincott, Williams & Wilkins, Two Commerce Square, 2001 Market street, Philadelphia, PA 19103.

Cramer GD, Gregerson DM, Knudsen JT, Hubbard BB, Ustas LM, Cantu JA. The effects of side posture positioning and spinal adjusting on the lumbar Z joints: a randomized controlled trial with sixty-four subjects. Spine. 2002;27(22):2459-2466.

Fairbanks J, Pynsent P. The Oswestry Disability Index. Spine. 2000;25(22):2940-52.

Fisher K. Assessing clinically meaningful change following a programme for managing chronic pain. Clin Rehabil. 2008;22(3):252-9.

Gardner A, Gardner E, Morley T. Cauda equina syndrome: a review of the current clinical and medico-legal position. Eur Spine J 2011;20(5):690-7.

Godolphin W. Shared decision-making. Health Q 2009;12 Spec No Patient:e186-90

Herzog W. The biomechanics of spinal manipulation. J Bodywork Mov Ther 2010;14(3):280-6.

Joines JD, McNutt RA, Carey TS, Deyo RA, Rouhani R. Finding cancer in primary care outpatients with low back pain: A comparison of diagnostic strategies. J Gen Intern Med. 2001;16(1):14-23.

Jordan K. A minimal clinically important difference was derived for the Roland-Morris Disability Questionnaire for low back pain. J Clin Epidemiol 2006;59(1):45-52.

Klineberg E, Mazanec D, Orr D, Demicco R, Bell G, McLain R. Masquerade: medical causes of back pain. Cleve Clin J Med 2007;74(12):905-13.

McKenzie RA, May S. The Lumbar Spine: Mechanical Diagnosis and Therapy. 2nd ed. Waikenae, NZ: Spinal Publications; 2003.

Nattrass CL, Nitschke JE, Disler PB, Chou MJ, Ooi KT. Lumbar spine range of motion as a measure of physical and functional impairment: an investigation of validity. Clin Rehabil 1999;13(3):211-8.

Newell D, Bolton JE. Responsiveness of the Bournemouth questionnaire in determining minimal clinically important change in subgroups of low back pain patients. Spine (Phila Pa 1976) 2010;35(19):1801-6.

Ostelo RW, Deyo RA, Stratford P, et al. Interpreting change scores for pain and functional status in low back pain: towards international consensus regarding minimal important change. Spine. 2008;33(1):90-4.

Papagoras C, Drosos AA. Seronegative Spondyloarthropathies: Evolving Concepts Regarding Diagnosis and Treatment. J Spine. 2011;1(1).

Parks KA, Crichton KS, Goldford RJ, McGill SM. A comparison of lumbar range of motion and functional ability scores in patients with low back pain: assessment for range of motion validity. Spine. 2003;28(4):380-384.

Pateder DB, Brems J, Lieberman I, Bell GR, McLain RF. Masquerade: Nonspinal musculoskeletal disorders that mimic spinal conditions. Cleveland Clinic J Medicine 2008;75(1).

Pickar JG. Neurophysiological effects of spinal manipulation. Spine J. 2002;2:357-371.

Rondinelli RD (ed). Guides to the Evaluation of Permanent Impairment. 6th Ed. Chicago: American Medical Association; 2008.

Siemionow K, Steinmetz M, Bell G, Ilaslan H, McLain RF. Identifying serious causes of back pain: cancer, infection, fracture. Cleve Clin J Med 2008;75(8):557-66.

Sloman R, Wruble AW, Rosen G, Rom M. Determination of clinically meaningful levels of pain reduction in patients experiencing acute postoperative pain. Pain Manag Nurs 2006;7(4):153-8.

Stratford PW, Gill C, Westaway MD, Binkley JM. Assessing disability and change on individual patients: a report of a patient specific measure. Physiother Can 1995;47:258-262.

Wideman TH, Hill JC, Main CJ, Lewis M, Sullivan MJ, Hay EM. Comparing the responsiveness of a brief, multidimensional risk screening tool for back pain to its unidimensional reference standards: the whole is greater than the sum of its parts. Pain. 2012 Nov;153(11):2182-91.

Section III:

Management Based on the Clinical Reasoning in Spine Pain™ Protocols

• CHAPTER 8 •
Principles of Effective Patient Management

For the practitioner-patient relationship to be of maximal benefit several principles should be followed. These principles not only apply to the patient but to the practitioner as well. And these principles apply not only to what the practitioner *says* and *does* but, more powerfully, to the *environment* in which the practitioner-patient relationship takes place. That is, the essence of a healing relationship is one in which empowering messages about overcoming low back disorders (LBDs) *permeates the entire patient care process.*

As has been discussed in previous chapters, psychological factors play an important role in the perpetuation of, and thus the recovery from, LBDs. The spine practitioner is in the optimal position to help with the majority of these psychological processes because the principles of cognitive-behavioral therapy and acceptance and commitment therapy are often most effective when incorporated into the process of managing the somatic and neurophysiologic components of the LBD. In most cases it is not necessary for the spine practitioner to provide direct one-on-one counseling in this regard. When the important messages that are discussed in this chapter are *fully ingrained in the practitioner* they can permeate every aspect of the practitioner-patient relationship. Therefore the practitioner must not only *understand* these principles, he or she must *live* them, and this must be brought to every aspect of the healing relationship. For this reason, this chapter starts with the practitioner because it is the practitioner who sets the tone and establishes the environment in which the practitioner-patient relationship takes place.

The Core Values of the Spine Practitioner and the Mindful Approach to Primary Spine Care

Virtually all people, whether they are aware or not, have a set of core values that are of utmost importance to them. These are the things that bring meaning to our lives and fill us with a sense of purpose.

Ideally, our core values inform everything we do. For the spine practitioner it is likely that one of the core values that led to his or her choice of a health care career is to help people to be healthier, particularly as it relates to the spine. Thus it is essential that the spine practitioner is always guided by this core value. The overriding purpose of the encounter between the spine practitioner and the patient is for this encounter to result in the patient overcoming the pain, disability and suffering related to the spine problem and, as a result, becoming a healthier, more fulfilled and productive individual. That is, healthier, more fulfilled and more productive in relation to *the patient's own core values*. At the heart of the patient-practitioner relationship is maximal benefit to the patient. If this core value can always be kept in mind, and can serve as the key guiding principle behind the entire process of care for patients with LBDs, a foundation is established upon which to build a healing relationship with all patients. However this is not always easy, as there are competing factors that can sometimes get in the way. These competing factors oftentimes are thoughts based on preconceived notions, judgments, fears and rules we have established for ourselves.

Mindfulness is a way of non-judgmentally observing our experiences, and our reactions to those experiences. Being mindful allows us to cultivate self-awareness as an objective observer of those experiences and reactions. As a result, we are able to make a determination as to whether the way in which we are thinking about and responding to any given circumstance is consistent with what is most important in life – our core values. This allows us to take charge of life rather than allowing ourselves to be at the mercy of the ever-chattering mind.

Thoughts, feelings, judgments and evaluative assessments naturally arise during the course of every-day activities – including patient care. For most of us these arise unconsciously (i.e., mindlessly) and they determine both our experience of life as well as our behaviors in response to the situations we encounter. Thus, the more "mindlessly" we live, the less ability we have to make choices regarding our experiences and behaviors. For spine practitioners, thoughts, feelings, judgments and evaluative assessments will arise related to patients, situations that come up in the office, clinic or hospital, situations with insurance companies and third-party payors, and with a whole variety of things that occur during the course of practice. When the practitioner is with the patient, he or she is able to be most helpful when fully engaged in the process of helping the patient overcome the LBD, being mindful and "in the moment." Everyone carries a great deal of "stuff" around – past events, current problems, future worries – that the mind is constantly chattering about (often under the guise of "working on them"). This takes us out of the present moment and diverts our full attention away from the task at hand. The tendency for most of us is to respond to this by trying to push this "stuff" out of the mind so that it will not interfere with present activities. Mindfulness takes a different and more effective approach. It teaches us to "go into" the "stuff", meaning to look directly at the thoughts, feelings, judgments and evaluative assessments, experience them fully and acknowledge their presence so we are able to then go about the business of caring for the patient *independent of the presence or absence of the "stuff."*

In order to connect with our core values as spine practitioners, and to ultimately base our clinical approach on these values, it is useful to observe the thoughts that run through our head in relation to our patient encounters in an objective, non-judgmental manner. Key questions to ask ourselves include:

"Are these thoughts consistent with my core values?"

"Are they useful in helping me care for the patient?"

"Do they potentially interfere with my ability to be of maximum benefit?"

By open-mindedly and non-judgmentally asking ourselves these questions we can establish an environment in which we can be most helpful to the patient. And we can bring that mindful awareness to our patient encounters, thus creating a healing framework through which we can engage in the process of helping each patient overcome his or her LBD. Finally, by taking a mindful approach to each patient encounter we set an example for the patient of how to mindfully live according to one's values. We become a beacon of light that can help guide the patient toward taking a mindful approach to overcoming his or her LBD.

Mindfulness will be discussed further in this chapter as well as Chapters 9 and 11 as it has great application for both the patient and the spine practitioner. Mindfulness allows the spine practitioner to develop an awareness of his or her thoughts, feelings, judgments and reactions during the course of patient care for the purpose of developing greater self-awareness and cultivating an identity as an "observer" of thoughts. Additionally, because mindfulness involves the practitioner non-judgmentally "observing" these mind activities, he or she can step back from them, determine whether they are providing useful information, and then go about the business, in the moment, of providing the best possible care for the patient.

The attitudes, beliefs and cognitions of the spine practitioner

"What are my beliefs and preconceived notions about LBDs? Are they conducive to helping my patients? Are they detrimental to my helping my patients?" These are critical questions the spine practitioner must ask. Research has shown that many doctors and therapists themselves have fear-avoidance beliefs about LBDs (e.g., Linton, et al – see Recommended Reading list). Everyone has attitudes, beliefs and cognitions about many aspects of life that they are unaware of. It is essential that the practitioner become mindful of the possibility that some of these may interfere with his or her ability to be of maximal benefit to the patient.

There is one way to find the answer to these questions. That is for the practitioner to look, listen and pay attention to the feelings and thoughts that arise during the course of everyday activities, particularly related to patient care. This allows the practitioner to develop an awareness of attitudes, beliefs and cognitions that may be of great benefit in patient care, or that may interfere with effective patient care. The most important aspect of this mindful approach is *non-judgment*. That is, allowing the attitudes, beliefs and cognitions to *be as they are*. They are not "good" or "bad", "right" or "wrong." They simply *are*. This allows the practitioner to make a determination as to, first, whether the attitudes, beliefs and cognitions are accurate and, second, whether they are helpful. Getting into the habit of being mindful of these mind activities is one of the most powerful things the spine practitioner can do in developing into the best practitioner possible.

A full exploration of using mindfulness in everyday life is beyond the scope of this book, but the reader is directed to the book by Hayes and Smith in the Recommended Reading list to learn more.

Being Fully Engaged in the Process of Patient Care and Detaching from the Outcome

Mindfulness helps the practitioner become aware of the thoughts and feelings that arise during the course of patient care, to allow the thoughts and feelings to "be there" and then to place maximum focus on *engaging in the process of helping the patient*. This means being fully alert and present in the moment during history taking and examination, when applying treatment methods, monitoring exercise and engaging in patient education or *whatever the practitioner is doing in any particular moment*. This allows the practitioner to avoid becoming *attached to the outcome* of care and to simply engage in the *process* of caring for the patient.

Being attached to outcome is far different from caring about obtaining a desired result. Therefore, detaching from outcome should not be seen as cold, callous or uncaring – in fact it is quite the opposite. Attachment to outcome results from the practitioner making an emotional investment in the care process "going well." Because of this investment the practitioner's emotional state is *dependent* on the outcome of care. Thus, attachment to outcome is about the *practitioner* and not the *patient*. Detaching from the outcome of care means caring so much about bringing about a favorable outcome for the patient that the practitioner is willing to let go of his or her own emotional investment and to focus on providing the best care possible *in each individual moment,* without demanding a certain result.

Detachment does not come easily for most people and it takes time to cultivate this skill. However as with any skill it becomes easier with time and practice. Pursuing the value of excellence in spine care is well worth the effort.

Connecting with the patient and establishing a healthy working relationship

The spine practitioner begins impacting the patient's pain, disability and suffering experience from the first encounter. From that point on, every encounter between the practitioner and the patient serves to either promote recovery from the LBD or promote perpetuation of the LBD. So it is essential that the practitioner establish a healing relationship right from the start. This begins with acceptance.

Acceptance is important for both the practitioner and the patient. The practitioner must accept the patient as he or she is. As was stated earlier, we all carry preconceived notions as to how we would like people and situations to be. Therefore it is essential that the practitioner recognize this by being aware of his or her reactions to the patient, and the preconceived notions that give rise to these reactions. Then, to allow these reactions and preconceived notions to be as they are. This allows the practitioner to move on from them if they are not useful for the healing encounter. The mind of the spine practitioner can then become open to seeing the patient as-is, without judgment.

There are many patients who have beliefs and cognitions about their LBD that are very different from the spine practitioner's understanding of these disorders. It is also common to encounter patients who appear to have issues of "secondary gain" or who perceive their suffering as being someone else's "fault." This is particularly common in patients whose LBD began during the course of employment or as a result of a motor vehicle collision or a slip-and-fall incident. It is tempting for the spine practitioner to find these things annoying and, as a result, to develop a feeling of animosity toward these patients.

The first important thing for the practitioner to recognize is that this is a normal reaction. The second important thing is for the spine practitioner to, as stated earlier, observe these reactions and feelings in a non-judgmental manner. This allows the practitioner to identify the thoughts behind the reactions and feelings. Finally, the practitioner can ask him- or herself "are these thoughts useful in helping me to be of maximal benefit to the patient?" If they are not, they should be gently set aside. That is not to say the practitioner should try to "push away" or "ignore" these thoughts but rather to allow them to be exactly as they are, and move on to the task of caring for the patient. By going through these steps the practitioner will be in a position to accept the patient and establish a healing environment that is most conducive to patient benefit.

Acceptance allows the practitioner to meet the patient where he or she is. As has been discussed throughout this book, it is common for patients with LBDs to develop fear, catastrophizing, poor self-efficacy, perceived injustice and other psychological responses that serve to perpetuate the pain, disability and suffering related to the LBD. These responses are often based on perceptions that are inconsistent with what is known about LBDs and about the spine in general. Commonly, these patients perceive the presence of pain to be an ominous sign that something is seriously wrong in the spine. Many patients perceive the spine to be a delicate organ that is highly susceptible to injury or "wear and tear." A common perception is that if someone with a LBD were to engage in normal activities, there would be considerable risk of furthering the "damage" in the spine. In addition, particularly in patients whose pain began following a work-related incident or a personal injury in which someone else is "at fault", perceived injustice leads to heightened pain, disability and suffering.

These beliefs and perceptions should not be judged as "good" or "bad" *per se*. They should be seen simply as they are – beliefs and perceptions that are either consistent or inconsistent with the reality of LBDs. This allows the practitioner to understand and accept the patient. Then the practitioner and patient together can examine these beliefs and perceptions. The examination should be carried out in light of, first, whether they are accurate and, second, whether they are useful in helping the patient overcome the problem or, conversely, whether they are more likely to perpetuate the problem. This will be explored further in Chapter 11.

Part of connecting with the patient is to understand what is most important to patients with LBDs. Laerum, et al (see Recommended Reading list) studied the characteristics of the consultation that LBD patients felt were most important to their satisfaction with the practitioner-patient encounter. These characteristics were:

- The patient being made to feel that he or she was taken seriously, i.e. that the practitioner placed the patient at the center of the consultation, sincerely listened to the patient's concerns and sincerely believed what he or she was saying.

- The patient being provided with a clear and understandable explanation of the problem.

- The practitioner taking a patient-centered approach, i.e., the practitioner seeking the patient's perspectives and preferences regarding the encounter.

- The patient receiving reassurance and, if possible, being given a positive prognosis.

- The patient being clearly told what can be done, both by the patient him- or herself and by the practitioner.

These characteristics must be kept in mind during every practitioner-patient encounter.

Promoting self-efficacy

One of the most fundamentally important goals of the practitioner-patient encounter is improving the patient's self-efficacy. That is, it is essential that as a result of the interaction between practitioner and patient, regardless of the diagnosis or the content of the management strategy, the patient is left with increased confidence in his or her ability to overcome or effectively cope with the LBD and to live a fruitful and productive life. This goal transcends all others and is more important than such measureable physical factors as muscle strength, endurance and range of motion. Therefore, every interaction between the practitioner and the patient should occur in the context of positive, empowering messages about LBDs in general and the patient's abilities in particular. In addition, the primary focus of the management strategy should be to provide self-care strategies the patient can employ to manage the pain and to improve functional abilities. Further, treatments that require application by the spine practitioner (or another professional) should be minimized and always used in the context of facilitating transfer of responsibility and capability toward the patient.

Providing healthy cognitive-behavioral, acceptance-commitment messages about LBDs

Every encounter between the practitioner and the patient is an opportunity to provide information regarding the realities of LBDs. This allows the practitioner to gently help the patient start to challenge his or her beliefs about the problem, particularly if these beliefs are inaccurate and/or likely to perpetuate the suffering. The following are the most important messages:

- The cognitions, beliefs and judgments that one has about LBD greatly influence its impact on one's ability to overcome the problem.

- In many cases the suffering arises not only from the actual nociceptive stimulus, but from one's judgments about and resultant emotional reaction to the stimulus.

- If one "looks at" the pain without judgment one can understand the pain for what it really is.

- A LBD is not a fearsome catastrophe. It is a very painful inconvenience that can at times have a great impact on one's life. But the impact largely depends on how the patient handles the problem. Handling the problem in a productive way can be learned and this is the central focus of the management strategy.

- Fear, catastrophizing and other psychological and emotional responses to the pain are understandable and normal. Given the intensity of the pain and the mysteriousness of the spine to most people, it is not at all surprising that one would react to a LBD with great emotional distress.

- The reason it is so important to address the psychological and emotional reactions to LBDs is not because these reactions are "bad" or "wrong" but because they can interfere with recovery, are very unpleasant and are not conducive to living a fruitful and productive life.

- The key to effectively dealing with a LBD is not to focus on "getting rid of" the pain but on "*overcoming*" the pain. Part of the management strategy focuses on reducing the intensity of the pain in whatever way possible. But ultimately the purpose of the management strategy is to help the patient move toward being able to live a fruitful and productive life *independent of the presence or absence of pain*. The nature of LBDs is that even when the pain "goes away" there is a good likelihood that it will "come back" at some point. Occasional back pain is common and is a normal part of life. If one develops the mindset that the only way to live a fruitful and productive life is to be pain-free, one places oneself on an emotional roller coaster ride that is controlled by the transient nature of LBDs. However, becoming independent of the presence

CLINICAL REASONING IN SPINE PAIN. VOLUME I

or absence of pain frees the individual to live life to the fullest regardless of what the back feels like at any given time.

- The best way to overcome the pain is to actively engage it through coping strategies that are focused on increasing one's ability to perform normal activities.

- Pursuing activity is conducive to recovery, avoiding activity interferes with recovery.

- The patient will be guided in gradually returning to activity.

- Overcoming a LBD is within the capability of virtually every patient. Even the patient with a chronic LBD who has been unable to cope effectively with the disorder can be taught how to overcome the problem and regain control of his or her life.

- Overcoming a LBD often requires time, work and patience. This need not be *overwhelming*, but it does require the patient to make a focused effort and commitment to taking on the problem in the most effective way possible.

- In cases of chronic LBD the intensity of the pain is largely due to nociceptive system sensitization (NSS). That is, with NSS the central nervous system receives pain signals from the spine and amplifies them several times before they reach the patient's conscious awareness. Thus, what starts out as a mild or moderate signal from the spinal tissues becomes severe pain by the time the signal reaches the brain. This is *good news* because it indicates that the actual disorder in the spine is not nearly as severe as it appears.

- Nociceptive system sensitization occurs in the lower part of the central nervous system, below the patient's conscious awareness. Therefore this process is not the patient's "fault." It is not *the patient* who is "exaggerating" the pain. The *central nervous system* is exaggerating the pain without the patient realizing this is happening.

- Getting in touch with one's most deeply held values can help provide a compass for recovery via goal setting. It also allows one to become aware of situations in which seeking pain relief in lieu of increased functional ability can interfere with the process of living a fulfilling life.

It must be noted that it is not always necessary to provide these messages directly and literally. There are many cases in which they can be gotten across indirectly, by example or as a result of the patient coming to these conclusions him- or herself through experiential training.

Promoting acceptance

As was discussed previously, self-efficacy is perhaps the most important psychological factor in the perpetuation of LBDs, in part because it mediates the effect of fear on ongoing disability. Someone with high fear beliefs who is confident in his or her ability to overcome the LBD is more likely to experience significant functional improvement than someone with high fear beliefs and little confidence in his or her ability to overcome the LBD. Similarly, acceptance mediates the relationship between catastrophizing and depression and avoidance of activities. In other words, the degree to which catastrophic thinking about pain leads to depression and avoidance is dependent on the degree to which the patient is able to *accept the presence of pain in the moment.*

From the very start it is essential that we guide the patient on the path of acceptance of the LBD. We do this by encouraging and teaching the patient to simply observe and experience the sensation of pain without judgment, analysis or labeling. Simply experiencing the actual sensation helps the patient gain a perspective on what pain really is – simply a sensory perception. In addition, the patient gains a greater identity as a dispassionate observer of the pain, as "the experiencer of the pain" rather than seeing the pain as all-encompassing of who he or she is. As the patient gets better at this, the realization arises that, first, the pain itself is not nearly as severe and overwhelming as it seemed to be and, second, overcoming the pain is well within the patient's capability. As a result, the pain becomes less fearsome and is seen as less of a catastrophe. This then leads a greater willingness to engage in active coping strategies and greater confidence in the ability to overcome the problem (i.e. the patient develops greater self-efficacy).

Minimalism – Less is more

To be maximally effective, primary spine care should be minimalist. That is, the less treatment that is "done to" the patient, the better. Minimalism increases the value of care by maximizing clinical outcome and minimizing cost. Further, while each patient is different, patients are often more satisfied with care that does not demand a great deal of their time and money.

Minimalism particularly applies to treatment modalities that are designed to reduce pain. Patients who seek to "get rid of" the pain by focusing on relief strategies actually experience amplified pain. Therefore, excessive focus on attempts to "get rid of" pain on the part of both the patient and the spine practitioner, in lieu of efforts to improve the patient's functional abilities, is counterproductive. The management strategy should concentrate on approaches that are most likely to effectively address the most important diagnostic factors identified by Clinical Reasoning in Spine Pain™ (the CRISP™ protocols). This means addressing the pain-producing factor(s) as quickly and expeditiously as possible but in the functional context that we have been discussing throughout this chapter. This allows both the spine practitioner and the patient to maintain a productive focus without being sidetracked by the perceived need to "make the pain go away."

Minimalism refers to the number of treatment modalities that are provided to the patient as well as the number of treatment sessions utilized. In addition, it applies to early and rapid transition away from approaches applied by the spine practitioner toward self-care strategies that are employed by the patient. Finally, the minimalism principle should be applied to exercise and self-care as well – only those strategies that are essential for self-treatment of the pain and prevention of recurrences should be provided. At the end of the treatment period, the patient should be left with a brief but focused exercise program as well as tools to address recurrences, should they arise. This maximizes the likelihood of compliance.

Of course, the spine practitioner must be aware that "doing enough" is essential. One has to be careful not to attempt to be so minimalist that the problem is not addressed appropriately. Again, the CRISP™ protocols provide the spine practitioner with guidance regarding this by helping to determine what specific treatment approaches should be applied for each individual patient.

Transitioning away from a passive care strategy toward an active care strategy

Passive approaches are treatment modalities that are *done to* the patient. In the early stages of care, passive approaches are sometimes useful to reduce the intensity of the pain as rapidly as possible. However, continued passive care beyond the very early stages can be detrimental. This is for several reasons:

- Passive approaches educate can the patient that pain relief is the ultimate goal of the management strategy, rather than improvement in functional abilities and self-efficacy. This, as was discussed earlier, promotes chronicity rather than recovery.

- Excessive emphasis on passive care disempowers the patient by placing him or her in a passive role, making the patient an uninvolved recipient of care rather than an active participant in his or her recovery.

- Passive care teaches the patient to emphasize passive coping strategies rather than to actively engage the pain.

- Passive approaches promote physical deconditioning.

Consequently passive treatment approaches should be used sparingly and strategically. The practitioner should choose those treatments that are best suited to address the source of the pain (i.e., diagnostic question #2) and use them only to the extent necessary to reduce the intensity of the pain and allow the patient to move on to active coping strategies. Pain-reducing modalities that can be self-applied by the patient, such as end range loading exercises (see Chapter 5), are always preferable over modalities that require practitioner application. Active approaches such as exercise should be incorporated as soon as possible; most patients can be provided with some type of home exercise right from the start.

Transitioning away from dependence on practitioner-driven processes toward self-reliance, self-efficacy and functional independence

There are many practitioner-driven methods that are effective in addressing the problems identified by diagnostic questions #2 and 3. These treatments, when applied skillfully and in the right circumstance, can be very powerful. However these methods must be used in the proper context in order for the practitioner to be maximally effective in helping the patient. There is a common tendency for professionals of all types to want to place themselves at the center of their work rather than placing their clients or patients at the center. Optimum management of LBDs requires establishing the patient as the central focus. This means empowering the patient to effectively overcome the problem. The best way to do this is to create a working environment in which it is clear from the beginning in the minds of both the practitioner and the patient that the plan is to move the patient away from dependence on professional services (i.e., those of doctors, therapists and others involved in the clinical care process) toward self-management and toward being able to engage in work, recreational and personal activities without depending on anyone else. For the practitioner, this will often mean becoming mindful of his or her natural desire to "be the hero" and "do things to the patient" in lieu of providing the patient with the knowledge and tools to self-manage the condition.

For some patients there is a tendency to want to be "taken care of" and to relinquish responsibility for recovery and transfer it to the practitioner. It is essential for the practitioner to take a leadership role in this regard and to make it clear from the very first contact that the purpose of the patient-practitioner relationship is to maximize the likelihood of the patient overcoming the LBD. This means helping the patient take charge rather than allowing the LBD to be in charge. This message must be clear and unequivocal.

Employing an aggressive stay-at-work/ return-to-work strategy

An aggressive stay-at-work/ return-to-work (SAW/RTW) strategy is important in all patients, particularly those with work-related LBD. One of the most therapeutic things a practitioner can do in helping a patient overcome a LBD is to help the patient remain at, or return to, some form of productive work activity.

It is common for practitioners and patients, particularly in situations in which the LBD started during the course of employment, to see SAW/ RTW as something that is "good for the insurance company" but that puts the patient at potential risk of "re-injury." The thought is (and on the surface this appears to be rational) that if a patient with a LBD returns to work "too soon", before tissue healing has fully taken place, he or she is vulnerable to experience worsening of the tissue damage that resulted from the injury. If this were to occur the patient would be at risk of developing an even more severe LBD, perhaps even developing long-term or permanent damage.

However, it is well known that the longer an individual remains out of work as a result of a LBD the more difficult it is to return to some form of gainful employment, independent of the severity of the initial injury. In fact, lack of effective SAW/ RTW is one of the most important predictors of failure to recover. What this means is that one of the biggest factors that places a patient at risk of developing chronic LBD is not returning to work "too soon", it is *not returning to work soon enough*!

There is growing evidence that work is not only necessary to allow one to support oneself and one's family, it is essential to living a fulfilling life (see the Waddell and Burton publications in the Recommended Reading list). Work has health benefits that extend well beyond any particular condition or body part. A person's total health and sense of wellbeing is enhanced by being involved in productive work. Work is therapeutic. Therefore, SAW/ RTW should be seen by the spine practitioner (as well as everyone else involved in helping the injured worker) not simply as a necessary nuisance but as a central component of care. Messages regarding SAW/ RTW should be provided to the patient from the very first encounter. These messages should include:

1. One of the most important aspects of care for LBDs is the SAW/ RTW process.

2. Work is healthy. To avoid potentially compromising recovery and general health, any time off work will be as brief as possible.

3. One of the key goals of care is for the patient to return to normal productive activities as quickly as possible. Work is one of the most important of these activities.

4. *"You don't get better in order to go back to work. You go back to work in order to get better."* This means that while there may be a brief period during which work activities will be modified, or even avoided completely, a gradual transition back to partial work duty, and ultimately full work duty, will not only be important for employment purposes, it will be *an essential part of therapy.*

5. Being afraid or apprehensive about returning to the environment in which the pain began is understandable and is a normal reaction. One should not feel guilty or "weak" because of this fear. However the fear itself can be an obstacle to recovery. This fear can be overcome with careful guidance.

6. The patient can expect to begin the RTW process while he or she is still symptomatic – waiting until the symptoms "go away" is not only unrealistic and unnecessary, it is detrimental to recovery.

7. The patient will be guided along the path to RTW. He or she is not alone in this process.

8. Patients who have been out of work for a long time can expect an increase in symptoms when they initially return to work. This is not usually a sign of "re-injury"; it is simply the awakening of "pain memory." That is, the pain pathway that was established during the early phase of the LBD is still present, and when the central nervous system experiences the normal "stresses" of the work environment, this pain pathway is sometimes activated.

9. If pain occurs upon RTW it will usually subside gradually as the work activities continue. This may require a few days or more. The gradual regression of the pain results from "habituation" in which the nociceptive system gradually desensitizes as it becomes accustomed to the new activity (see Chapter 11).

10. Pain upon RTW that persists and does not habituate, or that is very severe, will be evaluated and usually can be treated. It is not usually a sign of severe injury.

As with all of the empowering messages discussed in this chapter, the messages regarding SAW/ RTW do not all have to be provided to every patient, and they do not all have to be provided directly and verbally. Creating a SAW/RTW atmosphere in which the practitioner-patient relationship occurs is what is most essential.

Chapter 11 discusses, among other things, patient care approaches to the psychological factors that are identified with diagnostic question #3. There are particular "techniques" that can be utilized for this purpose. However, applying the general principles discussed in this chapter, and creating an environment in which mindfulness, acceptance, commitment and cognitive-behavioral messages permeate the entire practitioner-patient relationship, will allow the practitioner to address the psychological component of LBDs at every step along the care process. Establishing this healing environment makes the job of addressing the psychological factors far easier and more effective than simply applying specific techniques. This will be explored further in Chapter 11.

Recommended Reading

Dahl J, Lundgren T. Living Beyond Your Pain. Oakland; New Harbinger Publications, 2006.

Hayes SC, Smith S. Get Out of Your Mind and Into Your Life. The New Acceptance and Commitment Therapy. Oakland; New Harbinger Publications, 2005.

Kendall NAS, Burton AK, Main CJ, Watson PJ, on behalf of the Flags Think-Tank. Tackling musculoskeletal problems: a guide for the clinic and workplace - identifying obstacles using the psychosocial flags framework. London, The Stationery Office, 2009 [ISBN 9 780 11 703789 2] www.tsoshop.co.uk/flags

Laerum E, Indahl A, Skouen JS. What is "the good back consultation?" a combined qualitative and quantitative study of chronic low back pain patients' interaction with and perceptions of consultations with specialists. J Rehabil Med 2006;38(4):255-62.

Linton SJ, Vlaeyen J, Ostelo R. The back pain beliefs of health care providers: are we fear-avoidant? J Occup Rehab. 2002;12(4):223-232.

MacEachen E, Chambers L, Kosny A, Keown, K. A Guide to Identifying and Solving Return-to-Work Problems: Institute for Work and Health; 2009.

Smith M, Saunders R, Stuckhardt L, McGinnis JM, eds. Best care at lower cost: The path to continuously learning health care in America. IOM (Institute of Medicine), Washington, DC: The National Academies Press, 2012.

Vowles KE, McCracken LM, Eccleston C. Patient functioning and catastrophizing in chronic pain: the mediating effects of acceptance. Health Psychol 2008;27(2 Suppl):S136-43.

Waddell G, Burton AK, Kendall NAS. Vocational rehabilitation – what works, for whom, and when? London, The Stationery Office, 2008 [ISBN 0 11 7038615] http://www.dwp.gov.uk/docs/hwwb-vocational-rehabilitation.pdf

Waddell G, Burton AK. Is work good for your health and well-being? London, The Stationery Office, 2006 [ISBN 0 11 7036943]. http://www.dwp.gov.uk/docs/hwwb-is-work-good-for-you.pdf

Wager TD, Atlas LY, Lindquist MA, Roy M, Woo CW, Kross E. An fMRI-based neurologic signature of physical pain. New Engl J Med 2013 Apr 11;368(15):1388-97.

CHAPTER 9
General Management Strategies

There are several useful management strategies that are widely applicable to virtually all patients with low back disorders (LBDs) and are not necessarily diagnosis-specific. This chapter presents these general strategies. There may be certain patients whose specific needs necessitate a greater amount of time being spent on one or another strategy.

Patient education regarding the nature of low back disorders

There is a great deal of confusion among the lay public (and even health care practitioners!) regarding LBDs. Unfortunately, this confusion often leads to medicalizing or catastrophizing this group of disorders. The challenge with patient education in the field of LBDs is, as has been discussed in this book, threefold. First, in most cases the cause of the patient's pain, disability and suffering experience is multifactorial. Second, the contributing factors cut across different facets of "personhood" (somatic, neurophysiological, psychological and social). Finally, for most of the common factors that contribute to the LBD experience there is no definitive objective diagnostic test. Clinical Reasoning in Spine Pain™ (the CRISP™ protocols) helps the spine practitioner to provide a clear and concise multi-dimensional diagnosis while at the same time realizing that in most cases there is no way to be 100% certain of the etiology of the problem. This can inform not only the spine practitioner's diagnostic process but also but also patient education.

Telling the patient (as one possible example) "while there is no way to know with 100% certainty what causes most back pain, based on what is known about LBDs and my examination of you, your pain is most likely arising from one of your discs. And it appears that the problem is being perpetuated because the system that provides muscular support to your spine is not working at optimum" is a perfectly reasonable explanation that is acceptable to most patients. Obviously the explanation will differ depending on the specific diagnosis in each patient.

The patient should be provided with an explanation as to what the spine practitioner thinks is causing his or her pain, disability and suffering experience, based on the findings of the three questions of diagnosis, and that a trial of treatment will be carried out based on the diagnosis. The patient's response to this trial of treatment will be carefully monitored and alterations in the diagnosis and/or treatment approach will be made depending on the initial response.

The information the patient is provided should be based on evidence, rather than assumptions or preconceived notions, about LBDs. Too often patients are provided with "education" regarding their LBDs based solely on imaging findings. This can be a major cause of "iatrogenic imaging disability" if the imaging findings being communicated are common and benign but scary-sounding entities such as "disc bulge", "degenerative disc disease" or "spondylosis."

In addition, there are many patients for whom the explanation for the LBD is based on traditions or assumptions. For example it is common for patients to be told that their "pelvis is out of alignment." This is not an evidence-based explanation of spine pain (in fact, there is evidence that "misalignment" of the pelvis is normal! See Krawiec, et al in the Recommended Reading list). Telling a patient that the "pelvis is out of alignment" can serve to augment fear and catastrophizing by giving the patient the impression that the pelvis (or spinal vertebra) can mysteriously "misalign" without him or her knowing it, setting the stage for the development of pain. This reinforces the perception that the spine is a delicate and mysterious part of the body, in which sinister things can develop without one knowing about them.

Again, the CRISP™ protocols provide the spine practitioner with an evidence-based thought process upon which to base the diagnosis in each patient and allow the spine practitioner to appropriately educate the patient in an empowering and realistic manner.

It is essential to provide the LBD patient with correct information regarding the causes, risk factors and prognosis of LBDs and, in particular, the role that activity plays in perpetuation or recovery. Specifically, it should be made clear that little is known about the actual causes of LBDs. These types of disorders are so common (virtually everyone develops a LBD at some time during life) that it is difficult to pinpoint a specific activity or event that is causative. However in any individual case there may be elements in the patient's lifestyle that can factor in the development of a particular LBD. With regard to risk factors and prognosis, the patient should understand that back pain is a "normal" part of life in that virtually everyone is affected at some time. And it is not uncommon for back pain to return periodically. The important thing is that LBDs can be treated – oftentimes by the patient without the need to see a professional – and there are simple things the patient can do to lessen the frequency of recurrences. So while the periodic occurrence of back pain is virtually unavoidable, *chronic, disabling* back pain is *almost always* avoidable. This is a critical distinction as most people are not afraid of back pain itself, but many are afraid of being chronically disabled by back pain.

Chapter 2 contains information regarding the contributing factors of the LBD experience and can be used as the basis of patient education regarding the etiology of a particular patient's diagnosis.

Posture and Lifting

The most important consideration regarding maintaining a protective posture and proper lifting techniques for patients with LBDs is the lumbar lordosis. That is, maintaining the lumbar lordosis during static postures and dynamic movements is protective to the spine. Flexion of the spine increases intradiscal pressure and places the back extensors at a mechanical disadvantage in protecting against shear forces (see McGill in Recommended Reading list). Therefore patients should be taught to minimize repetitive or sustained flexion during everyday activities. This does not mean that the patient should become "flexion phobic" – in fact, it is essential that the spine practitioner be mindful not to promote fear of re-injury during all aspects of patient care. But because flexion is such a common static position and dynamic movement in everyday life, and is known to cause disc problems, it is important to minimize flexion whenever possible.

The training of posture and lifting starts with helping the patient become mindful of the normal lordotic position of the lumbar spine; this is often referred to as the "neutral spine." Teaching patients the neutral spine is perhaps most easily done in the supine, non-weight bearing position. The patient lies supine and the practitioner instructs him or her in the performance of a pelvic tilt movement, that is, moving the pelvis into posterior tilt (decreasing lumbar lordosis) and anterior tilt (increasing lumbar lordosis) (Fig. 9-1 and 9-2). In patients who have difficulty with this movement it is helpful for the practitioner to manually guide the movement.

As the patient becomes skilled with this movement identification of the neutral spine position can be trained. The patient moves into full anterior pelvic tilt, then backs just away from this to allow the spine to rest in a neutral position of lordosis.

The purpose of the pelvic tilt exercise is to help the patient gain an awareness of the neutral lordotic position of the spine. It should not be given as a home exercise in most circumstances as it involves repetitive flexion of the lumbar spine, which likely increases risk of both disc derangement and dynamic

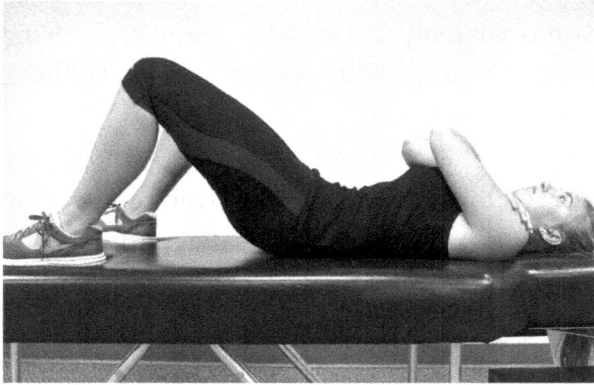

Figure 9-1. Posterior pelvic tilt.

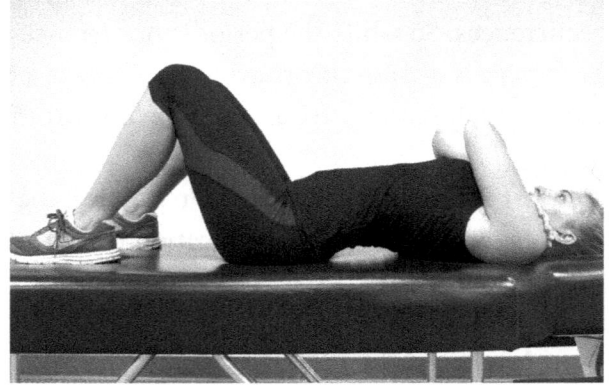

Figure 9-2. Anterior pelvic tilt.

instability. Also, a patient with an active disc derangement should not be instructed in posterior pelvic tilt (unless flexion has been determined to be the Direction of Benefit for exercise – see Chapter 5) until the derangement is resolved.

As the patient becomes aware of the neutral lordosis in the supine position he or she can be progressed to the seated position (Fig. 5-12). With patients who spend a great deal of time sitting, it is often beneficial to provide them with a lumbar support to help maintain the neutral lordosis when sitting.

Finally, the patient can be trained to maintain the neutral lordosis while bending and lifting. This is best done with the "Good Morning" exercise. The patient stands with the lumbar spine in the neutral lordotic position. The feet are placed slightly beyond shoulder width and the knees are slightly bent. The patient slowly bends forward, flexing at the hips rather than at the lumbar spine. The patient bends as far as possible without losing the neutral spine (Fig. 9-3) then returns to the starting position.

Many patients with LBDs will have a difficult time performing the Good Morning exercise without flexing the lumbar spine. A useful strategy in this case is to use a wooden dowel or broomstick as a tactile cue. The object is placed over the spine and contact is made with the sacrum, thoracic spine and head. The patient establishes a neutral lumbar lordosis and flexes forward while maintaining all 3 contact points. The patient bends as far as possible until no longer able to maintain contact at all three points (Fig. 9-4). The patient then returns to the starting position.

The Good Morning exercise should be done for 20 repetitions twice per day. Patients in whom the tactile cue is used should gradually be progressed to performing the exercise without the cue.

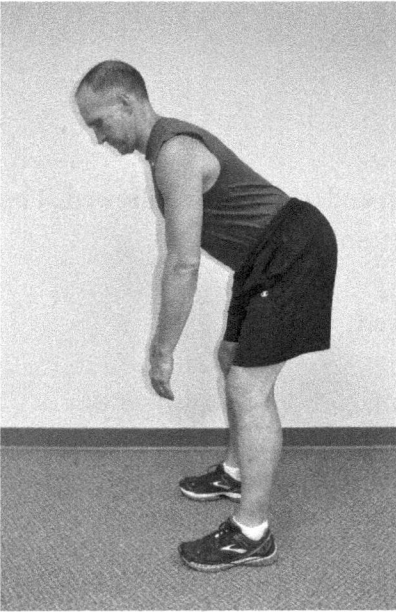

Figure 9-3. The "Good Morning" exercise. Note that the bending movement takes place at the hips while the neutral lumbar lordosis is maintained.

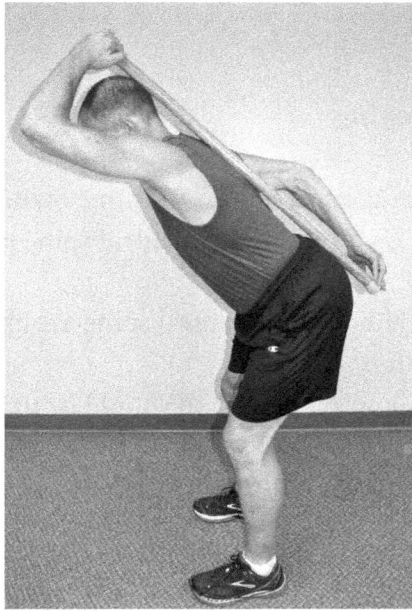

Figure 9-4. Bending forward at the hips using the tactile cue while maintaining a neutral lumbar lordosis.

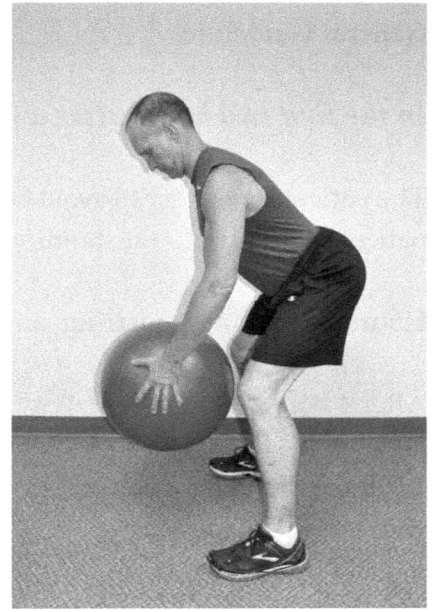

Figure 9-5. Lifting an object without flexing the lumbar spine.

Once the patient has mastered the ability to flex at the hips while maintaining a neutral lordosis he or she can be trained in lifting technique. This can be done by simply having the patient add knee flexion to the hip flexion movement to enable the patient to reach an object that is close to the ground. Depending on the size of the object the feet may have to be moved farther apart to allow the patient to get as close to the object as possible (Fig. 9-5).

Limiting early morning flexion

Snook, et al (see Recommended Reading) found that teaching patients how to minimize the magnitude and frequency of lumbar flexion in the morning is a useful strategy not only for treatment but to help maintain improvement after treatment ceases. Provided here is a simple approach that is particularly applicable in patients with disc derangements or who have increased pain in the morning. However, the approach can be applied to any patient.

General Guidelines

In the first two hours after awakening

The patient should try to avoid bending, squatting, and sitting. Standing and walking are allowed. The patient should try to eat standing or on a stool in the neutral spine position.

Hours 2-4: Sitting, squatting, or kneeling with a neutral spine are allowed.

After 4 hours: Moderate activity is allowed but flexion should be limited.

After 6 hours: Usual activities are allowed, but the principles of correct posture and lifting discussed above should be followed.

The following tips can be given to the patient for limiting flexion during activities of daily living:

Getting out of bed

- Roll completely onto one side with legs straight, facing the edge of the bed.

- While maintaining a neutral spine, push up with both arms and swing the legs off the bed to a seated position.

- Move to the edge of the bed.

- Maintain the neutral spine and stand without any forward bending.

Standing at the sink

- If there is a cupboard below the sink, open the door and place one foot on the threshold.

- Hold one hand on the lower back or one hand on the countertop with a straight arm to avoid any forward bending.

Showering

- Keep the soap and shampoo on a high shelf.

- While washing the feet or shaving the legs maintain a neutral spine and bend from hips (as in the "good morning" exercise).

Getting out of the car

- Swing both legs and the trunk so both feet can be placed on the ground.

- Move to the edge of the seat.

- Maintain the neutral spine and stand without any forward bending.

Vacuuming/Mopping

- Maintain a neutral spine.

- Keep the vacuum or mop directly in front of the body and not to the side.

- Do not reach far forward.

Anti-inflammatory nutrition for spinal pain – by David R. Seaman, DC, MS

The role that inflammation plays in LBDs is poorly understood. Many people, lay people and practitioners alike, view inflammation related to back pain either in terms of autoimmune processes, such as ankylosing spondylitis, or in terms of acute tissue injury. Given the fact that the cardinal signs of inflammation, which include redness, swelling, and heat, are rarely present in patients with LBDs, it is easy to assume that spine pain is not inflammatory. However, as was discussed in Chapter 2, inflammatory processes in LBDs involve more than just acute tissue inflammation.

The fact that spine pain may be inflammatory is evidenced by back pain patients who get relief when taking non-steroidal anti-inflammatory drugs (NSAIDs). It is often claimed that pain relief with NSAIDs reflects the analgesic actions of these medications, rather than an anti-inflammatory action. However this perspective on NSAID mechanisms is inaccurate. Pro-inflammatory chemicals are involved in pain both in the periphery and in the central nervous system. For example, glial cells in the spinal cord liberate cytokines and eicosanoids that excite nociceptive terminals and spinothalamic tract neurons. These are the same eicosanoids and cytokines that are released peripherally by macrophages, mast cells, and fibroblasts that stimulate the beginnings of nociceptive afferents in musculoskeletal tissues.

One of the effects of NSAIDs is to inhibit these eicosanoids. So when NSAIDs inhibit the peripheral release of eicosanoids it is termed an "anti-inflammatory" effect; however, when NSAIDs inhibit the central release of the exact same mediators, it is called "analgesia." In reality, the action is anti-inflammatory in both cases, as the mechanism of action is the inhibition of a pro-inflammatory chemical process. Thus, it is important to understand that the chemistry of inflammation and pain are identical and when NSAIDs provide pain relief, it is due to the peripheral and/or central inhibition of inflammatory chemicals.

Based on this introductory information, it is clear that an updated view of inflammation is needed. This section will describe inflammation in a clinical context that can be applied to patients with spinal and other musculoskeletal pains. Dietary and nutritional supplement applications are also discussed.

Inflammatory perpetuators of spinal pain

An elevated body mass index (BMI), depression, and poor self-rated health are all risk factors for pain chronicity. BMI is unique because some people may gain adipose tissue mass without becoming chronically inflamed while others will become chronically inflamed. This is the likely reason for the inconsistent correlations between BMI and spinal pain. The term "adiposopathy" ("sick fat" – see Recommended Reading list) has been used to refer to a situation in which elevated BMI is associated with inflammation and the expression of the metabolic syndrome.

The metabolic syndrome was given its name by Dr. Gerald Reaven in 1988 (see Recommended Reading list). Metabolic syndrome is synonymous with "syndrome X" and "insulin resistance syndrome." The metabolic syndrome is a systemic inflammatory state that is thought to promote a host chronic of inflammatory diseases such as cancer, heart disease, hypertension, diabetes and musculoskeletal pains such as tendinopathy and low back pain.

The metabolic syndrome is also associated with risk of depression and poor self-rated health, which are known promoters of chronic LBDs. Both depression and poor self-rated health are associated with elevated circulating inflammatory mediators, the most notable being high sensitivity C-reactive protein (hsCRP) and cytokines such as interleukin-1, interleukin-6, and tumor necrosis factor.

As obesity and the metabolic syndrome are associated with chronic LBDs and osteoarthritis, the emerging view is that the chronic systemic inflammation serves to seed local areas of tissue injury and prevent the resolution of inflammation. Poor nutrition can prevent the resolution of pain and inflammation.

Homeostatic challenges that create systemic inflammation and promote pain

Inadequate sleep and stress can lead to the release of the same inflammatory chemicals that are associated with the metabolic syndrome. The goal should be to get between 6-9 hours of sleep in a 24-hr cycle.

Inadequate sleep and stress also lead to the overconsumption of calorie-rich foods containing sugar, flour and fat, in part because inadequate sleep and stress each increases ghrelin levels. The average American's diet is characterized by the chronic consumption of what are known as "comfort foods", with approximately 60% of calories coming from sugar, flour, and refined oils.

The primary refined oils include corn, safflower, sunflower, cottonseed, and soybean oils, which contain an excessive amount of linoleic acid (an omega-6 [n-6] fatty acid), which the body converts into arachidonic acid. Arachidonic acid is the precursor to prostaglandin E2, which is pro-inflammatory and pain producing. In fact, NSAIDs and acetaminophen function to inhibit the production of PGE2. Thus, identifying that a patient gets relief from such medications suggests that dietary modifications are needed.

Another 15-20% of calories in the average American diet come from over-fat animal products, with 10% coming from dairy products. No more than 10% of calories come from fruits and vegetables. Herein, this diet is referred to as the pro-inflammatory diet.

The consumption of the pro-inflammatory diet leads to an immediate postprandial surge in blood sugar (hyperglycemia), free fatty acids, and triglycerides. The hyperglycemia in particular overwhelms mitochondria and causes them to generate an excess of free radicals. This induces systemic inflammation, endothelial dysfunction, hypercoagulability of the blood, and sympathetic hyperactivity. Fig. 9-6 illustrates the inflammatory response after a postprandial surge in blood sugar and lipids.

Free radicals activate nuclear factor kappa-B (NF-kB), which then translocates from the cytoplasm to the nucleus where protein synthesis is initiated. Phospholipase A2 (PLA2), cyclooxygenase (COX) and lipoxygenase (LOX) are produced, which act on dietary fatty acids. Consumption of an excess of n-6 fatty acids, including linoleic acid and arachidonic acid leads to the production and release of pro-inflammatory prostaglandin E2 (PGE2) and leukotriene B4 (LTB4). Activation of NF-kB also stimulates the production of pro-inflammatory cytokines such as interleukin-1 (IL-1), interleukin-6 (IL-6),

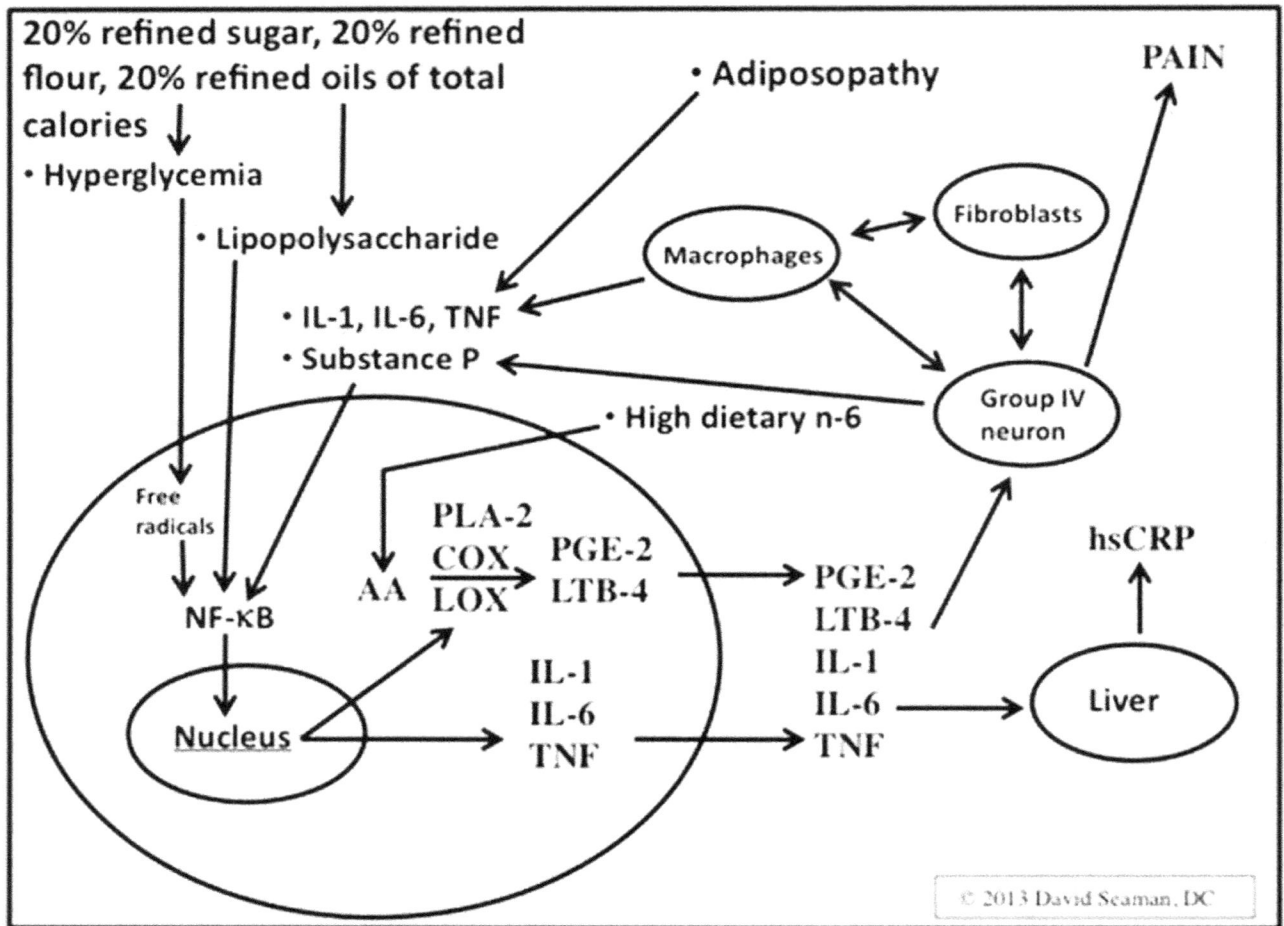

Figure 9-6. Inflammatory response after a postprandial surge in blood sugar and lipids.

and tumor necrosis factor (TNF). These are the same mediators identified in painful joints and discs. Eventually, the liver begins to overproduce C-reactive protein (hsCRP), which is a marker of systemic inflammation that is not specific to any one disease.

The pro-inflammatory diet acutely drives inflammation in a second fashion. This diet is devoid of anti-inflammatory phytonutrients from vegetation and spices; this allows for the postprandial absorption of lipopolysaccharide (LPS) from the gastrointestinal tract. LPS is also called bacterial endotoxin, which is derived from the cell wall of gram-negative bacteria. The absorbed LPS stimulates NF-kB to enter the nucleus to initiate the production of pro-inflammatory mediators. Thus, the consumption of the pro-inflammatory diet causes immune cells to act as if they are responding to an injury or infection, which leads to the systemic generation of essentially the same inflammatory mediators found locally in painful spinal tissues.

Regarding inflammation and pain, the human body is resilient. Each individual has a unique "envelop of tolerance" to various inflammatory stressors including the consumption of the pro-inflammatory diet. The diet-induced inflammatory state can remain a symptom-free state for years. In addition, the inflammatory state initially is primarily postprandial. However over time, as people continue to eat the pro-inflammatory diet and exercise less, adipose tissue mass increases and many develop adiposopathy along with the metabolic syndrome. This leads to chronic inflammation in the fasted state, which is further augmented by eating a pro-inflammatory meal. At some point during this process, patients begin to complain about low energy, depressed affect, feeling unwell, feeling old and various aches and pains. They typically do not associate these with their pro-inflammatory diet because the cause-effect relationship is protracted and less obvious than, for example, pain that starts after a lifting incident.

Regarding adiposopathy, as adipose tissue mass increases, chemotactic signals are released by adipocytes, leading to accumulation of excess immune cells, including monocytes, macrophages, lymphocytes and mast cells. Researchers now understand that in this adiposopathy state, adipose tissue behaves like an overactive immune organ that responds as if there were an infection or autoimmune disease, which results in the continuous release of inflammatory mediators into the systemic circulation. Not surprisingly, a substantial number of overweight individuals suffer with depression, fatigue, poor self-perceived health and pain. They are also at greater risk of diabetes, cancer, heart disease and other chronic illnesses.

All musculoskeletal and visceral tissues are of the same mesodermal origin and have the same metabolic needs, so it is reasonable to assume that degenerative and inflammatory changes would occur in both tissue types when systemic inflammation develops. For this reason chronic LBDs are commonly seen as a generalized pattern of ill-health that includes obesity, the metabolic syndrome, diabetes, tension-type or migraine headache, fibromyalgia, abdominal pain, and chronic widespread pain. In addition, both elevated BMI and hsCRP have been implicated in the development of LBDs.

Which spinal pain patients need dietary changes?

From the perspective of pure pain relief, not all patients with spinal pain need to change their diet as a treatment for their pain. Those who have adequate improvement in pain as a result of treatment for the findings related to diagnostic question #2 do not need to make dietary changes for pain relief. However, from the perspective of overall health and longevity, all patients should endeavor to follow the anti-inflammatory diet to prevent chronic disease (see Table 9-1).

An excellent example of the anti-inflammatory diet has been referred to as the ketogenic Mediterranean diet. This is not the typical high fat ketogenic diet but rather is a diet that includes olive oil, moderate red wine, green vegetables and salads and fish as the primary protein, as well as lean meat, fowl, eggs, shellfish and cheese. Nuts and fruit can also be added to this diet. Conspicuously absent are sugar, refined grains, whole grains, and legumes. This is because refined carbohydrates such as sugar and refined grains are overtly inflammatory and whole grains and legumes are all far less nutrient dense per calorie than fruits and vegetables.

Table 9-1. The anti-inflammatory diet

Fish, lean meat, skinless chicken, n-3 eggs
Vegetables
Fruit
Sweet potatoes and other tubers
Raw nuts
Dark Chocolate (75% or more cocoa)
Red wine and stout beer
Coffee and tea
Ginger, turmeric, garlic, and other spices
Olive oil, coconut oil, butter

Patients who are inflamed especially need to adhere to the anti-inflammatory diet. During history taking, patients who are inflamed due to an excessive consumption of omega-6 fatty acids will state that NSAIDs and acetaminophen give them pain relief (as stated earlier, although acetaminophen is not considered an "anti-inflammatory" medication its mechanism of action, like that of NSAIDs, relates to its effects on pro-inflammatory chemicals in the CNS).

Inflamed patients can also be identified through specific history and physical exam information. Table 9-2 lists the criteria for the pro-inflammatory metabolic syndrome. While each should be viewed as a marker of chronic inflammation, 3/5 markers must be present in order to satisfy the criteria for making the diagnosis.

Table 9-2. Metabolic syndrome

Markers	Abnormal value
1. Fasting blood glucose	≥ 100 mg/dL
2. Triglycerides	≥ 150 mg/dL
3. HDL cholesterol	< 50 for women; < 40 men
4. Blood pressure	≥ 130/85
5. Waist circumference	> 35" women; > 40" men

Table 9-3 lists additional markers of inflammation. As a single marker, BMI is the least reliable. This is because people with a normal BMI can have the inflammatory metabolic syndrome. Additionally, well-muscled athletes and exercisers commonly have a BMI above 25, which should not be interpreted as inflammatory. Well-muscled individual with a high BMI will typically have a low waist/hip ratio, which suggests a low inflammatory state.

Thus, BMI must be considered in the context of the other markers listed in Table 9-3. This is because BMI, weight, waist circumference, hip circumference, and waist-hip ratio are significantly correlated to circulating inflammatory mediators, such as of hsCRP, TNF and IL-6.

Table 9-3. Pro-inflammatory markers

Marker	Parameters
Regular use of NSAIDs or acetaminophen	If medication use reduces pain – indicates diet-induced inflammation
Body mass index (BMI)	18.5-24.9 = normal 25-29.9 = overweight ≥30 = obese
Waist/hip ratio women (risk factor for diabetes)	< 0.80 = low risk 0.81-.85 = moderate risk > 0.85 = high risk
Waist/hip ratio men (risk factor for diabetes)	< 0.95 = low risk 0.96-1.0= moderate risk > 1.0 = high risk
2-hour postprandial glucose	< 140 mg/dl = normal 140-199 = prediabetes 200+ = diabetes
Fasting triglycerides	< 90 mg/dl predicts controlled postprandial response
hsCRP in mg/L (marker of chronic inflammation)	< 1.0= normal 1.0-3.0= moderate > 3.0 = high
25(OH)D	32-100 ng/ml (goal >40 ng)
Fasting blood glucose	³ 100 mg/dL
2-hour postprandial glucose	<140 mg/dl = normal 140-199 = prediabetes 200+ = diabetes
Lack of sleep	Less than 6 hrs or more than 9 hrs
Stress	Self-perceived stress is associated with systemic inflammation
Sedentary living	A lack of exercise promotes systemic inflammation

Depression	Depression is associated with systemic inflammation
Self-rated health	Low self-rated health is associated with systemic inflammation

Nutritional supplements for inflammation and pain

The nutritional approach to inflammation reduction is to drastically modify dietary behavior, the primary issue being the avoidance of sugar, flour, and n-6 fatty acids and increased consumption of vegetables, fruit, and spices. This leads to a normalization of NF-kB, PLA2, COX, LOX and cytokines and the relative disappearance of the dietary promoters of inflammation. Supplements should be taken to support or "supplement" the anti-inflammatory diet. Table 9-4 outlines key supplements that support normal metabolism by influencing inflammation, free radicals, and ATP synthesis.

Table 9-4. Supplements for inflammation

Supplement	Dose	Mechanism of action	Clinical consideration
For short term use			
Proteolytic enzymes (bromelain, trypsin, and chymotrypsin)	1000-2000 mg per day taken on an empty stomach	Antagonizes fibrin and cytokines	Acute inflammation after obvious injury
White willow bark	1000-4000 mg per day	Antagonizes free radicals, NF-kB, PLA2, COX, LOX, collagenase	Pain exacerbation without obvious injury
For long term use			
Ginger, turmeric, boswellia, and other botanicals	1000-2000 mg per day	Antagonizes free radicals, NF-kB, COX, LOX	Chronic inflammation/ pain management
Magnesium	400-1000 mg per day	Involved in 100s of enzymes; reduces inflammation and regulates central nociception	Chronic inflammation/ pain management

Omega-3 fatty acids	1000-3000 mg per day	Precursor for anti-inflammatory mediators	Chronic inflammation/ pain management
Vitamin D	1000-10,000 IU based on blood levels	Regulates 2000 genes including pro- and anti-inflammatory cytokines	Chronic inflammation/ pain management
Probiotics	Depends on product	Reduces gut inflammation and associated systemic inflammation	Chronic inflammation/ pain management
Coenzyme Q10	100 mg per day or more	ATP production, antioxidant, regulates skeletal muscle gene expression	Chronic inflammation/ pain management
μ-Lipoic acid	200 mg bid	ATP synthesis, antioxidant, insulin sensitivity	Chronic inflammation/ pain management

At present, data are lacking regarding the precise identification of which supplements or regimen is most appropriate for specific patients. Proteolytic enzymes and white willow bark can be helpful for acute injuries and pain exacerbation. The remaining supplements in Table 9-4 should be viewed in the context of the long-term maintenance of anti-inflammatory metabolic function.

While this recommendation may appear to be very general, it is similar to the recommendation for adequate sleep, proper stress management, regular exercise and the anti-inflammatory diet. The goal is to create a systemic anti-inflammatory state that does not seed and perpetuate local areas of injury and inflammation.

Further information and resources regarding the anti-inflammatory diet can be found at www.deflame. com [accessed 6 August 2013].

Mindfulness, Acceptance, Commitment and Values

Mindfulness, acceptance, commitment and values are part of a psychotherapeutic modality that has wide application in both mental and physical health called Acceptance and Commitment Therapy (ACT - see Hayes and Smith and Dahl and Lundgren in the Recommended Reading list). Their application by the primary spine practitioner for patients with LBDs need not be complicated or time-consuming; rather than being applied as a therapeutic "technique", it should inform and be weaved through all aspects of patient care.

Mindfulness

Mindfulness was discussed in the previous chapter and the concepts and methods related to mindfulness permeate many parts of this book. Through mindfulness patients can learn to become an objective observer of their pain as well as their fears, cognitions, beliefs and emotional reactions to their pain. As has been discussed throughout this book, much of what produces the disability and suffering in patients with spine related disorders is not the pain itself, i.e., the nociceptive stimulus, but the emotional and behavioral response to the pain. The way in which a patient responds to a LBD is based on his or her beliefs and cognitions about the pain. These beliefs and cognitions may accurately reflect the reality of LBDs but, as discussed earlier, they are usually inaccurate. Even more important, the patient's reactions and the motivations behind them may appear "automatic" and beyond the patient's control.

It is "normal" for people, in response to an unpleasant feeling or situation, to want to "get rid of" the problem or to "wish it would just go away." The common thought is that in order to live a full, productive life one has to first get rid of his or her problems. While this is understandable and "natural", it is a mistake that actually inhibits a person's ability to live a full, productive life. However it is important that, when addressing this belief with a patient, the practitioner make it clear that the patient is simply engaging in a response that we all engage it at various times. The issue is not that the patient is "weak" or "deficient" in some way because of this belief, or any of the other numerous counterproductive beliefs patients have about their pain. The issue is that this belief is not accurate and will interfere with the patient's ability to overcome the LBD and return to a healthy, productive and fulfilling life. So while working on reducing the nociception is a worthwhile goal, and one that usually can be accomplished to a greater or lesser degree, the primary focus of care should be on helping the patient *overcome* the LBD and take charge of his or her life. Focusing on trying to "make the pain go away" actually strengthens the pain and gives it more power than it would otherwise have.

It is not always necessary for the spine practitioner to train the patient in mindfulness techniques directly. First, the practitioner can point the patient to resources for learning these methods, such as the Hayes and Smith book and the Dahl and Lundgren book that can be found in the Recommended Reading list. Second, and more powerfully, the practitioner can teach patients to be mindful of the pain and of their reactions to the pain indirectly by example, by taking the mindful approach to the practitioner-patient relationship that was discussed in the previous chapter. Further, the practitioner can bring mindfulness to each therapeutic interaction. For example, the process of end range loading, both as an examination procedure and a treatment procedure (see Chapter 5) can serve not only as a diagnostic and therapeutic tool, but as a mindfulness tool as well. As was discussed in Chapter 5, when the patient is guided through end range loading maneuvers to identify characteristics of the pain generating tissue, he or she is asked to *observe the pain* and *describe what the pain is doing*, i.e., if it is increasing in intensity, decreasing in intensity, centralizing into the back, peripheralizing into the extremity, etc. This process provides important diagnostic information, but at the time trains the patient to become an *objective observer of the pain*. Rather than being enveloped by all the judgments, beliefs and fears the patient has regarding the pain, the patient is trained to simply observe the actual sensation itself. This can be applied during any examination or treatment encounter. Any time a particular diagnostic test, exercise, or therapeutic maneuver is applied that provokes a certain amount of pain, the patient can be asked to fully experience the sensation, and observe the thoughts and emotions that arise at that moment. This can be a form of mindfulness training.

Acceptance and Commitment

Acceptance can be very difficult for patients to understand and, well, *accept* but it is one of the most powerful skills that one can develop when working on overcoming any problem. Another term that has been used for acceptance is *surrender.* Acceptance means *acknowledging the fact that the pain is what it is and being willing to experience the pain in this moment.* It is *not* accepting a life of misery or accepting being a slave to the pain. And it is not accepting that the pain will never go away and will always be in charge of the patient's life. Acceptance is not about the future. It is about *this moment only. Acceptance* is simply coming to terms with reality as it is and then making a *commitment* to taking steps in the direction of overcoming the LBD and returning to a healthy, productive and fulfilling life.

Values

One of the most important questions the practitioner can ask a patient is, "Are there any activities or any aspect of your life that is really important to you that you are avoiding, are afraid to try or feel you cannot do because of this LBD?" This helps patients get in touch with their most deeply held *values.*

As was discussed in the previous chapter regarding the spine practitioner's most deeply held values, we all have things that are most important to us, that we would most like our life to be about. Getting in touch with these values and making a commitment to live a life that is consistent with them can be a powerful motivator for overcoming any obstacle, including a LBD, which may be interfering with a patient living a *valuing* life.

As was stated earlier, different patients will require a greater or lesser focus on incorporating the principles of Acceptance and Commitment Therapy (ACT) into the practitioner-patient relationship. The spine practitioner should not feel obligated to spend an inordinate amount of time on these principles. On the level of primary spine care, providing these concepts as discussed here during the course of patient care will be adequate for the vast majority of patients and can easily be incorporated into a busy practice environment. For patients who require more intensive training in this regard, the first step should be to introduce them to resources, such as the Hayes and Smith book and the Dahl and Lundgren book that can be found in the Recommended Reading list, and the second step can be referring the patient to a psychologist trained in ACT.

Motivational Interviewing

Motivational interviewing (MI) grew out of work with substance abuse problems. It is a useful method for eliciting behavior change in patients. Basic changes in health behaviors can be of great usefulness in helping patients overcome LBDs. These changes include those related to exercise, diet, self-care strategies, smoking, sleep hygiene and generally living a healthy lifestyle.

Behavior change is not easy, as inertia and conflicting desires often leads to *ambivalence* to change, i.e., for many people there is a part of them that wants very much to change health behaviors yet there is another part that is very resistant to such change. MI is a method by which the practitioner can help the patient become mindful of this ambivalence and connect with his or her deepest held values to gain a greater identification with the inner desire to live a healthy, productive and fulfilling life.

Resources for learning more about MI are provided in the Recommended Reading list. Discussed here is an overview of how MI applies to the management of patients with LBDs.

MI emphasizes the collaborative nature of the practitioner-patient relationship. That is, as discussed in Chapter 1, establishing a healing environment in which behavioral change can blossom involves creating a partnership in which each partner (practitioner and patient) has a role to play, with the ultimate goal being to help the patient overcome the LBD.

MI is also designed to be evocative in nature. That is, it is designed to bring out the patient's own motivations and skills in changing behavior, rather than forcing change on the patient.

Finally, it is important in MI to recognize and honor the patient's autonomy. When all is said and done, it is the patient's life, and the patient is free to live it as he or she sees fit. The patient does not *have to* change behavior; he or she does not *have to* overcome the LBD. The role of the practitioner is simply as "helper", "guide" and "coach" in the process of overcoming LBDs, if the patient chooses this path. This can be challenging to the practitioner because it is tempting to want to tell the patient what to do, coerce the patient to make needed changes, and become irritated if the patient does not comply (i.e., to become attached to the outcome). As was discussed in Chapter 8, the practice of detachment from the outcome is very useful in applying MI.

The four guiding principles of MI can be remembered by the acronym RULE:

1. *Resist the righting reflex:* Again, it is very tempting, when a practitioner encounters a patient who is engaging in unhelpful beliefs or behaviors, to want to "correct" the patient or "set the patient right." This involves "doing something *to*" the patient. It is important for the practitioner to recognize this temptation, forgive him- or herself for doing this (as this is practically a universal temptation), self-congratulate for caring so much, and then *let go of this temptation.* The reason the righting reflex must be resisted is that it is counterproductive. It is the natural tendency for most people to resist being coerced. So trying to force a patient to change will often have the effect of activating the side of the patient's ambivalence that wants to stay the same and resist change.

2. *Understand the patient's motivations:* The two sides of the coin of ambivalence are motivation to change and resistance to change. The purpose of MI is to understand and cultivate the motivational side of the patient's ambivalence. This means that it is the *patient's* reasons for wanting to change that are important, *not* the practitioner's (though, of course, these may be similar).

3. *Listen to the patient:* When it comes to behavior change, the patient often already has the answer. By "telling" the patient what to do the practitioner loses the opportunity to uncover the patient's own solutions to the ambivalence that is interfering with the change to healthy behaviors. By listening to the patient the practitioner can learn a great deal about the motivations and

fears that underlie the patient's ambivalence and to help the patient discover how to rise above these fears and bolster the motivation.

4.   *Empower the patient:* As discussed in Chapters 1, 2, 6 and 8, self-efficacy is a critically important factor that can determine whether patients recover quickly or become chronic sufferers. Empowering patients to develop strategies for behavioral change leads to increased confidence in their ability to effectively overcome LBDs. In addition, it makes it more likely that the behavior change will be lasting, as it was brought out from within rather than forced from outside.

Cultivating "Change Talk" in MI

"Change talk" occurs when the patient makes statements that reflect the consideration of, motivation for and commitment to engaging in behavior change. The practice of MI involves eliciting change talk through empathic listening, encouragement, empowerment and the asking of open-ended questions.

Change talk can be elicited by engaging in a conversation with the patient that is open-ended and non-judgmental and that encourages the patient to explore the natural ambivalence that most people have about behavior change. Having the patient explore the pros and cons, or the challenges and benefits, of the change in behavior and asking the patient to elaborate on these in an open-ended fashion is useful. Also, self-efficacy can be explored by having the patient rate his or her confidence with regard to the ability to make the behavior change on a scale of 0 (no confidence) to 10 (supreme confidence). Perhaps most useful is to encourage the patient to get in touch with his or her innermost values and to think about how the behavior change would be helpful in living according to these cherished values.

Incorporating MI into a Busy Practice Environment

The utilization of MI may seem to be quite time-consuming, but it need not be. In fact, spending a lot of time talking can be detrimental in many cases. As was discussed with regard to cognitive-behavioral and acceptance-commitment messages, MI should be incorporated into the process of patient care; the use of MI in primary spine care is not about engaging in "counseling" sessions, it is about allowing the process of patient care be informed by MI principles and methods. This means limiting the amount of time that is spent on "small talk" and keeping the focus of communication on the process of helping the patient overcome the LBD. At times, utilizing the assistance of other practitioners that may be involved in the care of the patient may be useful. This can be done through electronic health record, written communication or a phone call.

A useful way to initiate the process of helping the patient identify the motivation for behavior change is to utilize the Patient-Specific Functional Scale discussed in Chapter 7. With this measure, the patient comes up with two or more valued activities that the patient would like to engage in or return to. Reminding the patient of the activities included on this scale can help the patient get in touch with the inner values behind the desire to participate in these activities. This, then, will make it easier to help the patient with the behavioral changes that are necessary to be able to return to a fulfilling, active and productive life.

A detailed exploration of MI is beyond the scope of this book but the reader is encouraged to read the book by Rollnick, Miller and Butler and to visit the MI website. Both are provided in the Recommended Reading list.

This chapter presents a number of general methods that are helpful in a wide variety of patients with LBDs, independent of diagnosis. All of the methods presented do not have to be provided to all patients – it is up to the spine practitioner to use clinical reasoning to determine which methods should be provided for any given patient. At the heart of effective management of patients with LBDs is the delicate balance between comprehensiveness and efficiency, between "less is more" and "doing everything that is needed." Negotiating this balance is an art that cannot be learned from a book, but should be developed and refined through keen, mindful observation and hands-on training such as is provided by the Primary Spine Provider Network. Details can be found at www.primaryspineprovidernetwork.com.

The coming two chapters will get into more specifics by presenting treatment procedures that can be applied in response to diagnostic questions #2 (Chapter 10) and 3 (Chapter 11).

Recommended Reading

Bays HE. Adiposopathy: is sick fat a cardiovascular disease? J Am Coll Cardiol 2011;57:2461-73.

Bogduk N. Pharmacological alternatives for the alleviation of back pain. Expert Opin Pharmacother. 2004;5(10):2091-98.

Dahl J, Lundgren T. Living Beyond Your Pain. Oakland; New Harbinger Publications, 2006.

Hayes SC, Smith S. Get Out of Your Mind and Into Your Life. The New Acceptance and Commitment Therapy. Oakland; New Harbinger Publications, 2005.

http://www.motivationalinterview.org/ [accessed 23 July 2013]

Krawiec CJ, Denegar CR, Hertel J, Salvaterra GF, Buckley WE. Static innominate asymmetry and leg length discrepancy in asymptomatic collegiate athletes. Manual Therapy. 2003;8(4):207-213.

McGill S. Low Back Disorders. Evidence-Based Prevention and Rehabilitation. Champaign, IL: Human Kinetics; 2002.

Reaven GM. Banting Lecture 1988: Role of insulin resistance in human disease. Diabetes. 1988;37:1595-1607.

Rollnick S, Miller WR, Butler CC. Motivational Interviewing in Health Care: Helping Patients Change Behavior. New York; The Guilford Press, 2008.

Seaman DR. A sports nutrition: a biochemical view of injury care and prevention. In Hyde TE, Gengenbach MS. Eds. Conservative management of sports injuries. 2nd ed. Boston: Jones and Bartlett; 2007: p.1067-1092.

Seaman DR. Anti-inflammatory diet for pain patients. Pract Pain Management. 2012;12(10)36-46. http://www.practicalpainmanagement.com/issue/1210

Seaman DR. Body mass index and musculoskeletal pain: is there a connection? Chiropractic Man Ther. 2013;21:15

Seaman DR. Nutritional considerations for pain and inflammation. In Liebenson CL. Ed. Rehabilitation of the spine: a practitioner's manual. Baltimore: Williams & Wilkins; 2006: p.728-740.

Seaman DR. Nutritional considerations in the treatment of soft tissue injuries. In Hammer WI. Editor. Functional soft-tissue examination and treatment by manual methods. Boston: Jones & Bartlett; 2007: p.717-734.

Snook SH, Webster BS, McGorry RW, et al. The reduction of chronic nonspecific low back pain through control of early morning lumbar flexion: A randomized controlled trial. Spine 1998; 23(23):2601-2607.

Snook SH, Webster BS, McGorry RW. The reduction of chronic, nonspecific low back pain through the control of early morning lumbar flexion: 3 year follow up. J Occup Rehabil 2002; 12:13-19.

· CHAPTER 10 ·

Treatment Approaches for Diagnostic Question #2

The second question of diagnosis is "Where is the pain coming from?" Another way to ask this question is "Are there characteristics of the pain generating tissue or tissues that can be identified and that allow treatment decisions to be made?" As has been stated repeatedly throughout this book, in the majority of patients it is not possible to determine with absolute certainty what the pain generating tissue is. But based on signs and symptoms it is possible to develop a reasonable diagnostic hypothesis that can aid in the development of a management strategy.

The clinical entities considered under diagnostic question #2 are:

1. Disc derangement

2. Joint dysfunction
   a. Lumbar facet
   b. Sacroiliac

3. Radiculopathy

4. Myofascial pain

It is possible for more than one of these to be present at the same time, although this is not typical. The exception to this is myofascial pain, which often develops in response to one of the other pain generators. There are treatment approaches that can be applied to each of these disorders that can be tailor-made for each individual patient.

Disc derangement

End range loading (ERL) strategies to detect disc derangement were presented in detail in Chapter 5. The reader is encouraged to seek hands-on training, as can be obtained through the McKenzie Institute International (see Recommended Reading list).

As was iscussed in Chapter 5, in many patients, particularly those with antalgia, the treatment is inherent in the assessment process. In patients with disc derangement who do not exhibit antalgia, the treatment is determined by the results of the ERL exam. If a direction of movement is identified that produces centralization or decreased intensity of pain along with easing of obstruction of movement (which identifies disc derangement as well as the Direction of Benefit), the primary treatment is ERL exercises in that direction. These exercises are described in detail in Chapter 5. In most patients, the exercises should be performed for 10 repetitions four to six times per day.

There are some patients in whom the practitioner may want to provide sustained positioning in the Direction of Benefit for up to a minute, rather than or in addition to repetitive movements. One example would be a patient with disc derangement for whom the ERL examination identified the Direction of Benefit to be extension, but in whom the increase in proximal symptoms associated with movement in this direction prevents full extension. This patient may have to be provided with sustained positioning in the Reclining on Elbows position (Fig. 5-6), with gradual relaxation and "settling into" this position prior to the institution of prone extension exercises.

Distraction manipulation (aka Cox technique – see recommended reading list) is helpful in many patients with disc derangement. This manipulative method decreases intradiscal pressure, thus relieving disc pain. The reader is encouraged to obtain training in this method. Details can be found at http://www.coxtechnic.com/ [accessed 28 June 2013].

Joint dysfunction

The treatment for joint dysfunction is manipulation. The purpose of manipulation is to apply movement to a spinal joint. Manipulation causes gapping of the zygapophyseal joints and induces neural responses that reduce pain intensity. There are a variety of different methods of applying manipulation to the spinal joints. The purpose of this chapter is not to provide an exhaustive review of all the various techniques but rather to present some general concepts and applicable techniques of manipulation.

There are good resources for a more detailed understanding of manipulative techniques such as the text by Peterson and Lawrence that can be found in the Recommended Reading list. It is important for the spine practitioner to master a wide variety of manipulative techniques and to be able to choose the best technique in any given situation.

It must be noted that the proper utilization of manipulation requires great skill that comes from extensive training. This training cannot be obtained from a book. Therefore this section should not be mistaken for a substitute for hands-on training in the art of manipulation. The purpose of presenting the techniques found in this chapter is to provide individuals who are already trained in manipulation, or are undergoing such training, some common maneuvers that are generally applicable to a variety of patients. However each patient is different and it is expected that the well-trained and experienced practitioner will be familiar with dozens of methods of applying manipulation to each area of the spine. People with no training or inadequate training should not attempt the maneuvers presented here.

General principles regarding manipulation

For the purpose of this book, the term "manipulation" is used as the general term for application of manual maneuvers to the spine for the purpose of introducing motion to a joint and, ultimately, the relief of joint-related pain. As stated earlier, there are a wide variety of methods that fall under this general description. In this book the methods will be divided into those that target the lumbar facet joints and those that target the sacroiliac (SI) joints. The methods will also be divided into high-velocity, low amplitude (HVLA) techniques (sometimes referred to a "thrust" techniques) and low velocity, low amplitude techniques (LVLA) (sometime referred to as "mobilization" techniques). The low velocity, low amplitude techniques will be further divided into oscillatory mobilization techniques and muscle energy techniques. In the majority of cases the practitioner and patient positioning is the same with HVLA and LVLA techniques. The difference is in the application of the therapeutic movement.

The barrier

All tissues, when lengthened, allow for a certain amount of increased length while providing little or no resistance. There then reaches a point at which internal resistance can be perceived by the practitioner. This point is known as the *barrier of resistance*, or just *the barrier*. When applying manipulation it is important to move the involved joint to the barrier and then to apply the manipulative maneuver, be it HVLA or LVLA, from the barrier. While the importance of the barrier has not been specifically subjected to rigorous scientific investigation, it is likely that attention to the barrier during manipulation maximizes the therapeutic benefit of this method.

High-Velocity, Low Amplitude Manipulation

With HVLA manipulation, the patient is positioned in a manner that allows the practitioner to bring the targeted joint to the barrier. At that point the practitioner applies a quick (high-velocity) and short (low amplitude - some have estimated this to be about 3 millimeters) maneuver designed to move the joint just beyond the barrier. Most commonly, this maneuver is accompanied by an audible release, or "click" sound although this sound is not always necessary for therapeutic benefit. Typically only one maneuver is necessary.

Muscle Energy Manipulation

Muscle energy technique (MET) is a general term for a method that uses reflexes to elicit relaxation of muscles and, where appropriate, allow for the lengthening of tissues. What is described here is the application of MET to joint manipulation. The theory behind the use of MET for joint manipulation is that the MET procedure relaxes the muscles that would limit joint movement, thus allowing for easier mobilization of the involved joint.

The practitioner and patient positioning is the same as with HVLA manipulation and oscillatory mobilization (see below). The joint is moved to the barrier as with the other methods. But with MET an isometric contraction is elicited in a direction opposite that in which the joint is being moved. The patient then takes an in-breath. During this time, the practitioner maintains the positioning at the barrier. The patient then ceases the isometric contraction, relaxes and breaths out. At this point the practitioner continues to feel the barrier and as the barrier releases, the practitioner gently guides the joint to a position in which the barrier is again met. Once the barrier is again reached, the isometric contraction and in-breath are repeated, followed by relaxation and out-breath. As the barrier releases, the joint is again moved until a new barrier is reached. The maneuver is then repeated again. Typically, three repetitions of the maneuver are sufficient.

Oscillatory Mobilization

With oscillatory mobilization (OM) the practitioner and patient positioning is the same as with HVLA manipulation and MET. The targeted joint is moved to the barrier as with the other methods. However with OM, instead of the practitioner applying a high-velocity, low-amplitude maneuver or an MET procedure, an oscillatory motion is applied to the joint. To do this the practitioner moves the joint away from the barrier, and then returns back to the barrier. This is done repeatedly. As the repetitions are being applied the practitioner feels the barrier. It is expected that the barrier will gradually be perceived later in the movement, i.e., it will take longer to reach the point of the perceived barrier. However, the important thing is for the practitioner to continually engage the barrier on each repetition of the oscillatory maneuver, regardless of at what point in the movement the barrier is reached.

The specificity of manipulation

As of this writing, research on the mechanics of manipulation is still in its infancy. Physiologic and anatomical evidence, at least in the lumbar spine, does not support the contention that a practitioner can consistently target an individual joint with manipulation. In addition, it is not known whether the therapeutic effect of manipulation is to "correct" a "lesion" in the spine or whether there is another explanation for this effect. There is good evidence, however, that manipulation is a useful tool in patients with low back disorders (LBDs), that it causes gapping of the zygapophyseal joints and that it has segmental and central nervous system neurologic effects. Further research should shed light on the mechanisms by which manipulation is helpful. In the meantime, it seems sensible for the practitioner to try to be as precise as possible when applying manipulation while realizing that absolute specificity may not be realistic.

Lumbar facet joints

A common manipulative technique that is applied to the lumbar facet joints is one that is applied in the side posture position. The patient is placed on his or her side with the involved side (i.e. the side of the symptomatic facet joint) up. The practitioner applies counter-rotation to the spine by pulling the downside arm forward (Fig. 10-1). The practitioner then places one forearm in the axilla of the patient with the fingers of this hand on the up side of the superior vertebra. At that same time the other forearm is placed on the patient's posterolateral pelvic region while the fingers of that hand are placed on the down side of the spinous process of the inferior vertebra (Fig. 10-2). The spine is further counter-rotated until the barrier is met. At that point the practitioner can apply an HVLA maneuver.

MET can be applied from this position as well. The set-up is exactly the same as that described above. However once the barrier is met, rather than applying an HVLA maneuver the practitioner asks the patient to press his or her leg up against the practitioner's thigh as if trying to raise the leg toward the ceiling. The practitioner then asks the patient to breathe in. After the patient fully inhales the practitioner asks the patient to stop pushing, breathe out and completely relax. The practitioner then feels

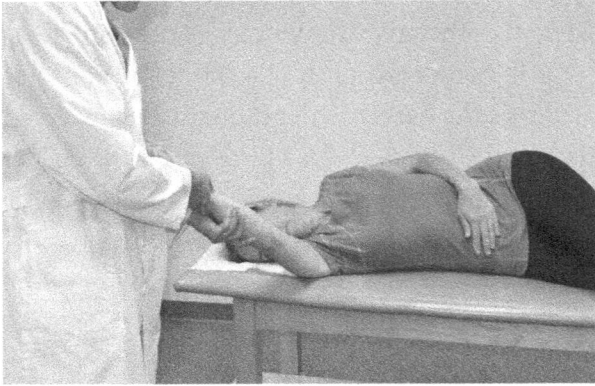

Figure 10-1. Counter-rotating the spine by pulling the downside shoulder forward.

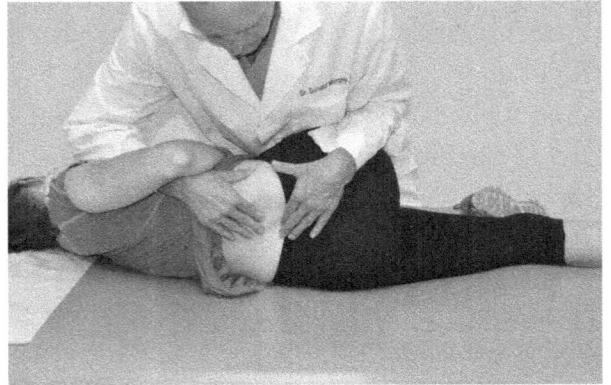

Figure 10-2. Practitioner positioning for lumbar facet manipulation. Note the practitioner finger positioning designed to counter-rotate the involved segment.

for the release of the barrier. Once the release of the barrier is perceived, the practitioner gently guides movement of the lumbar facet joints further into rotation until the barrier is once again met. The procedure is then repeated twice more.

To apply OM, again the set up is identical to that described above. Once the barrier is met the practitioner backs away from the barrier slightly then moves to the barrier again. This is repeated several times in an attempt to gently mobilize the lumbar facet joints.

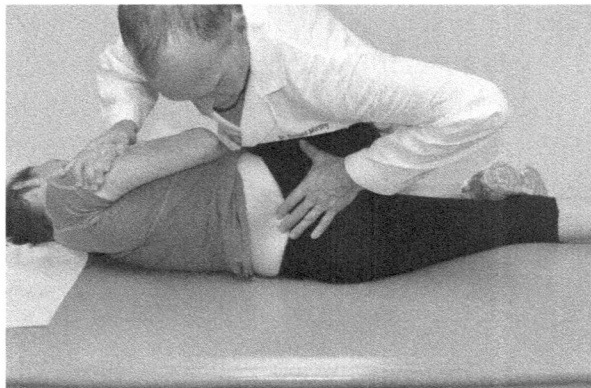

Figure 10-3. Alternate positioning for lumbar facet manipulation in the side posture position.

An alternate method is for the patient to be placed in the same position, with the same counter-rotation movement applied. But rather than the practitioner's superior forearm being placed in the patient's axilla, the hand on the patient's shoulder to counter-rotate the spine and meet the barrier (Fig. 10-3). From this position an HVLA, MET or OM maneuver can be applied.

Patient-generated movements for the lumbar facet joints

Cat and Camel

The patient is in the quadruped position and first simultaneously moves the lumbar and cervical spine into flexion (Fig. 10-4). This movement is then reversed and the patient moves the lumbar and cervical spine into extension (Fig. 10-5). This is done repetitively.

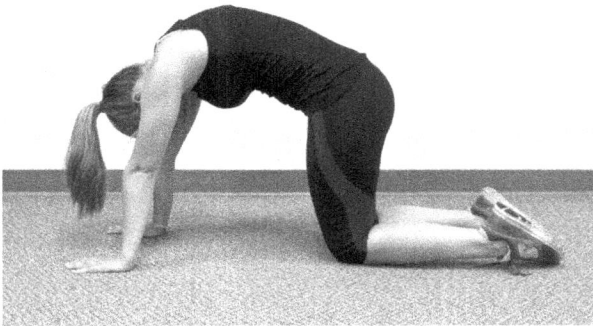

Figure 10-4. Cat and camel flexion phase.

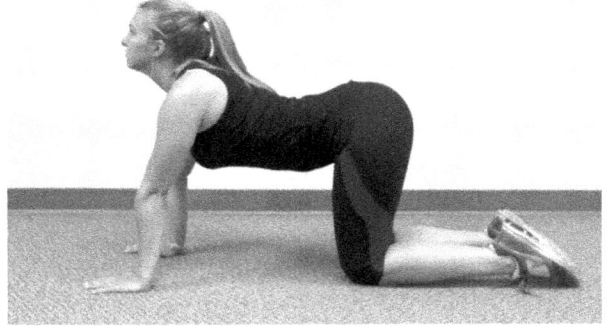

Figure 10-5. Cat and camel extension phase.

Side gliding

This exercise is the same as that described for patients with disc derangement in whom the ERL exam has identified side gliding as the Direction of Benefit. By definition, a patient with facet joint dysfunction is one in whom the end range loading examination did not identify a clear Direction of Benefit. However the side gliding maneuver can be used as a general exercise for self-generated mobilization of the facet joints. For this purpose it is performed bilaterally, unless on ERL exam it was found that this maneuver caused peripheralization of symptoms in one or both directions. If so, the direction of movement that caused peripheralization should be avoided, at least until subsequent testing fails to reveal peripheralization.

Sacroiliac joint

The SI joint can be treated with the patient in the side posture position in a similar manner as was demonstrated for the lumbar facet joints. The patient is placed in the side posture position with the involved side up and counter-rotation is applied as it was with lumbar facet manipulation. The practitioner sets up in the same manner as with lumbar facet manipulation, with the forearm of the superior upper extremity in the patient's axilla and forearm of the inferior upper extremity on the patient's posterolateral pelvic region. However with SI joint manipulation the superior hand is placed on the sacrum in an attempt to limit its movement (Fig. 10-6). From this position, an HVLA maneuver, MET maneuver or OM maneuver can be applied using the same methodology as that used for facet manipulation.

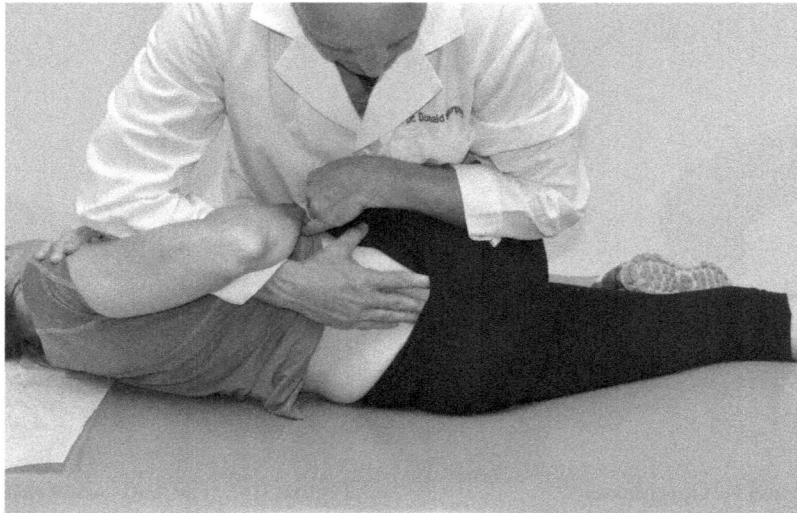

Figure 10-6. Positioning for SI joint manipulation in the side posture position.

Another way to apply OM to the SI joint is with the patient in the prone position. Wedges (also called blocks) are placed under the anterior superior iliac spine on the involved side and slightly below this point on the uninvolved side (Fig. 10-7). The purpose of this is to attempt to gap the SI joint on the involved side. The practitioner then places one hand over the posterior superior iliac spine on the involved side and the other hand on the sacrum at approximately the S2 level. Oscillatory mobilization maneuvers are applied in a direction that attempts to separate the ilium from the sacrum.

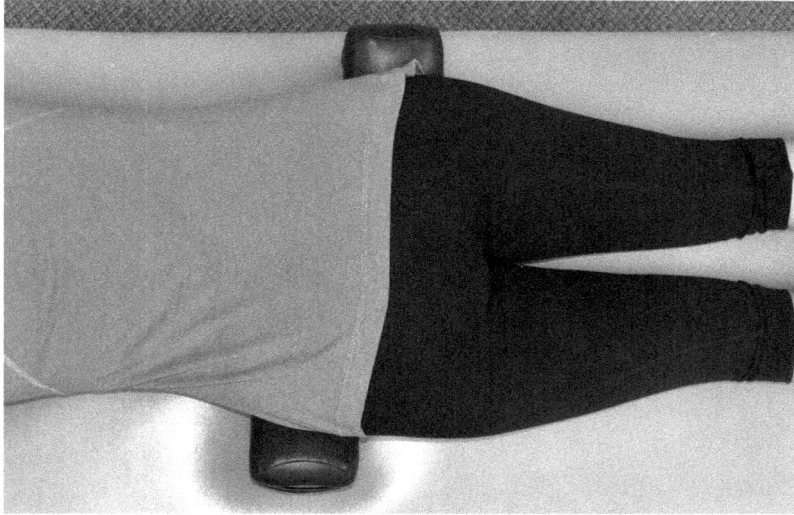

Figure 10-7. Block placement for oscillatory mobilization of the SI joint in the prone position.

A further method of SI manipulation can be performed with the patient in the supine position. Patient and practitioner positioning is the same as described for the Thigh Thrust test in Chapter 5 in which the hip on the involved side is flexed to 90 degrees and the practitioner places one hand on the sacrum to attempt to hold it in place (Fig. 5-25). The practitioner places the other hand on the patient's knee and applies gentle pressure straight downward along the long axis of the femur. From this position an HVLA, ME or OM maneuver can be applied. With the ME maneuver the patient is asked to gently push the knee forward into the practitioner's hand and then breathe in. The patient is then asked to stop pushing and breathe out and when the practitioner senses the release the barrier he or she guides the SI joint to move to a new barrier. This is repeated two more times.

Patient-generated movements for the SI joint

Side-lying SI joint self-mobilization

The patient is side-lying with the arm on the downside supporting the head. Keeping the upper part of the body relatively straight, the patient raises the feet in the air, rotating the pelvis forward (Fig. 10-8). The patient then lowers the feet to the floor. This is done repetitively. The exercise should be performed bilaterally regardless of side of sacroiliac involvement.

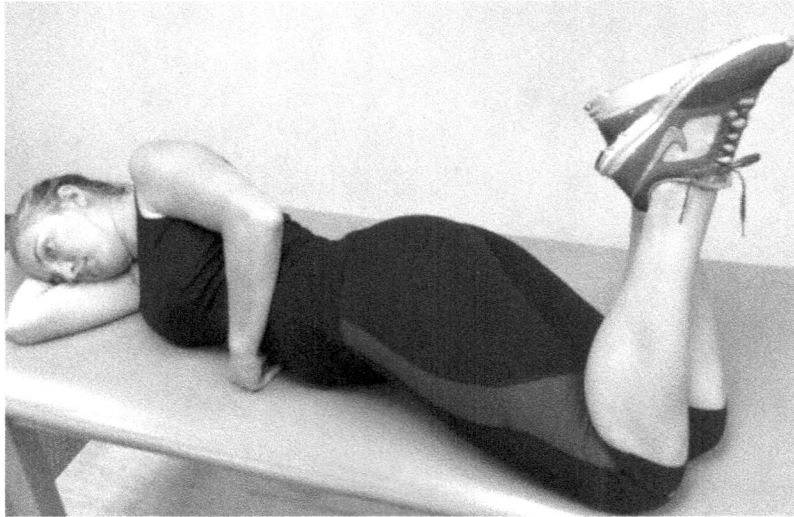

Figure 10-8. Side-lying SI joint self-mobilization

Standing SI joint self-mobilization

The patient is standing with the foot on the involved side on a block or a stair step. The other leg is hanging free. The patient gently lowers the free-hanging side a few inches (Figure 10-9), then returns to the starting position. This is done repetitively.

Manual SI joint self-mobilization

The patient is seated and crosses the leg of the involved side over the other leg. The patient grasps the knee, and then pulls that leg toward the opposite shoulder until a gentle "pull" is felt in the buttock or SI joint (Fig. 10-10). The patient gently moves the knee back and forth (i.e., toward the shoulder and away from the shoulder) in an oscillatory manner. This is done repetitively.

As was discussed in Chapter 5, some patients with SI area pain may not have pain from the joint itself but rather from the dorsal SI ligament. In these patients, SI joint manipulation may not be helpful. Friction massage is often useful in these patients. With the patient lying prone, the dorsal SI ligament is identified by palpating just inferior to the posterior superior iliac spine as a hard ridge. Transverse friction massage can be applied by massaging back and forth approximately perpendicular to the direction of the fibers of the ligament. This can be done for 5-10 minutes. Often the patient can be taught to

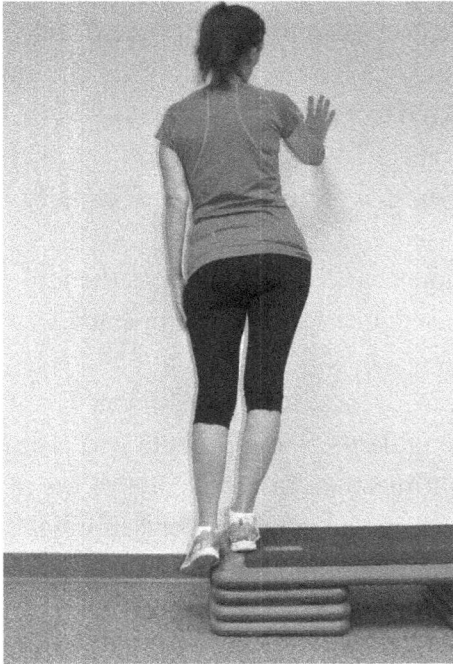

Figure 10-9. Standing SI joint self-mobilization

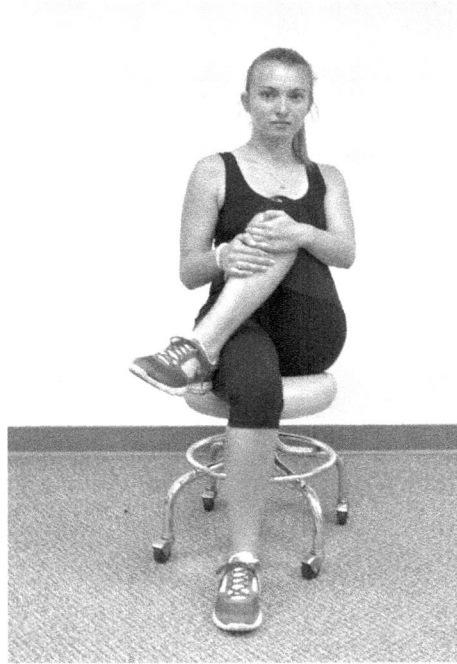

Figure 10-10. Seated manual SI joint self-mobilization.

perform friction massage at home. The massage may be followed by cold application for approximately 10 minutes.

As stated earlier, there are many other techniques that can be used for both manipulation and patient-generated mobilization of the lumbar facet or SI joints. The practitioner is encouraged to be knowledgeable and skilled in a wide variety of methods.

Anyone who does not have adequate training in manipulation should not attempt this form of treatment.

Joint injections are sometimes used for patients with joint pain. With these injections, anesthetic, with or without steroid, is injected into the joint for the purpose of relieving pain and/ or suspected inflammation. As discussed in Chapter 5, these are useful at times for diagnostic purposes, as substantial temporary relief (i.e., 80% improvement in pain) after injection suggests that the injected joint is the primary pain source. If this is the case, pain improvement should be experienced shortly after the injection, during the period in which the anesthetic is expected to exert its anesthetic effect. Occasionally, longer lasting improvement occurs as a result of the steroid. Lasting benefit is "hit or miss" – some patients experience improvement in pain for extended periods of time. However most do not.

While complications, including allergic reaction, infection and bleeding, are rare, the limited benefit of therapeutic joint injections is such that they should be used judiciously and sparingly.

Joint injections should be avoided in patients with systemic or local infection, history of allergy to anesthetic or steroid, bleeding disorder or who are on anticoagulants. Some patients with severe degenerative changes in the facet joint are not candidates for joint injection. In these patients the primary spine practitioner should discuss the case with the interventionalist who would be performing the procedure.

In those patients who do experience substantial temporary relief from joint injection, manipulation under joint analgesia may be worthwhile. The theory behind this approach is that a joint that is resistant to manipulation due to pain-related muscle tension may respond better to manipulation after it is anesthetized. It is useful for the interventionalist and primary spine practitioner to coordinate their activities in this regard.

Radiculopathy

Acute – anti-inflammatory measures

With acute radiculopathy, the pathophysiology is primarily related to acute inflammation. Therefore, anti-inflammatory measures are most important. This can be in the form of non-steroidal anti-inflammatory medication (NSAIDs), oral steroid medication or epidural steroid injection. Many NSAIDs can be obtained by patients over-the-counter. For spine practitioners who are not licensed to prescribe medications or do not perform injections, these will have to be obtained by referral.

Oral medications

The oral medications most commonly used to treat an acute inflammatory process such as acute radiculopathy are non-steroidal anti-inflammatory drugs (NSAIDs) and oral steroids. NSAIDs include medications that can be obtained over-the-counter such as aspirin, ibuprofen and naproxen and prescription-only medications such as diclofenac, etodolac, fenoprofen, flurbiprofen, oxaprozin and celecoxib. Side effects and complications of NSAIDs include gastrointestinal (GI) disorders such as ulcers and high blood pressure. A type of NSAID known as a Cox-II inhibitor (celecoxib) reduces the likelihood of GI disturbance but this medication carries a risk of myocardial infarction and stroke.

Oral steroids are more powerful anti-inflammatory medications and are designed to be used for a brief period. Examples of oral steroids include prednisone, cortisone, methylprednisolone and triamcinolone. They are commonly administered in a tapered fashion, with a gradually decreasing dosage schedule over the course of days. Side effects and complications of oral steroids include glaucoma, fluid retention, elevated blood pressure, mood swings, weight gain and elevated blood sugar.

Both NSAIDs and oral steroids should only be used under close supervision. Particularly in the case of prescription medications, the patient must be under the supervision of a practitioner who is licensed to prescribe these medications.

Epidural steroid injection

Epidural steroid injection (ESI), as with joint injection, is a procedure most commonly performed by anesthesiologists or physiatrists although some spine surgeons perform these as well. It usually involves the injection of a combination of a steroid such as cortisone and either a short-acting analgesic, such as lidocaine or a long-acting analgesic, such as bupivacaine. Sometimes saline is included for the purpose of "flushing" the area or diluting chemicals around the nerve root that promote inflammation. The injection needle is inserted into the epidural space in order to place the injectate as close to the involved nerve root as possible. This procedure is best performed under fluoroscopic guidance to ensure proper placement. Typically a contrast dye is injected first to confirm that the needle is properly placed. This is followed by injection of the solution.

Serious complications of ESIs are very uncommon. Infection can occur in approximately 0.1% to 0.01% of ESIs and dural puncture in approximately 0.5%. Bleeding or nerve root injury, as a result of the needle contacting the nerve root itself, can also occur. Less severe side effects may also occur, including temporary local pain, temporary headache, nausea and vomiting, temporary fever, facial flushing, anxiety, sleep disturbance, blood sugar elevation and temporary immunosuppression. Other side effects have been reported as well.

ESI should be avoided in patients with systemic or local infection, a bleeding disorder or those on anticoagulants or a history of allergy to contrast material, anesthetic or corticosteroid.

Subacute or chronic – neural mobilization

In subacute and chronic cases acute inflammation plays a less prominent role in the pathophysiology of radiculopathy. At this stage, congestion, ischemia, intraneural edema and periradicular fibrosis dominate the pathophysiological picture. Therefore in patients with subacute or chronic radiculopathy neural mobilization should be incorporated into the management strategy. This involves applying maneuvers that are designed to improve the mobility of the involved nerve root and theoretically to improve circulation in and around the nerve root. This can be done through manual procedures and exercises, most of which the patient can perform at home.

In addition to neural mobilization, distraction manipulation (aka Cox technique) should be utilized in patients with subacute or chronic radiculopathy. See Murphy, et al in the Recommended Reading list. Distraction manipulation is often helpful in patients with acute radiculopathy as well, although neural mobilization should be avoided in these patients until the acute inflammation has resolved.

General principles regarding neural mobilization

A number of descriptions of neural mobilization can be found in various books and seminars (see Recommended Reading list). Presented here is a streamlined approach that can be applied in virtually any patient with subacute or chronic lumbar radicular pain. Neural mobilization can be applied to a variety of problems in which neural structures are involved, including the peripheral nerves, nerve roots and, occasionally, the spinal cord. For the purpose of this book, only maneuvers that are designed to target the lumbar and sacral nerve roots are presented.

Of course, the nerve root cannot be moved in isolation. Any mobilization maneuver applied to neural structures moves an entire neural tract. The particular part of the nervous system that is moved is determined by patient positioning. For example, as was discussed in Chapter 3, the Straight Leg Raise test is designed to apply tension to the lumbosacral nerve roots. It does this via dorsiflexion of the ankle and flexion the lower extremity at the hip while the knee remains extended. This maneuver applies tension to the sciatic nerve, lumbosacral nerve roots and the central nervous system. Likewise, therapeutic mobilization maneuvers move not only a targeted structure but the entire neural tract of which the targeted structure is a part.

In general there are two different types of maneuvers involved in neural mobilization:

1. Flossing (sometimes called gliding) maneuvers: These are maneuvers that are designed to move the nerve root back and forth within the lateral canal. This is done by slackening the neural tract at one end and tensioning the neural tract on the other.

2. Tensioning maneuvers: These are maneuvers that are designed to apply tension to the nerve root. This is done by keeping one end of the neural tract stationary and applying tension to the other end.

Flossing and tensioning maneuvers can be applied both by the practitioner and by the patient. It is important to emphasize patient-generated neural mobilization maneuvers in all cases. This allows the maneuvers to be applied daily and also promotes self-efficacy and active coping.

Both flossing and tensioning maneuvers can be performed from three different locations:

1. Distal: The emphasis of the movement is on the distal end of the neural tract.

2. Intermediate: The emphasis of the movement is somewhere in the middle of the neural tract.

3. Proximal: The emphasis of the movement is on the proximal end of the neural tract

All three flossing or tensioning locations (distal, intermediate and proximal) can be performed on the same visit. Because flossing maneuvers are generally better tolerated than tensioning maneuvers, it is often useful to start with flossing maneuvers and later transition to tensioning maneuvers.

Neural mobilization maneuvers are to be done repetitively with little or no pause. These are mobilization maneuvers, not stretches. In most cases 10-30 repetitions of the movement is adequate although the number may vary based on patient comfort, symptom production and relative acuteness of the condition.

The barrier phenomenon as applied to neural mobilization

The barrier phenomenon that was discussed in the section on manipulation should be applied to neural mobilization as well. Mobilization maneuvers should be performed at the barrier. This means that when setting up the neural mobilization maneuver the practitioner should move the extremity in the direction required to elicit tension on the neural structure being targeted and should feel for the initial onset of resistance to this movement. This serves as the starting point for neural mobilization, be it flossing or tensioning. In most cases it can be expected that the point at which the practitioner perceives the barrier will also be the point at which the patient initially perceives symptoms. This will be felt by the patient as mild tension or "pulling" or sometimes mild discomfort. However there are some patients who will report significant discomfort before the point at which the barrier is perceived by the practitioner. It is best in these cases for the practitioner to start neural mobilization at the point at which initial symptom production is reported by the patient rather than trying to start at the barrier. Generally, as desensitization occurs it will be easier for the practitioner to work from the barrier. However, patient symptoms should take priority over the practitioner's perception of the barrier – it is better to work at a level that is well tolerated by the patient than to attempt to work at the barrier.

It is important that the practitioner carefully monitor symptoms while performing neural mobilization. A certain amount of mild pain and/or paresthesia is normal and should not cause alarm or lead to alteration of the technique. However, if significant pain and/or paresthesia should occur, particularly if the elicited symptoms cause the patient distress, the amplitude of the movement should be reduced, i.e., tension should be taken off the involved neural structure so the maneuver can be applied with minimal to mild symptoms.

The principle of centralization and peripheralization, as discussed with regard to end range loading (see Chapter 5) should apply to neural mobilization. That is, if the pain or paresthesia that is elicited gradually moves toward the axial spine (i.e., "centralizes") with repeated movements, even if the central pain increases, the maneuver should be continued, with careful monitoring of symptoms. However, if the pain or paresthesia moves further down into the lower extremity (i.e., "peripheralizes") with repeated movements, the maneuver should be stopped or the amplitude should be reduced.

A wide variety of practitioner-generated and patient-generated maneuvers can be used for neural mobilization. Presented here are a number of manual procedures and exercises that are widely applicable to the vast majority of patients with lumbar radiculopathy. This is by no means an exhaustive examination of all the various maneuvers that are available. Readers who are interested in learning additional maneuvers are directed to Butler, Shacklock, Neurodynamic Solutions and the NOI Group, listed under Recommended Reading.

L4 through S1 radiculopathy – sciatic nerve mobilization

Mobilization maneuvers that utilize the sciatic nerve are applied to patients with subacute or chronic radiculopathy involving the L5, S1 and occasionally L4 nerve roots. Less commonly, the sacral nerve roots may be involved. These are cases in which the neurodynamic examination reproduces the patient's pain with the straight leg raise and/ or the slump test, and structural differentiation confirms this pain to be of neural origin (see Chapter 5).

Sciatic nerve flossing – practitioner-generated movement

As was stated earlier, flossing maneuvers are designed to move the nerve root back and forth within the lateral canal, much like dental floss is moved back and forth between two teeth. This is done by applying tension to one end of the neural tract while slackening the other end, followed by a reverse of this – applying tension to the end of the neural tract that had previously been slackened and slackening the end of the neural tract that had previously been tensioned. This flossing movement is performed repetitively.

Distal flossing: The patient is supine and the practitioner dorsiflexes the ankle on the involved side and flexes the hip while maintaining knee extension to the point at which the barrier is met and/or symptoms are mildly elicited (Fig. 10-11). The patient is asked to flex the cervical spine, bringing the chin toward the chest while at the same time the practitioner plantar flexes the ankle (Fig. 10-12). Cervical flexion causes tension on the nervous system while ankle plantar flexion slackens the nervous system. The patient then lowers the head back to the table while the practitioner dorsiflexes the ankle (Fig. 10-11). This maneuver is performed repetitively, each repetition involving coordinated movement of cervical flexion/ extension with ankle plantar flexion/ dorsiflexion.

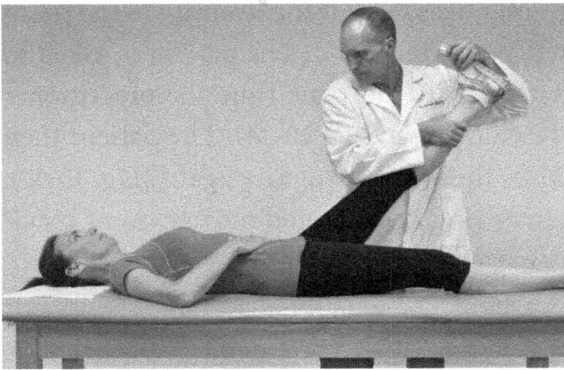

Figure 10-11. Start and finish position for practitioner-generated distal sciatic nerve flossing in the supine position.

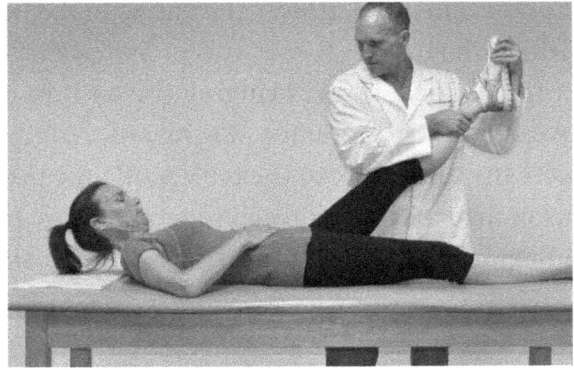

Figure 10-12. Flexion of the cervical spine with plantar flexion of the ankle for practitioner-generated distal sciatic nerve flossing in the supine position.

Intermediate flossing: The patient is supine and the practitioner dorsiflexes the ankle on the involved side and raises the lower extremity to the point at which the barrier is met and/or symptoms are mildly elicited (Fig. 10-11). The patient is asked to flex the cervical spine, bringing the chin toward the chest while at the same time the practitioner flexes the knee (Fig. 10-13). The patient then lowers the head back to the table while the practitioner extends the knee (Fig. 10-11). It is important that the practitioner maintain dorsiflexion of the ankle while performing this movement. This maneuver is performed repetitively, each repetition involving coordinated movement of cervical flexion/ extension with knee flexion/ extension.

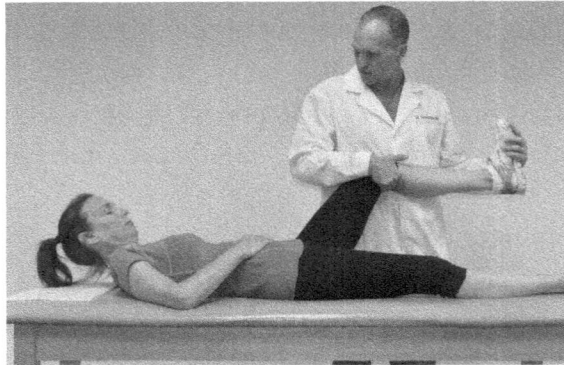

Figure 10-13. Flexion of the cervical spine with flexion of the knee for practitioner-generated intermediate sciatic nerve flossing in the supine position.

Proximal flossing: As with the distal and intermediate flossing maneuvers, the patient is supine and the practitioner dorsiflexes the ankle on the involved side and raises the lower extremity to the point at which the barrier is met and/or symptoms are mildly elicited (Fig. 10-11). The patient is asked to flex the cervical spine, bringing the chin toward the chest while at the same time the practitioner moves the lower extremity downward, reducing the hip flexion angle (Fig. 10-14). The patient then lowers the head back to the table while the practitioner raises the lower extremity again (Fig. 10-11). This maneuver is performed repetitively, each repetition involving coordinated movement of cervical flexion/ extension with lowering and raising the lower extremity.

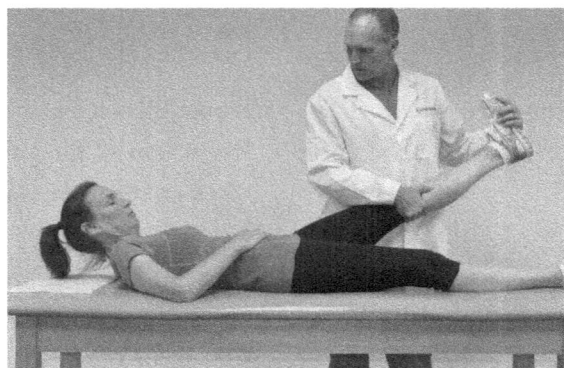

Figure 10-14. Flexion of the cervical spine with lowering of the extremity for practitioner-generated proximal sciatic nerve flossing in the supine position.

In patients who have difficulty with flexing and extending the head during the performance of flossing maneuvers, an assistant can be used for the purpose of providing the head movement. If an assistant is not available, the patient can use his or her hands to provide the head movement.

Sciatic nerve flossing – patient-generated movement

The basic patient-generated exercise for flossing of the lumbosacral nerve roots is performed in the seated position. The patient is seated, preferably on a surface high enough for the feet to be suspended off the floor. It is important for the patient to maintain a normal lumbar lordosis during the performance of this maneuver. The patient flexes the cervical spine while keeping the knee in the flexed position (Fig. 10-15). The patient then extends the cervical spine while at the same time extending the knee and dosiflexing the ankle on the involved side (Fig. 10-16). The patient then flexes the head and returns the lower extremity to the starting position (Fig. 10-15). This is done repeatedly.

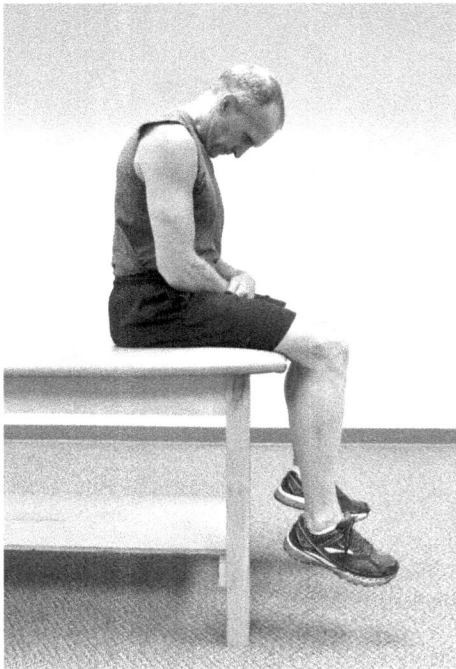

Figure 10-15. Flexion of the cervical spine without movement of the lower extremity for patient-generated sciatic nerve flossing in the seated position.

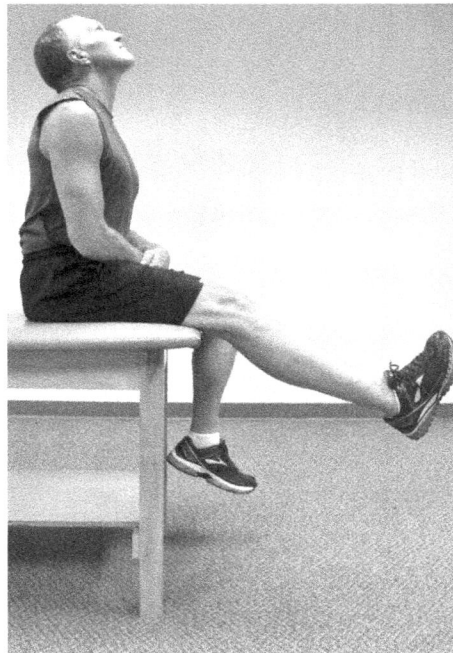

Figure 10-16. Extension of the cervical spine with extension of the knee and dorsiflexion of the ankle for patient-generated sciatic nerve flossing in the seated position.

Sciatic nerve flossing can also be performed in the seated position by having the patient sit with one leg on a surface such as a bed or bench. The foot should be hanging off the end (Fig. 10-17). It is important for the patient to maintain the lordosis of the lumbar spine. A distal flossing maneuver can be performed by the patient flexing the cervical spine while at the same time plantar flexing the ankle (Fig. 10-18). The patient then extends the cervical spine while at the same time dorsiflexing the ankle (Fig. 10-19). This is done repetitively.

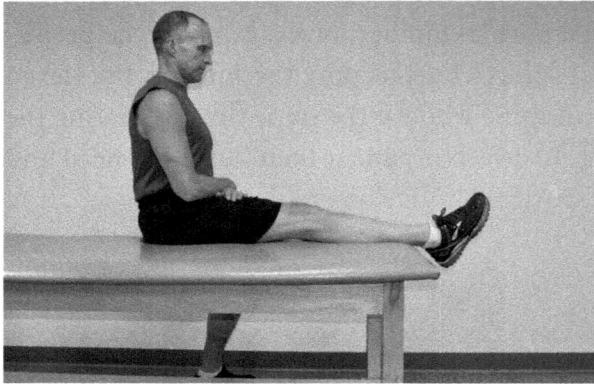

Figure 10-17. Starting position for patient-generated distal sciatic nerve flossing in the seated position.

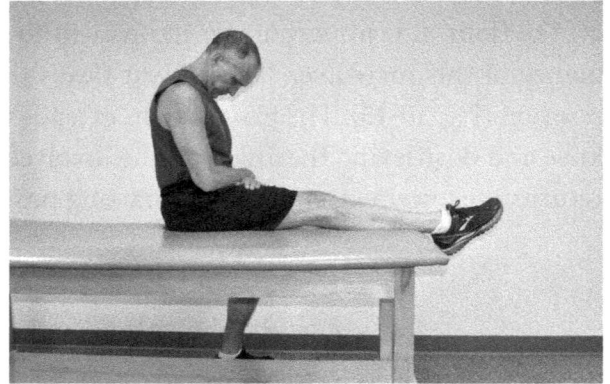

Figure 10-18. Flexion of the cervical spine with plantar flexion of the ankle for patient-generated distal sciatic nerve flossing in the seated position.

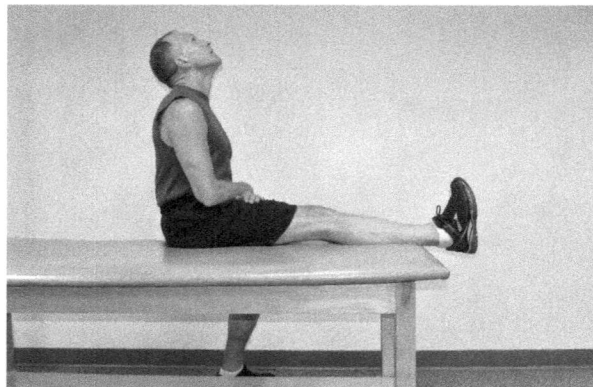

Figure 10-19. Extension of the cervical spine with dorsiflexion of the ankle for patient-generated distal sciatic nerve flossing in the seated position.

Sciatic nerve tensioning – practitioner-generated movement

As was stated earlier, tensioning maneuvers are designed to apply tension to a neural structure. This is done by keeping one end of the neural tract stationary while tension is applied to the other end of the neural tract. Tensioning maneuvers are performed at the barrier, i.e., when setting up the maneuver the neural tract is tensioned to the point at which the barrier is engaged or until mild symptoms are elicited. In most cases, the practitioner will perceive the barrier at the same point at which the patient will experience mild symptoms. However, patient comfort must always be respected and if the patient feels significant symptoms before the point at which the practitioner perceives the barrier, the maneuver should be performed at the point at which mild symptoms are produced.

Distal tensioning: The patient is supine and, as with distal flossing, the practitioner dorsiflexes the ankle on the involved side and flexes the hip while maintaining knee extension to the point at which the barrier is met and/or symptoms are mildly elicited (Fig. 10-11). The practitioner then moves the foot into plantar flexion, moving slightly away from the barrier (Fig. 10-20). This is followed by the practitioner moving the foot into dorsiflexion, again to the point at which the barrier engaged (Fig. 10-11). This movement is performed repetitively, with the practitioner always moving the foot just to the barrier and then away from the barrier.

Intermediate tensioning: The patient is supine and the practitioner dorsiflexes the ankle on the involved side and flexes the hip while maintaining knee extension to the point at which the barrier is met and/or symptoms are mildly elicited (Fig. 10-11). While maintaining hip flexion and ankle dorsiflexion, the

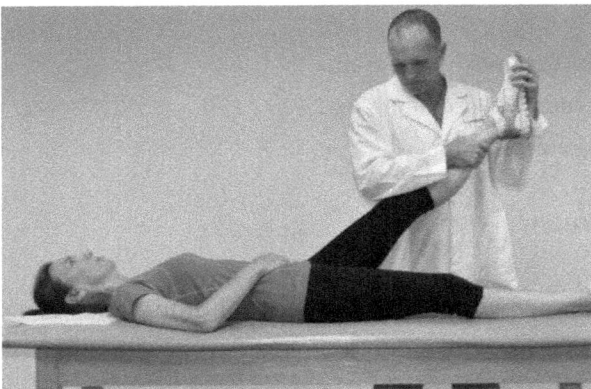

Figure 10-20. Plantar flexion of the ankle away from the barrier for practitioner-generated distal sciatic nerve tensioning in the supine position.

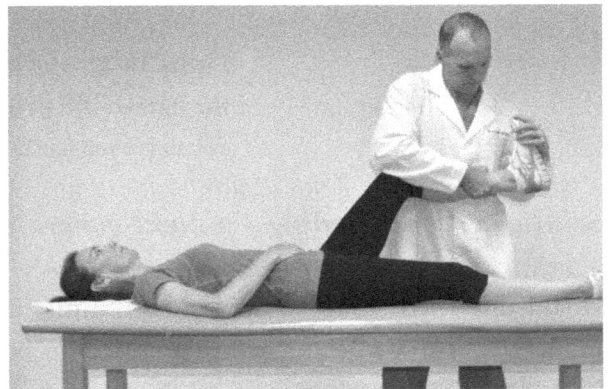

Figure 10-21. Flexion of the knee away from the barrier for practitioner-generated intermediate sciatic nerve tensioning in the supine position.

practitioner flexes the knee, moving slightly away from the barrier (Fig. 10-21). This is followed by the practitioner moving the knee into extension, again to the point at which the barrier is engaged. This movement is performed repetitively, with the practitioner always moving the knee just to the barrier and then away from the barrier.

Proximal tensioning: As with the distal and intermediate tensioning maneuvers, the patient is supine and the practitioner dorsiflexes the ankle on the involved side and flexes the hip while maintaining knee extension to the point at which the barrier is met and/ or symptoms are mildly elicited (Fig. 10-11). While maintaining knee extension and ankle dorsiflexion, the practitioner moves the entire lower extremity downward, moving slightly away from the barrier (Fig. 10-22). This is followed by the practitioner moving the hip into flexion, again to the point at which the barrier is engaged (Fig. 10-11). This movement is performed repetitively, with the practitioner always moving the hip just to the barrier and then away from the barrier.

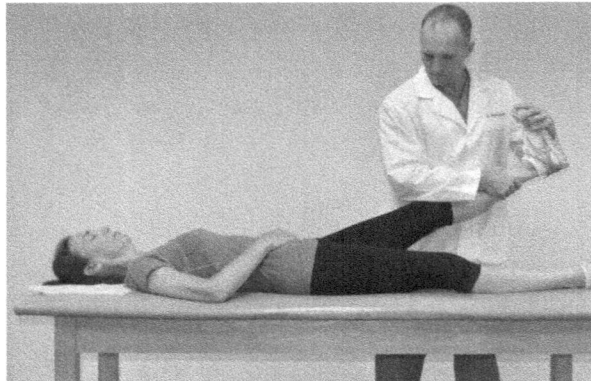

Figure 10-22. Moving the lower extremity away from the barrier for practitioner-generated proximal sciatic nerve tensioning in the supine position.

Sciatic nerve tensioning – patient-generated movement

Distal, intermediate and proximal tensioning can easily be performed by the patient at home. Tensioning maneuvers can be performed in a variety of positions. The most basic maneuvers can be done seated or supine.

Distal tensioning in the seated position: The patient is seated with one leg on a surface such as a bed or bench. The foot should be hanging off the end (Fig. 10-17). It is important for the patient to maintain

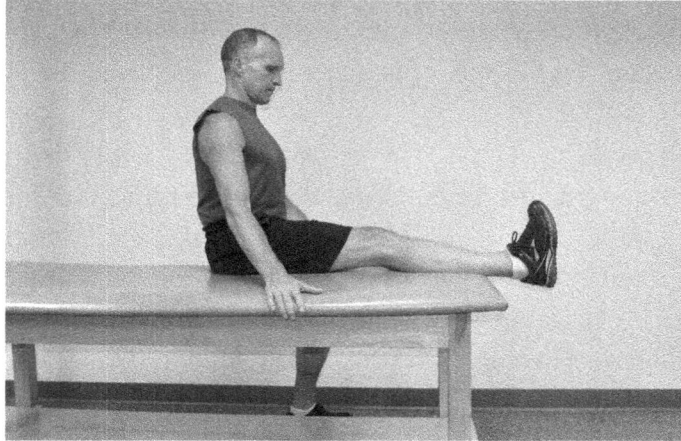

Figure 10-23. Dorsiflexion of the ankle to the barrier for patient-generated distal sciatic nerve tensioning in the seated position.

the lordosis of the lumbar spine. The patient moves the ankle into dorsiflexion to the point at which he or she feels tension in the distribution of the sciatic nerve (Fig. 10-23) followed by return to the starting position (Fig. 10-17). This maneuver is performed repetitively.

Intermediate tensioning in the seated position: The patient is seated on a bed or bench with the lower legs hanging off the end. It is important for the patient to maintain the lordosis of the lumbar spine. The patient dorsiflexes the ankle and then moves the knee into extension to the point at which he or

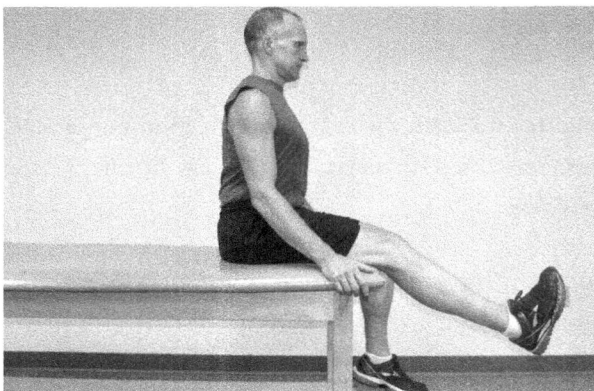

Figure 10-24. Extension of the knee with ankle dorsiflexion for patient-generated intermediate sciatic nerve tensioning in the seated position.

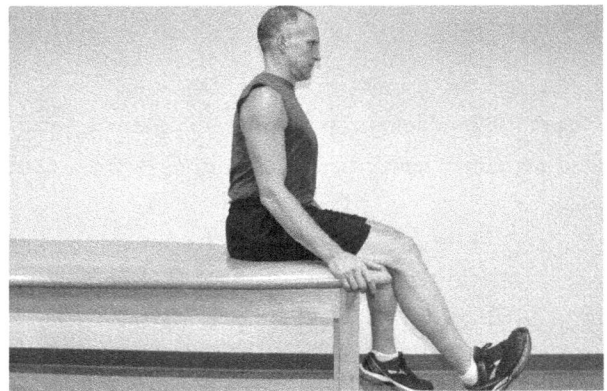

Figure 10-25. Flexion the knee away from the barrier during patient-generated intermediate sciatic nerve tensioning in the seated position.

she feels tension in the distribution of the sciatic nerve (Fig. 10-24). The patient then flexes the knee away from the point of tension (Fig. 10-25). This maneuver is performed repetitively.

Proximal tensioning in the seated position: The patient is seated with one leg on a surface such as a bed or bench with the foot hanging off the end (Fig. 10-17). It is important for the patient to maintain the lordosis of the lumbar spine. The patient dorsiflexes the ankle and then moves the trunk forward while maintaining ankle dorsiflexion, flexing at the hip to the point at which he or she feels tension in the distribution of the sciatic nerve (Fig. 10-26). The patient then returns to the starting position while maintaining ankle dorsiflexion. This maneuver is performed repetitively.

Some patients' sciatic nerve complex will be too sensitive to perform sciatic nerve tensioning maneuvers while seated in a completely upright position. These patients should be instructed to lean backward, supporting themselves with their hands, to the point at which they can comfortably perform the maneuvers, while still feeling tension at the barrier (Fig. 10-27).

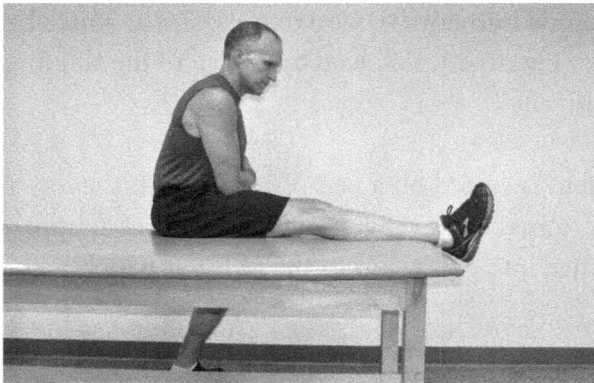

Figure 10-26. Flexion at the hip for patient-generated proximal sciatic nerve tensioning in the seated position.

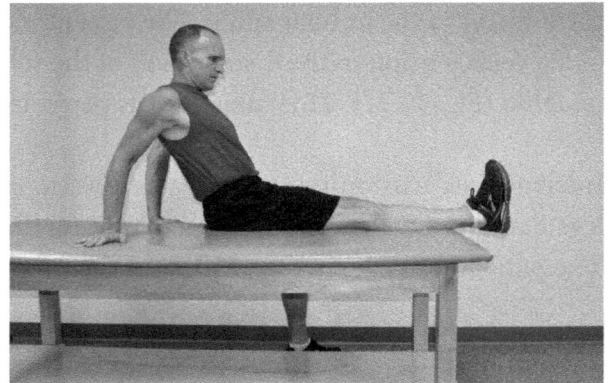

Figure 10-27. Alternate starting position for patient-generated sciatic nerve tensioning in the seated position.

Distal tensioning in the supine position: The patient is lying supine with the knee extended and the hip held in flexion (Fig. 10-28). The patient moves the ankle into dorsiflexion to the point at which he or she feels tension in the distribution of the sciatic nerve (Fig. 10-29) then returns to the starting position (Fig. 10-28). This maneuver is performed repetitively.

Intermediate tensioning in the supine position: The patient is lying supine with the hip held in flexion and the ankle dorsiflexed (Fig. 10-30). The patient extends the knee to the point at which he or she feels

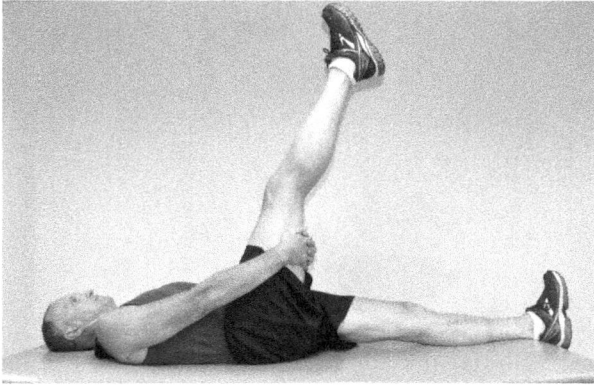

Figure 10-28. Start and end position for patient-generated distal sciatic nerve tensioning in the supine position.

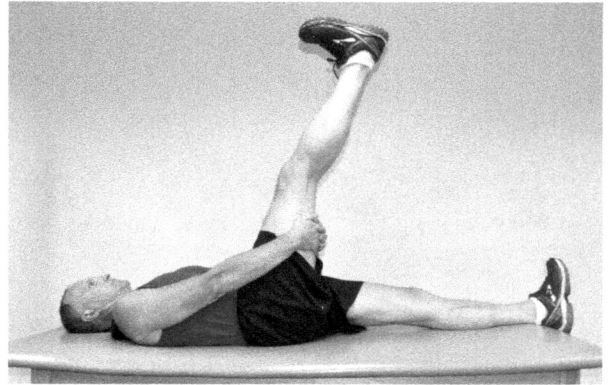

Figure 10-29. Dorsiflexion of the ankle for patient-generated distal sciatic nerve tensioning in the supine position.

tension in the distribution of the sciatic nerve (Fig. 10-31). This is followed by flexion of the knee away from the point of tension. This maneuver is performed repetitively.

Proximal tensioning in the supine position: The patient is lying supine with the knee extended and the ankle dorsiflexed (Fig. 10-32). The patient flexes the hip to the point at which he or she feels tension in the distribution of the sciatic nerve (Fig. 10-33). This is followed by lowering of the extremity away from the point of tension. This maneuver is performed repetitively.

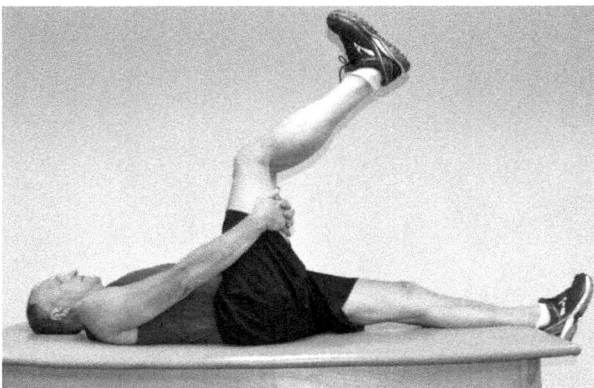

Figure 10-30. Starting position for patient-generated intermediate sciatic nerve tensioning in the supine position.

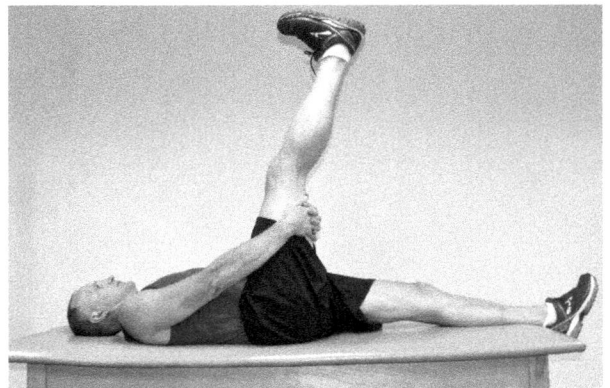

Figure 10-31. Extension of the knee for patient-generated tensioning in the supine position.

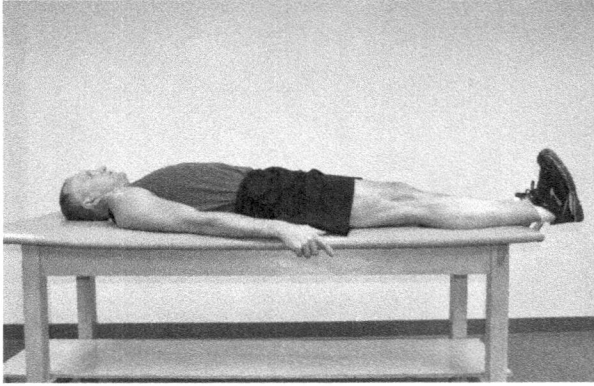

Figure 10-32. Starting position for patient-generated proximal sciatic nerve tensioning in the supine position.

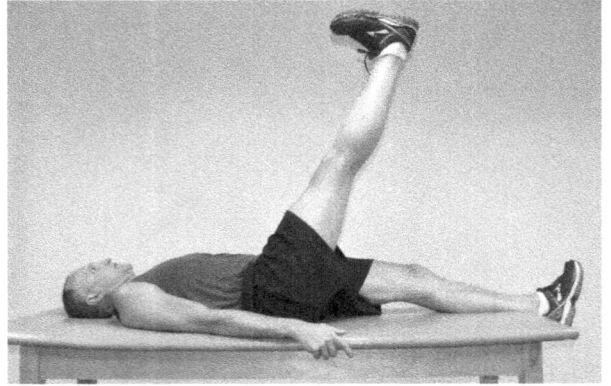

Figure 10-33. Flexion of the hip for patient-generated tensioning in the supine position.

A general sciatic nerve tensioning maneuver can be performed in the standing position. The patient stands next to a wall or some other object that they can use for support. With the ankle dorsiflexed and the knee extended, the patient flexes the hip to the point at which he or she feels tension in the distribution of the sciatic nerve (Fig. 10-34), and then lowers the extremity. This maneuver is performed repetitively.

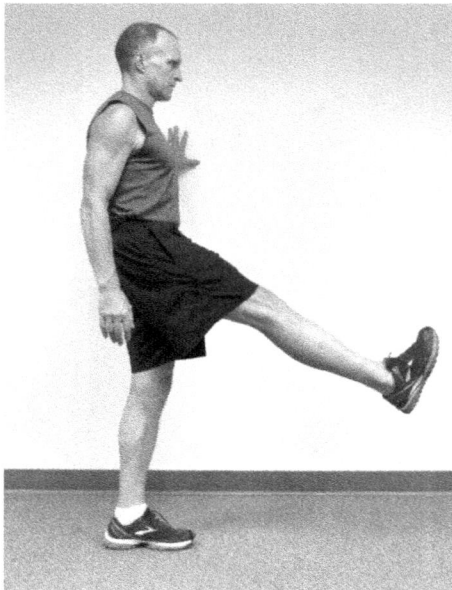

Figure 10-34. Patient-generated general sciatic nerve tensioning in the standing position.

L2 through L4 radiculopathy – femoral nerve mobilization

Mobilization maneuvers that utilize the femoral nerve are applied to patients with subacute or chronic radiculopathy involving the L2 through L4 nerve roots. These are cases in which the neurodynamic examination reproduces the patient's pain with the Femoral Nerve Stretch Test, with structural differentiation confirming this pain to be of neural origin (see Chapter 5). Neural mobilization maneuvers for the femoral nerve can be performed distally or proximally. Because the femoral nerve crosses the knee but does not extend below the ankle, there are no neural mobilization maneuvers that involve the foot. Therefore for the purpose of femoral nerve mobilization distal maneuvers are those that involve movement at the knee and proximal maneuvers are those that involve movement at the hip.

Femoral nerve flossing – practitioner-generated movement

Distal flossing: The patient is in the side-lying position with the involved side up and moves into the slumped position, as with the Femoral Nerve Slump Test (Fig. 5-40). The practitioner holds the patient's thigh with the superior hand and the patient's ankle with the inferior hand. The practitioner moves the knee into flexion and the hip into extension to the point at which the barrier is engaged (Fig. 5-40). The patient is asked to extend the cervical and thoracic spine while the practitioner flexes the knee (Fig. 10-35). The patient is then asked to flex the cervical and thoracic spine while the practitioner extends the knee (Fig. 10-36). This maneuver is performed repetitively, each repetition involving coordinated movement of cervical and thoracic flexion/ extension with knee extension/ flexion.

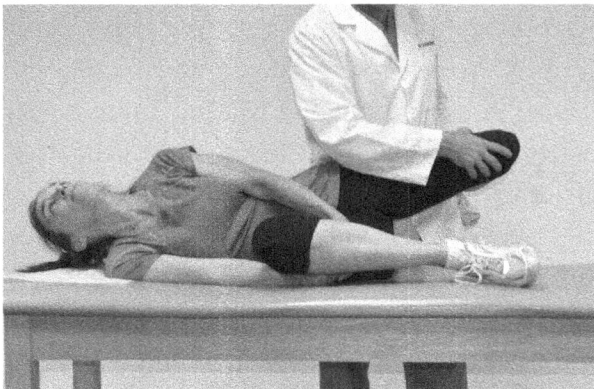

Figure 10-35. Cervical and thoracic extension with knee flexion for practitioner-generated distal femoral nerve flossing in the side-lying position.

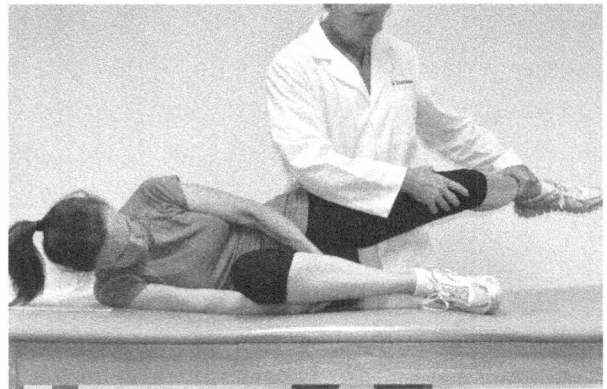

Figure 10-36. Cervical and thoracic flexion with knee extension for practitioner-generated distal femoral nerve flossing in the side-lying position.

Distal flossing can also be performed with the patient in the prone position. The patient lies prone with the head hanging off the end of the table. The practitioner supports the pelvis with the superior hand and holds the patient's ankle with the inferior hand and flexes the patient's knee to the point at which the barrier is engaged. The patient is asked to flex the cervical spine by lowering the head toward the floor while at the same time the practitioner extends the knee, moving away from the barrier (Fig. 10-37). The patient then extends the cervical spine by raising the head while at the same time the practitioner flexes the knee (Fig. 10-38). This maneuver is performed repetitively, each repetition involving coordinated movement of cervical flexion/ extension with knee extension/ flexion.

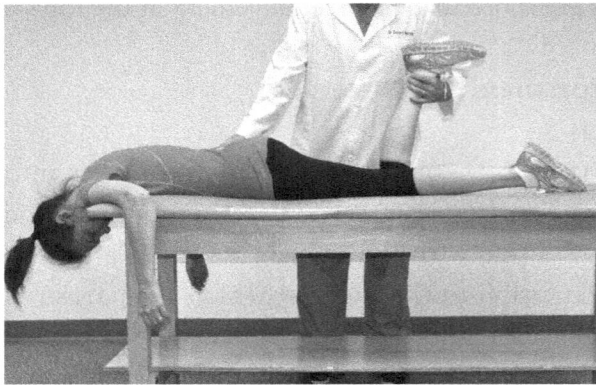

Figure 10-37. Cervical flexion with knee extension for practitioner-generated distal femoral nerve flossing in the prone position.

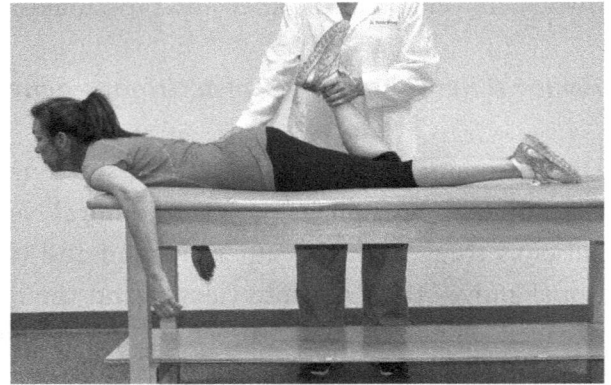

Figure 10-38. Cervical extension with knee flexion for practitioner-generated distal femoral nerve flossing in the prone position.

Proximal flossing: The patient is in the side-lying position with the involve side up and moves into the slumped position, as with distal flossing. The practitioner holds the patient's thigh with his or her superior hand and the patient's ankle with his or her inferior hand. The practitioner moves the knee into flexion and the hip into extension to the point at which the barrier is engaged. The patient is asked to extend the cervical and thoracic spine while the practitioner while extends the hip (Fig. 10-39). The patient then moves the cervical and thoracic spine into flexion while the practitioner flexes the hip (Fig. 10-40). This maneuver is performed repetitively, each repetition involving coordinated movement of cervical and thoracic flexion/ extension with hip flexion/ extension.

As with distal flossing, proximal femoral nerve flossing can be performed with the patient in the prone position. The practitioner supports the pelvis with the superior hand and with the inferior hand

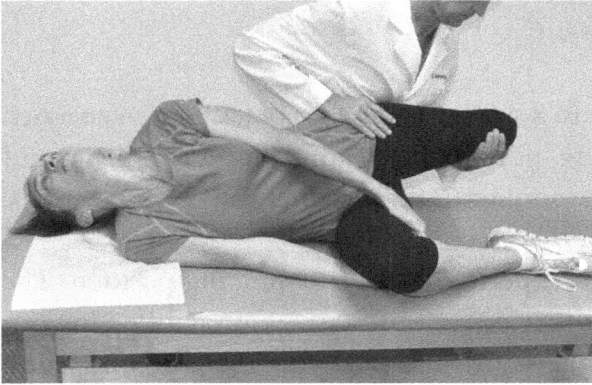

Figure 10-39. Cervical and thoracic extension with hip extension for practitioner-generated proximal femoral nerve flossing in the side-lying position.

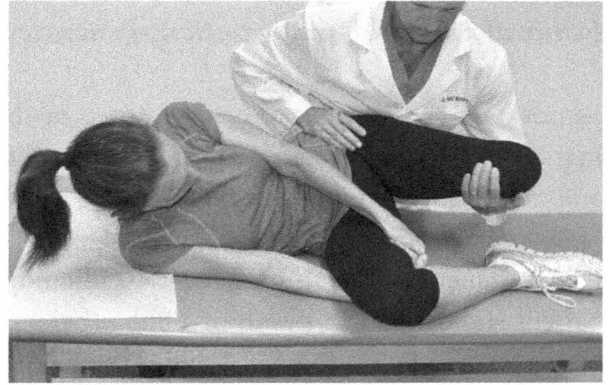

Figure 10-40. Cervical and thoracic flexion with hip flexion for practitioner-generated proximal femoral nerve flossing in the side-lying position.

grasps the patient's thigh just above the knee while the patient's knee is flexed. The hip is extended to the point at which the barrier is engaged. The patient is asked to flex the cervical spine by lowering the head toward the floor while at the same time the practitioner flexes the hip, moving away from the barrier (Fig. 10-41). The patient then extends the cervical spine by raising the head while at the same time the practitioner extends the hip (Fig. 10-42). This maneuver is performed repetitively, each repetition involving coordinated movement of cervical flexion/ extension with hip flexion/ extension.

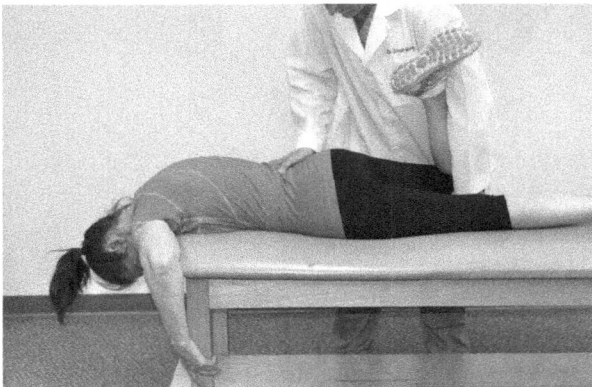

Figure 10-41. Cervical flexion with hip flexion for practitioner-generated proximal femoral nerve flossing in the prone position.

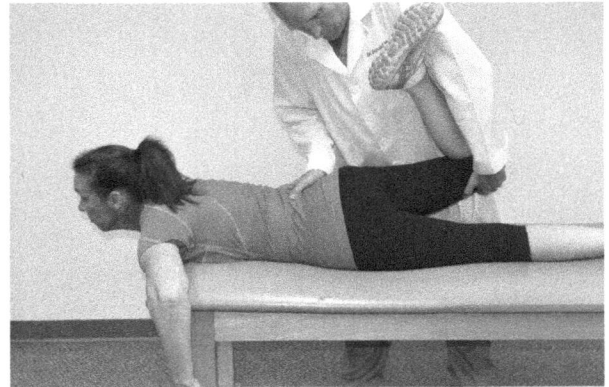

Figure 10-42. Cervical extension with hip extension for practitioner-generated proximal femoral nerve flossing in the prone position.

Femoral nerve flossing – patient-generated movement

Femoral nerve flossing can be performed by the patient in a similar manner as practitioner-generated maneuvers. Exercises can be performed in the side lying, prone and standing positions. The easiest and most widely applicable exercises are those that are performed in the standing and prone positions.

Patient-generated flossing for L2-L4 radiculopathy can be performed in the standing position. The patient stands next to a wall of some other solid object they can use for balance. Distal flossing can be performed by the patient flexing the knee while at the same time extending the head and trunk (Fig. 10-43). The patient then extends the knee while at the same time flexing the head and trunk (Fig. 10-44). This maneuver is repeated, each repetition involving coordinated movement of head and trunk extension/ flexion with knee flexion/ extension.

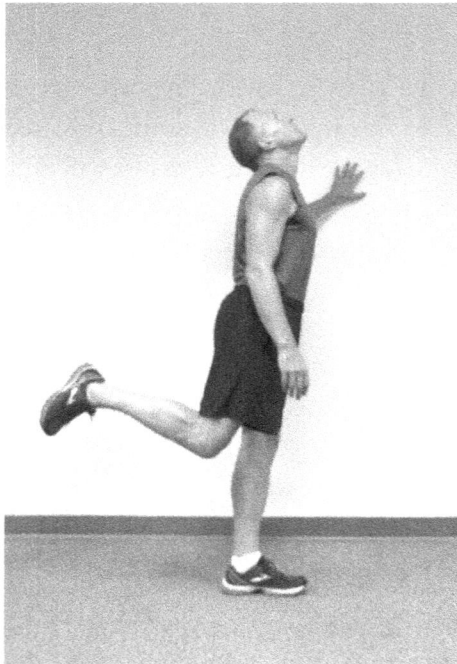

Figure 10-43. Knee flexion and cervical and thoracic extension for patient-generated distal femoral nerve flossing in the standing position.

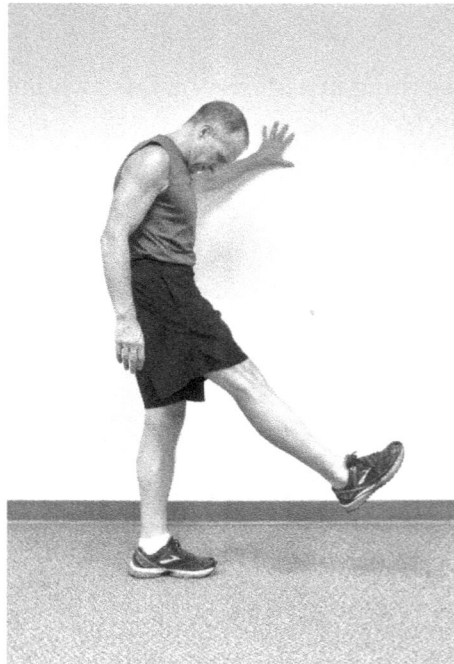

Figure 10-44. Knee extension and cervical and thoracic flexion for patient-generated distal femoral nerve flossing in the standing position.

Proximal flossing in the standing position can be performed by the patient maintaining a flexed knee and extending the hip while at the same time extending the cervical and thoracic spine (Fig. 10-45). The patient then flexes the hip while at the same time flexing the cervical and thoracic spine (Fig. 10-46). This maneuver is repeated, each repetition involving coordinated movement of hip extension/ flexion with head and trunk extension/ flexion.

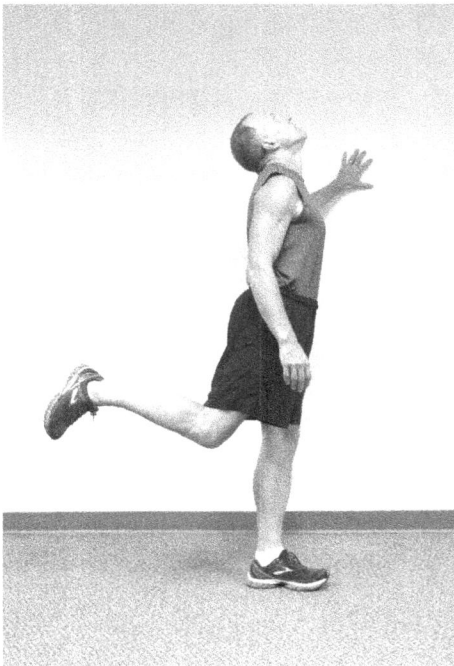

Figure 10-45. Hip extension with cervical and thoracic extension for patient-generated proximal femoral nerve flossing in the standing position.

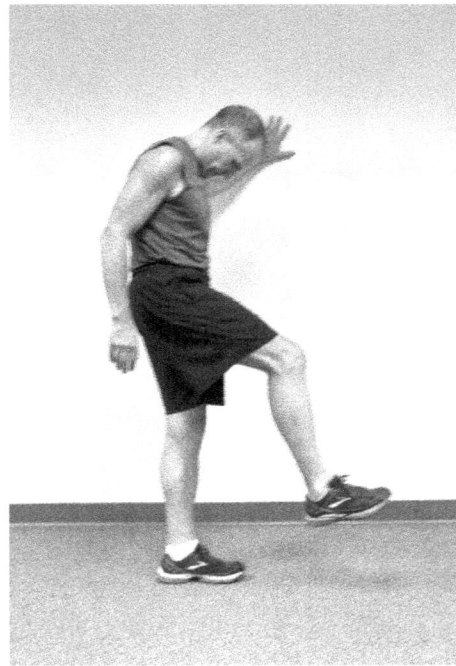

Figure 10-46. Hip flexion with cervical and thoracic flexion for patient-generated proximal femoral nerve flossing in the standing position.

Patient-generated flossing for L2-L4 radiculopathy can also be performed in the prone position. The patient lies prone with the arms under the chest so that the head is raised slightly. The patient flexes the knee while at the same time extending the cervical spine (Fig. 10-47). The patient then lowers the leg, moving away from knee flexion while at the same time flexing the cervical spine (Fig. 10-48). This maneuver is performed repetitively, each repetition involving coordinated movement of knee flexion/ extension with cervical extension/ flexion.

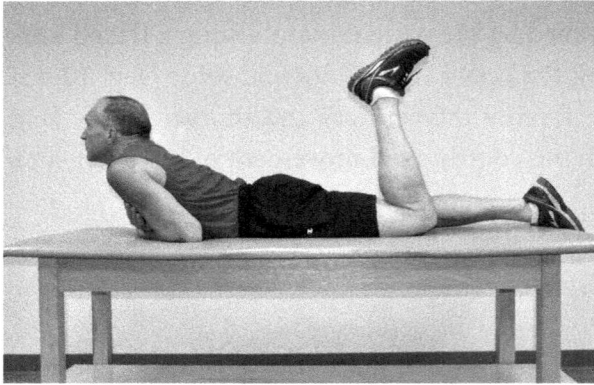

Figure 10-47. Knee flexion with cervical and thoracic extension for patient-generated femoral nerve flossing in the prone position.

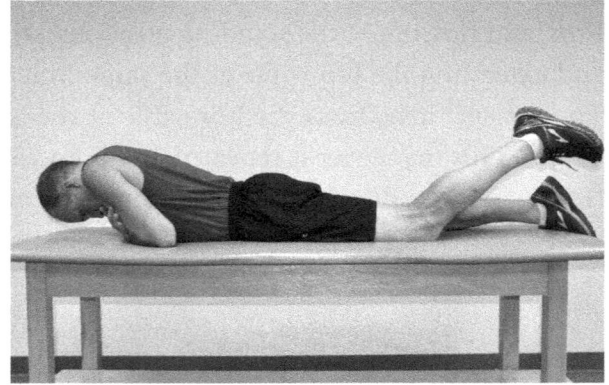

Figure 10-48. Knee extension with cervical and thoracic flexion for patient-generated femoral nerve flossing in the prone position.

Femoral nerve tensioning – practitioner-generated movement

Practitioner-generated tensioning maneuvers for the L2 through L4 nerve roots are most easily performed in the prone position.

Distal tensioning: The patient lies prone and the practitioner supports the pelvis with the superior hand while grasping the patient's ankle with the inferior hand. The practitioner flexes the patient's knee to the point at which the barrier is engaged, as with the Femoral Nerve Stretch Test (Fig. 5-37). The practitioner then moves the knee slightly away from the barrier (Fig. 10-49). This is followed by the practitioner again moving the knee into flexion to the point at which the barrier engaged (Fig. 5-37). This movement is performed repetitively, with the practitioner always moving the leg to the barrier and then away from the barrier.

Proximal tensioning: The patient lies prone and the practitioner supports the pelvis with the superior hand while grasping the patient's thigh just above the knee with the inferior hand while the patient's knee is flexed. The hip is extended to the point at which the barrier is engaged (Fig. 10-50). The practitioner then moves the thigh slightly away from the barrier (Fig. 10-51). This is followed by the practitioner again extending the hip to the point at which the barrier is engaged (Fig. 10-50). This movement is performed repetitively, with the practitioner always moving the thigh to the barrier and then away from the barrier.

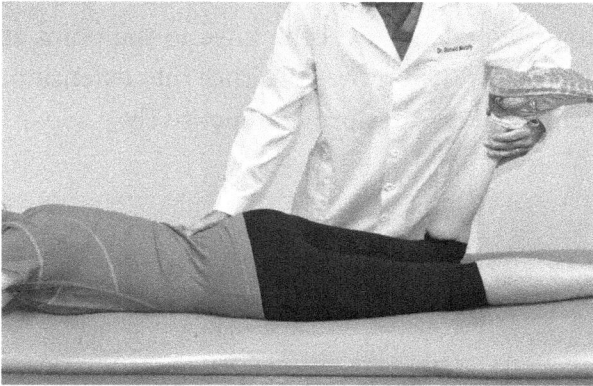

Figure 10-49. Moving the lower leg away from the barrier for practitioner-generated distal femoral nerve tensioning in the prone position.

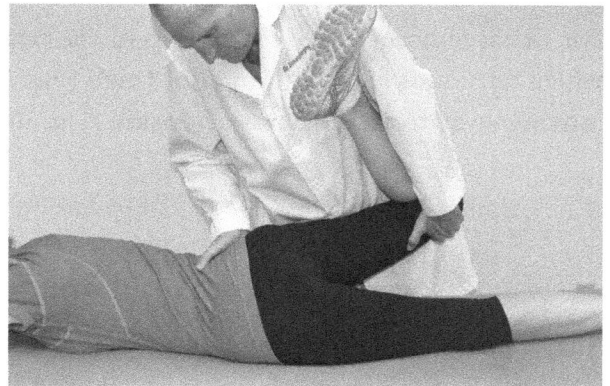

Figure 10-50. Knee flexion and hip extension to the barrier for practitioner-generated proximal femoral nerve tensioning in the prone position.

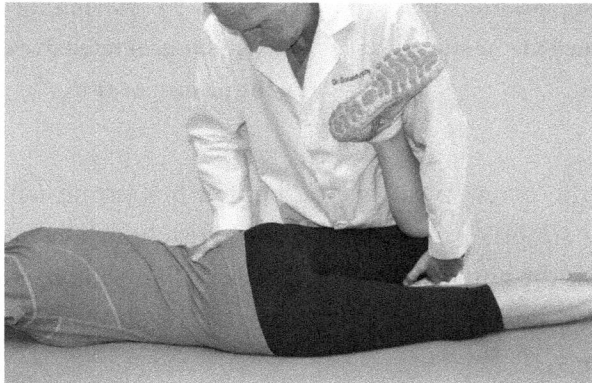

Figure 10-51. Lowering the thigh away from the barrier for practitioner-generated proximal femoral nerve tensioning in the prone position.

Femoral nerve tensioning – patient-generated movement

As with patient-generated flossing maneuvers, the easiest and most widely applicable exercises for femoral nerve tensioning can be performed in the standing and prone positions. The maneuvers can be performed distally, intermediate and proximally.

For distal femoral nerve tensioning in the prone position the patient flexes the knee to the point at which tension is felt in the anterior thigh (Fig. 10-52). The patient then moves the knee into extension, moving away from the point of tension (Fig. 10-53). This maneuver is performed repetitively.

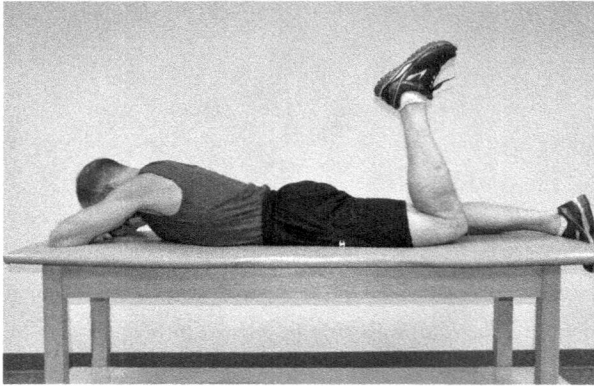

Figure 10-52. Starting and finishing position for patient-generated distal and intermediate femoral nerve tensioning in the prone position.

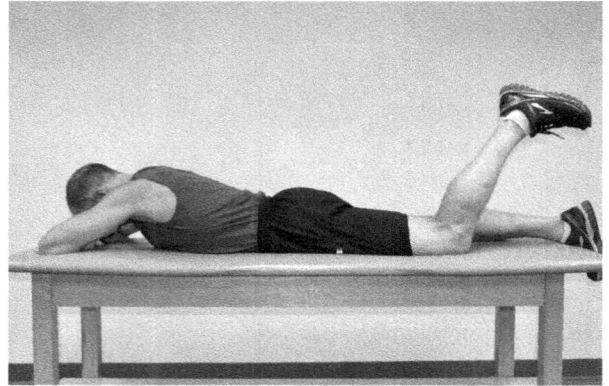

Figure 10-53. Moving the leg away from the barrier for patient-generated distal femoral nerve tensioning in the prone position.

For intermediate tensioning in the prone position the patient lies prone with the knee flexed. The patient flexes the knee to a point slightly before the barrier is reached. The patient extends the hip to the point at which tension is felt in the anterior thigh (Fig. 10-54). The patient then flexes the hip, moving away from the point of tension and returning the thigh to the starting position (Fig. 10-52). This maneuver is performed repetitively.

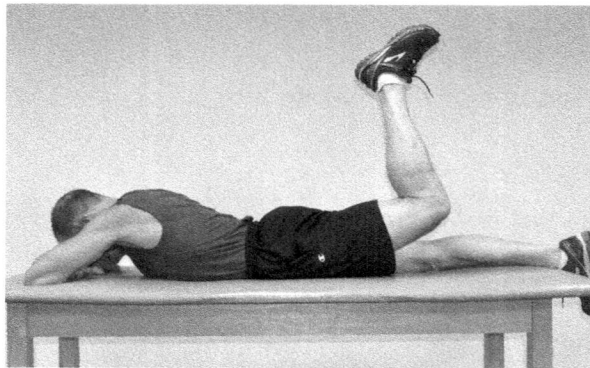

Figure 10-54. Patient-generated intermediate tensioning of the femoral nerve in the prone position.

Proximal femoral nerve tensioning utilizes movement of the spinal cord to create tension on the nerve roots. The patient lies prone with the arms under the chest so that the head is raised slightly. The patient flexes the knee to a point slightly before the barrier is reached. With the knee flexed the patient flexes the cervical spine to the point at which he or she feels tension in the anterior thigh (Fig. 10-55). The patient then extends the cervical spine, moving away from the point of tension (Fig. 10-56). This maneuver is performed repetitively.

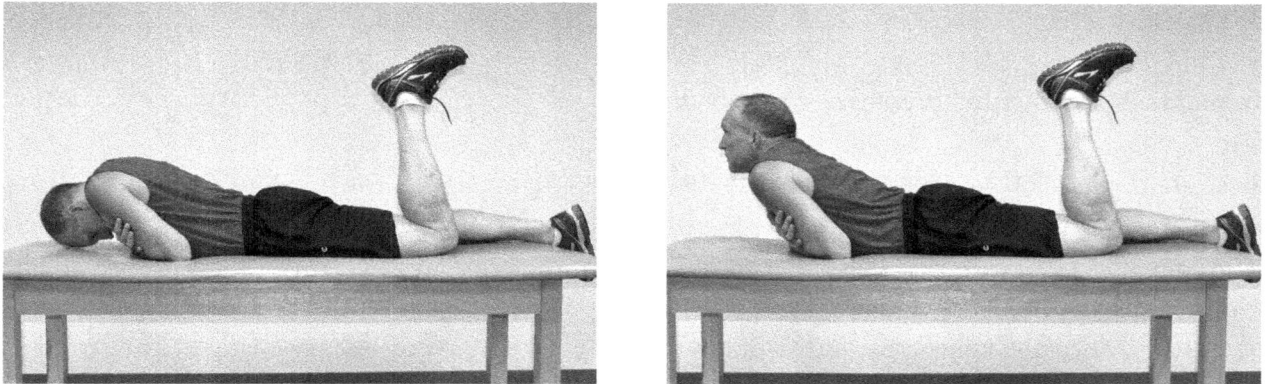

Figure 10-55 and 10-56. Patient-generated proximal femoral nerve tensioning in the prone position.

For patient-generated femoral nerve tensioning maneuvers in the standing position, the maneuvers are exactly the same as those for femoral nerve flossing in the standing position (see Figs. 10-43 through 10-46) except that the patient only moves one body part at a time. For distal femoral nerve tensioning, movement occurs at the knee only. For intermediate femoral nerve tensioning, movement occurs only at the hip. For proximal femoral nerve tensioning movement occurs only at the head and trunk.

In patients for whom non-surgical management fails to resolve the problem, surgery is an option. See Chapter 12 for discussion of surgical decision making.

Myofascial pain

As discussed in Chapter 5, trigger points (TrPs) are very common in patients with LBDs but usually develop in response to one of the other pain generators (disc derangement, joint dysfunction or radiculopathy). It is unusual for a TrP to be the primary pain generator. Thus, TrPs typically resolve when the primary pain generator has been appropriately addressed. However, there are some patients in whom residual myofascial pain remains after the primary pain generator has resolved. In these patients, myofascial therapy is necessary.

There are a wide variety of methods that are used to treat myofascial pain and it is beyond the scope of this book to present an exhaustive review of all methods. As with the other manual methods presented here, it is important for the spine practitioner to be able to apply various methods and to be able to adapt those methods to any given clinical situation.

Methods for treating TrPs can be separated into those that focus on muscle lengthening, those that focus on manual or instrumented pressure release and those that focus on a combination of both these approaches.

Manual or instrumented pressure release techniques

These are myofascial treatments that utilize direct pressure applied to the involved myofascial tissues. Techniques for manual pressure release have been referred to by a variety of names such as Nimmo Technique and ischemic compression. The mechanism of action of these methods is not clear. They involve using the hands or a manual instrument to apply direct pressure to the TrP. A useful way to apply this treatment is to use the thumb or another finger in the same way as when palpating for diagnosis (Fig. 5-43) and gradually press deep into the TrP until the patient's pain is reproduced. Some techniques involve the use of a manual tool to apply pressure to the TrP. The pressure can then be maintained and the patient is asked to identify when the pain starts to diminish or centralize (i.e., when the pain starts to occupy a smaller area). The pressure is further maintained for up to approximately one minute, or until the pain disappears.

This method can be applied to any muscle that can be reached by the hands, which includes most of the common muscles that are involved in patients with LBDs. The application of the treatment simply requires locating the TrP that reproduces the patient's pain. Once the TrP is identified, pressure release treatment can be applied. See Chapter 5 for description of the identification of TrPs in the most common muscles involved in patients with LBDs. Once the practitioner has a clear understanding of how to palpate for TrPs in any spinal muscle, he or she can easily apply manual pressure release techniques.

Muscle lengthening procedures

The purpose of muscle lengthening procedures in the treatment of myofascial pain is to lengthen the muscle fibers that are involved, thereby releasing the TrPs. There are a variety of methods that can be used for this purpose. One simple and useful technique is postisometric relaxation (PIR). With this method, isometric contraction and breathing are utilized in the same way described earlier in the section on muscle energy technique for joint manipulation. First, the patient is positioned in a way that lengthens the muscle being treated. The muscle is then lengthened to the point at which the barrier is engaged, in the same may as described for muscle energy technique for joint manipulation. The patient is then asked to isometrically contract the muscle while the practitioner maintains positioning at the barrier. The patient inhales to further facilitate the isometric contraction. The patient is then asked to stop the isometric contraction and exhale. The practitioner feels for the release of the barrier. When the release of the barrier is perceived the practitioner gently lengthens the muscle to the point at which the barrier is again engaged. The process is then repeated. A total of three repetitions is usually sufficient.

1. Lumbar erector spinae: The patient is in the side-lying position with the involved side up. The arm on the down side is placed behind the patient and the arm on the up side is placed in front of the patient. The lower extremity on the down side is placed in a position of hip flexion while the lower extremity on the up side is placed in a position of hip extension. The practitioner then lengthens the muscle by moving the trunk on the upside into rotation away from the side of involvement and moving the pelvis into rotation toward the side of involvement (Fig. 10-57). The patient is asked to isometrically contract the muscle by pressing against the practitioner's superior hand, attempting to rotate the trunk toward the side of involvement. At the same time, the patient is asked to look up toward the ceiling. The patient is asked to inhale. The practitioner then asks the patient to stop pushing, look down to the floor and exhale. The practitioner waits to feel the barrier release. When this occurs, the practitioner gently lengthens the muscle by moving the trunk further into rotation.

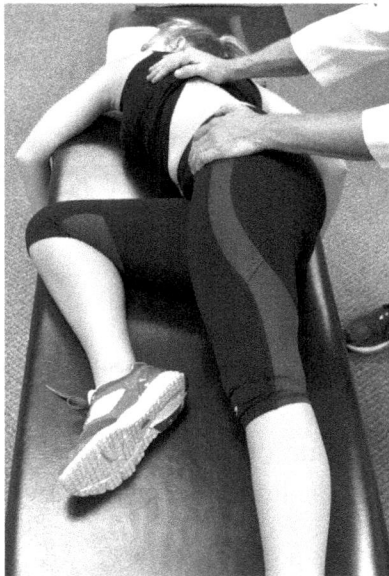

Figure 10-57. PIR for the lumbar erector spinae muscles.

2. Lumbosacral multifidis: The positioning and procedure for PIR to the lumbar multifidis muscles is identical to that for the lumbar erector spinae muscles except that the patient is positioned so that the targeted muscles are on the down side, rather than the up side.

3. Quadratus lumborum: The patient is in the side-lying position with the involved side up. It is best to peak the table if this is possible or to place a pillow, a foam roll, or something similar underneath the patient to laterally flex the lumbar spine away from the side that is being treated. The patient is positioned with the arm on the up side overhead and the lower extremity on the up side behind the other lower extremity. The practitioner places one hand on the iliac crest and the other on the lower rib cage and applies pressure inferiorward on the iliac crest and superiorward on the lower rib cage in order to lengthen the quadratus lumborum to the barrier (Fig. 10-58). The patient is asked to isometrically contract the muscle by trying to elevate the iliac crest. The patient is asked to inhale. The patient is then asked to stop pushing and exhale. The practitioner waits to feel the barrier release. When this occurs, the practitioner gently lengthens the muscle by moving the iliac crest inferiorward and the rib cage superiorward.

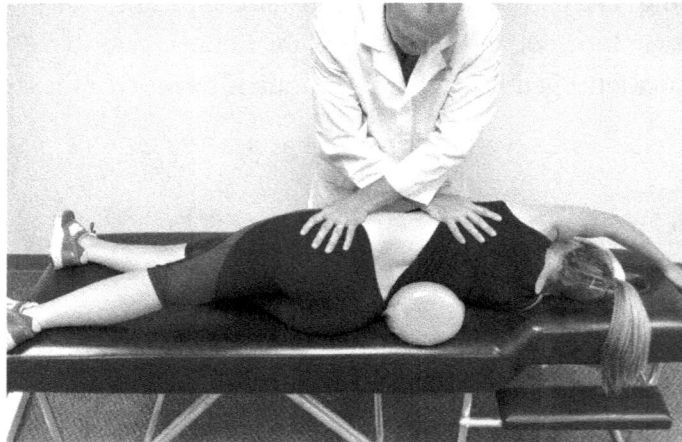

Figure 10-58. PIR for the quadratus lumborum muscle.

4. Gluteus maximus: The gluteus maximus is less amenable to muscle lengthening procedures than the other major muscles of the lumbopelvic area and is best treated with manual release techniques.

5. Piriformis: The patient lies supine and the practitioner stands on the side of involvement. The practitioner moves the lower extremity into hip flexion to slightly below 90 degrees and then

adducts and externally rotates the hip. The knee is maintained in a position of 90 degrees of flexion. The practitioner then applies pressure along the long axis of the femur from the knee toward the hip (Fig. 10-59). The practitioner feels for the barrier. From the barrier the patient is asked to press his or her ankle against the practitioner's inferior hand and to inhale. The patient is then asked to stop pushing and exhale. The practitioner waits to feel the barrier release. When this occurs, the practitioner gently lengthens the muscle by moving the lower extremity further into adduction and external rotation.

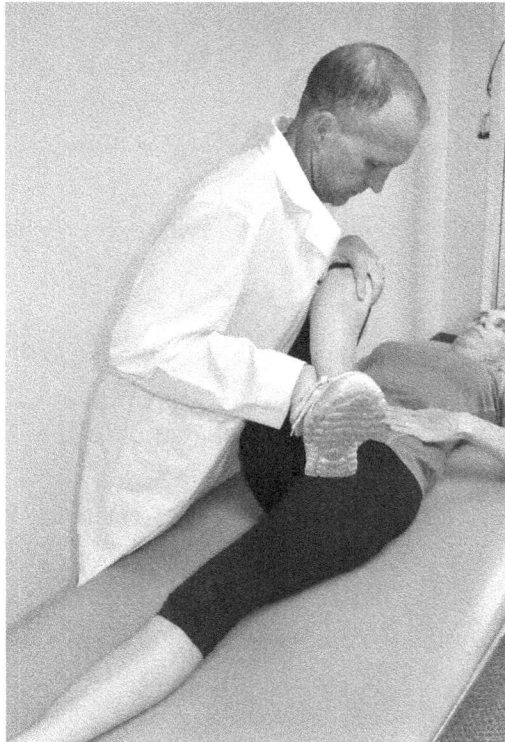

Figure 10-59. PIR for the piriformis muscle.

Methods that combine manual release with muscle lengthening

There are other methods of treating myofascial pain that combine manual release with muscle lengthening. With these techniques a contact is made in the vicinity of the TrP and the muscle lengthened in a similar manner as demonstrated here. While the muscle is lengthening the trigger point passes beneath the manual contact in an attempt to manually release the trigger point while the involved muscle fibers are lengthening.

TrP injection may be useful in certain circumstances. This involves injecting a local anesthetic, such as lidocaine or procaine and occasionally a steroid, non-steroidal anti-inflammatory medication or botulinum toxin. The risk of TrP injection is very small but it is very uncommonly necessary.

Appropriately identifying the answer to diagnostic question #2 allows the practitioner to choose methods of treating the primary pain generator that will bring about rapid reduction of pain. While this is an important part of the overall management of the patient, there still remains the aspect of the clinical picture identified by diagnostic question #3. Strategies to address the perpetuating factors of LBDs are presented in the next chapter.

Recommended Reading

Bergmann T, Peterson D. Chiropractic Technique Principles and Procedures; 3rd Ed. St. Louis: Elsevier, Mosby, 2011.

Butler DS. The Sensitive Nervous System. Adelaide, Australia: Noigroup Publications; 2000.

Chaitow. Muscle Energy Techniques. 4th ed. Edinburgh: Churchille Livingstone; 2013.

Cox, JM. Low Back Pain: Mechanism, Diagnosis, and Treatment, 7th edition, 2011, Philadephia: Lippincott, Williams & Wilkins.

http://emedicine.medscape.com/article/1820854-overview [article on spine injections accessed 28 June 2013]

http://emedicine.medscape.com/article/325733-overview [article on ESI accessed 28 June 2013]

Lewit K. Manipulative Therapy in the Rehabilitation of the Locomotor System. 3rd Ed. Oxford: Butterworth-Heinemann Ltd., 1999

McKenzie RA, May S. The Lumbar Spine: Mechanical Diagnosis and Therapy. 2nd ed. Waikenae, NZ: Spinal Publications; 2003.

Murphy DR, Hurwitz EL, Gregory AA, Clary R. A non-surgical approach to the management of patients with lumbar spinal stenosis. Biomed Central Musculoskel: 2006;7:16.

Murphy DR, Hurwitz EL, McGovern EE. A non-surgical approach to the management of patients with lumbar radiculopathy secondary to herniated disc: A prospective observational cohort study with follow up. J Manipulative Physiol Ther 2009;32(9):723-33.

Neurodynamic Solutions: http://www.neurodynamicsolutions.com (accessed 27 June 2013)

Shacklock M. Clinical Neurodynamics. A New System of Musculoskeletal Treatment. Edinburgh: Elsevier; 2005.

Simons DG, Travell JG, Simons LS. Myofascial Pain and Dysfunction: The Trigger Point Manual. Volume 1. Baltimore: Williams and Wilkens; 1999

The McKenzie Institute International: http://www.mckenziemdt.org/ [accessed 27 June 2013]

The NOI Group: http://www.noigroup.com (accessed 27 June 2013)

· CHAPTER 11 ·

Treatment Approaches for Diagnostic Question #3

The third question of diagnosis is "What has happened with this person as a whole that would cause the pain experience to develop and persist?" Another way of asking this question is, "what factors are present in this patient that are perpetuating the ongoing pain, disability and suffering experience or are causing recurrent episodes?" As discussed in Chapters 2 and 6, the factors that are thought to perpetuate the pain, disability and suffering experience encompass somatic, neurophysiological and psychological processes. Thus, it is essential for the spine practitioner to have a well-rounded understanding of the pathophysiology and psychology of low back disorders (LBDs) (see Chapter 2) in order to help patients overcome the problem and get back into the driver's seat of life.

Also as was discussed in Chapter 6, from a diagnostic standpoint question #3 is important in the subacute or chronic LBD patient (in addition to diagnostic questions #1 and 2). In the acute LBD patient, questions #1 and 2 are paramount. The more longstanding the LBD, the more significant diagnostic question #3 becomes. Nevertheless, from a management standpoint it is still important to start sowing the seeds of prevention of somatic, neurophysiological and psychological perpetuating factors in the acute stage, as these often have their genesis early on.

Dynamic instability

Dynamic instability is believed to result from impairment of the motor control system that serves to provide protection to the spine. The inclusion of dynamic instability in the diagnosis is made based on the combination the historical factors and examination procedures that were presented in detail in Chapter 6.

The treatment for dynamic instability is stabilization exercise. A variety of approaches to stabilization exercise have been developed and there is no clear evidence that one approach is better than another.

Presented here is a basic approach that is consistent with the literature, has been found to be beneficial to patients with LBDs, and is applicable to a primary spine care environment.

There are a variety of different exercises and challenge strategies that can be applied depending on the individual needs of the patient. For example, rehabilitating high-level athletes may require the addition of more advanced exercises than those presented here. On the other hand for patients whose stability requirements are smaller, a simple and basic approach can be used.

The principle of minimalism applies here – the patient should be placed on the simplest exercise program necessary to respond to his or her needs. In addition, emphasis should always be on transitioning the patient away from in-clinic rehabilitation and toward an independent home exercise program. As the focus of this book is clinical excellence in primary spine care, an approach to stabilization training designed for the majority of patients with LBDs is presented.

Some practitioners might want to delve further into spine rehabilitation or get involved with specialized rehabilitation such as that of elite athletes. These readers are encouraged to seek out sources of information such as the textbook by Liebenson (see Recommended Reading list). However for the vast majority of patients with LBDs the approach presented here is more than enough to improve dynamic stability.

Very few patients will require all of the exercises presented here. A variety of exercises, organized according to tracks, are presented so the practitioner can design an individualized program that best meets the needs of each patient.

It appears from experimental studies that when dynamic instability develops in the spine, the transverse abdominis (TrA) and multifidis (MULT) muscles tend to become inhibited while the rectus abdominis and other superficial muscles tend to become hyperactive.

Some have misinterpreted this phenomenon as suggesting that the TrA and MULT are more important in spine stability than other muscles, or that patients need to be taught to consciously co-contract these muscles in isolation during the performance of everyday activities in order to increase spine stability. This is a mistake. However, it is important to train co-contraction of these muscles in as focused a fashion as possible during the early stages of stabilization training. This is because, as stated earlier, these muscles, for reasons that are currently unknown, tend to become inhibited. So training co-contraction of the TrA and MULT in the early stages helps ensure that these muscles participate in the more complex and challenging exercises to which the patient is progressed later on. So when the patient is being trained to challenge the motor control system as a whole, it is essential to make sure the TrA and MULT are participating in the exercises. Therefore, the first stage in the process of stabilization training is co-contraction of these muscles. This is done with the co-contraction maneuver.

Co-contraction maneuver: The co-contraction maneuver is performed with the patient lying supine with the hips and knees flexed. To co-contract the TrA and MULT the patient gently draws the umbilicus straight backward, as if moving it toward the spine. This maneuver has sometimes been referred to as an "abdominal hollow" but this term is not being used here because it creates the image of causing the abdomen to take on a concave configuration (Fig. 11-1). This is improper technique and will decrease, rather than increase, trunk muscle activity.

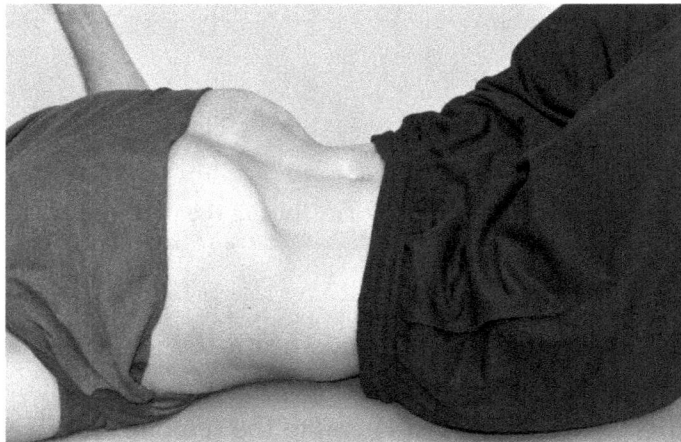

Figure 11-1. Incorrect performance of "abdominal hollowing."

It is important for the practitioner to make sure the patient is properly recruiting the TrA and MULT during the performance of the co-contraction maneuver. This can be done via palpation. To palpate the TrA the fingers are placed on the patient's anterior superior iliac spine and then moved approximately 1 inch medial and slightly inferior to this landmark (Fig. 11-2). The palpating fingers should apply gentle pressure deep into this part of the abdomen. When the patient performs the co-contraction maneuver, the practitioner should be able to feel the muscle contract under the fingers. The contraction of the TrA should feel like a flat band becoming tense. This should be distinguished from contraction of the internal oblique, which is perceived as a "bulging out" of the muscle. If the practitioner is not sure whether TrA contraction is occurring it is sometimes useful to have the patient release the maneuver so the practitioner can feel the muscle relax. When the patient then performs the maneuver again it is easier to sense the muscle contraction. If the contraction clearly feels like a "bulging out" (i.e., internal oblique activation), the patient should be instructed to repeat the maneuver but at approximately half the intensity. This usually causes the TrA to activate rather than the internal oblique.

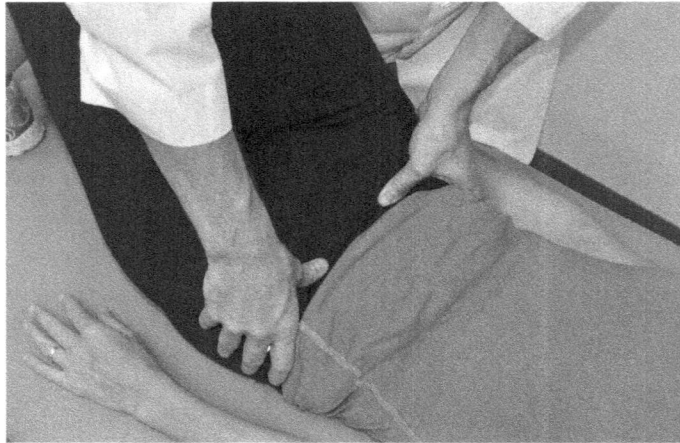

Figure 11-2. Palpation of the TrA during the performance of the co-contraction maneuver.

To palpate the MULT the practitioner reaches underneath the patient and places the hand on the patient's lower back. The fingers are placed on the far side and the thumb on the near side. Both contact points should be in the lumbosacral spine just lateral to the spinous processes (Fig. 11-3). The patient performs the co-contraction maneuver and the practitioner feels the contraction of the MULT. As was stated regarding the TrA, if the practitioner is not sure if the MULT is activating it is sometimes useful to have the patient release the maneuver so the practitioner can feel the relaxation of the muscle and then perform the maneuver again so the practitioner can feel the contraction.

The TrA and MULT can both be palpated at the same time by the practitioner placing one hand on the TrA and the other on the MULT.

If the patient is not able to co-contract the TrA and MULT and the practitioner is confident that the palpation technique is correct, there are "tricks" the practitioner can use to train the central nervous system to activate these muscles. One "trick" is to teach the patient to co-contract the TrA and MULT indirectly. This is done by activating the pelvic floor muscles.

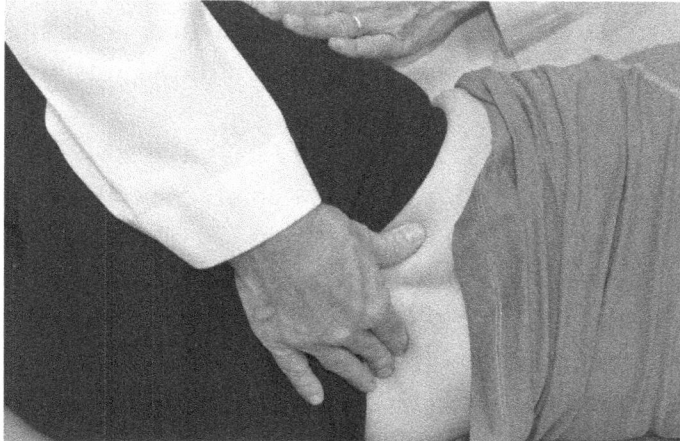

Figure 11-3. Hand positioning for palpating the MULT. For illustration purposes the patient is side-lying in the figure. However, for clinical application the patient should be supine.

The patient is in the supine position as when performing the co-contraction maneuver. The practitioner palpates the TrA and MULT. The patient is instructed to imagine that he or she were urinating and to tense the pelvic muscles as if gently trying to stop the flow of urine. This is similar to the well-known "Kegel exercise." The practitioner palpates for activation of the TrA and MULT during this maneuver. Typically the practitioner will feel a very gentle contraction of these muscles. The patient may have to do this exercise at home for a few days prior to advancing to the full co-contraction maneuver. However, other patients will be able to superimpose the co-contraction maneuver on top of the pelvic floor activation right away. To do this the patient activates the pelvic floor muscles as described and then, while holding this contraction, draws the umbilicus toward the spine. The practitioner should be able to feel increased activation of the TrA and MULT.

Another "trick" is to have the patient perform the co-contraction in the quadruped position. The movement is performed in the same manner as in the supine position, the patient gently drawing the umbilicus toward the spine while the practitioner palpates the TrA and MULT.

There are some patients who will be able to activate the TrA during the performance of the co-contraction maneuver but not the MULT. In these cases one "trick" that can be used is to instruct the patient to imagine there is a cable attached from the umbilicus to the spine. The patient is asked to imagine tension building in the cable while the practitioner palpates the MULT. In most cases the practitioner will feel activation of the MULT. This can be performed as a home exercise, with gradual transition to the co-contraction maneuver as activation of the MULT improves.

Once the patient is able to perform the co-contraction maneuver, it should be performed as a home exercise. The patient holds the co-contraction for 10 seconds and then lets it go. This is repeated 10 times.

As stated earlier, the purpose of starting the process of stabilization training with co-contraction of the TrA and MULT is to ensure that these muscles are participating in motor control responses during subsequent exercises as well as during daily activities. Once the ability to co-contract these muscles is established the patient can be progressed on a series of exercises that provide increasing challenge to the motor control system. Where the patient starts on this progression and how quickly the patient moves along the progression will be determined on an individual basis. The exercise progressions are designed for the patient to start at a level that is challenging but that can be performed with relative ease. The patient can perform the exercises in the clinic but it is important that the exercises are maximally conducive to performance at home or at a health club, as this builds self-efficacy. With each exercise the patient first performs the co-contraction maneuver in order to ensure that the TrA and MULT are participating in the exercise. The patient maintains co-contraction of the TrA and MULT during the performance of each exercise. Ideally, the patient should not let go of the co-contraction between repetitions of each exercise.

If the patient is not able to maintain the co-contraction during an exercise, the practitioner should have the patient stop between each repetition and perform the co-contraction maneuver again prior to the next repetition. Gradually, the patient should be progressed to holding the co-contraction for two repetitions, then three repetitions, and so on until he or she can maintain the co-contraction during a full set of an exercise.

For ease of application the exercises are organized along tracks. The tracks start with exercises that are low-load and low complexity and gradually progress to become more challenging to the motor control system. It is not necessary for every patient to perform every exercise. The practitioner should try to find the best starting point for each patient on each track, depending on the individual abilities of each patient. As the patient masters each exercise from a motor control standpoint (i.e., the patient can perform the exercise for 20 repetitions while maintaining good motor control) he or she can be progressed to the next exercise. The patient can be progressed along multiple tracks at the same time.

Supine Track

Supine Single Arm Raise: The patient lies supine with the knees and hips flexed and the arms extended toward the ceiling. The patient performs the co-contraction maneuver and then moves one arm overhead toward the floor while the other arm remains in place (Fig. 11-4). The patient returns this arm to the starting point and then moves the other arm toward the floor. This is repeated for 10-20 repetitions. As this is a motor control exercise it is important that the movement is carried out slowly and deliberately with the uninvolved arm remaining perfectly stationary as the involved arm is moving. The patient should maintain the co-contraction throughout the set.

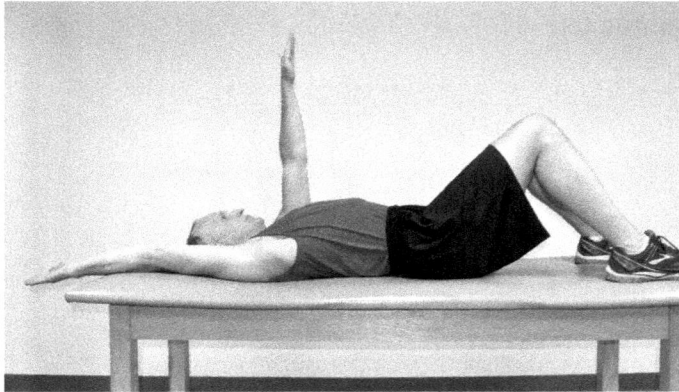

Figure 11-4. Supine Single Arm Raise.

Supine Single Leg Raise: The patient lies supine with the hips and knees flexed and the arms extended toward the ceiling. The patient performs the co-contraction maneuver and then raises one lower extremity in the air, maintaining knee flexion (Fig. 11-5). The patient returns the extremity to the starting position and then raises the other lower extremity. This is repeated for 10-20 repetitions with the patient maintaining the co-contraction throughout the set. As was stated with the single arm raise, it is important that the movement is carried out slowly and deliberately and that the uninvolved lower extremity remains stationary while the involved lower extremity is moving.

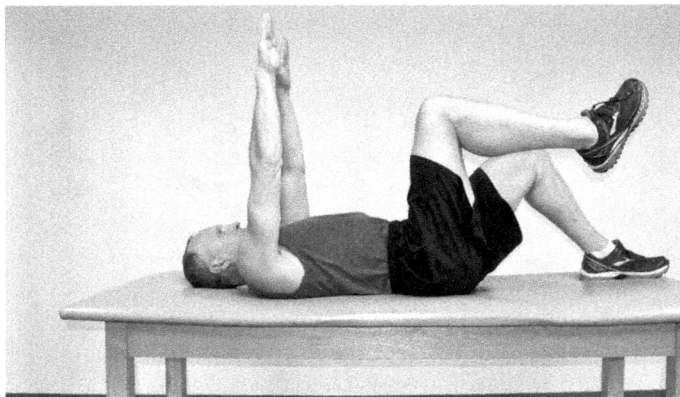

Figure 11-5. Supine Single Leg Raise.

Supine Single Arm and Leg Raise: The patient lies supine with the knees and hips flexed and the arms extended toward the ceiling. The patient performs the co-contraction maneuver and then slowly and deliberately moves one arm overhead toward the floor while simultaneously raising the opposite lower extremity (Fig. 11-6). The patient returns to the starting position and then simultaneously raises the other upper and lower extremities. This is repeated for 10-20 repetitions with the patient maintaining the co-contraction throughout the set.

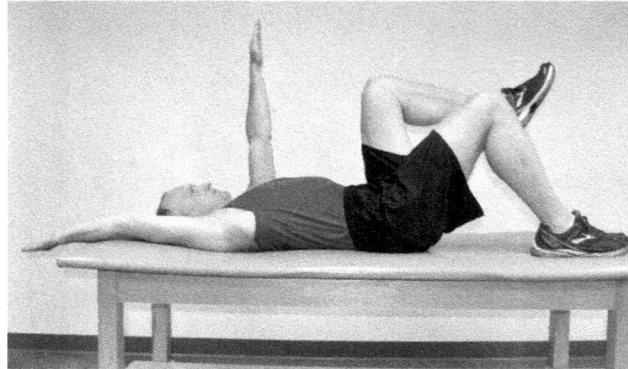

Figure 11-6. Supine Single Arm and Leg Raise.

Supine Alternating Kicks: The patient lies supine with the knees and hips both flexed to 90 degrees so that the feet are in the air. The patient performs the co-contraction maneuver and then slowly and deliberately moves one lower extremity forward while the other remains stationary (Fig. 11-7). The patient returns to the starting position and then repeats the movement with the other lower extremity. This is repeated for 10-20 repetitions with the patient maintaining the co-contraction throughout the set.

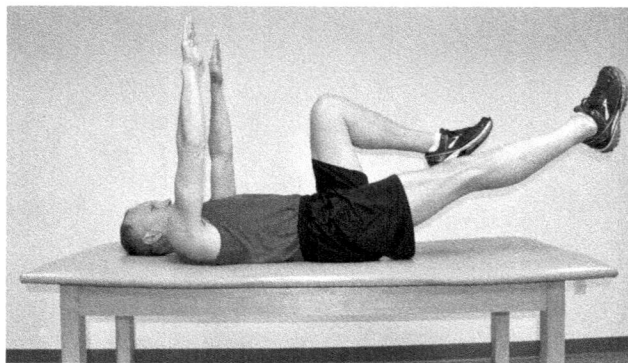

Figure 11-7. Supine Alternating Kicks

Dead Bug: The patient lies supine with the arms extended toward the ceiling and the knees and hips both flexed to 90 degrees so that the feet are in the air. The patient performs the co-contraction maneuver and then slowly and deliberately moves one arm overhead toward the floor while simultaneously moving the opposite lower extremity forward. The other upper and lower extremities remain stationary (Fig. 11-8). The patient returns to the starting position and then repeats the movement with the other upper and lower extremities. This is repeated for 10-20 repetitions with the patient maintaining the co-contraction throughout the set.

Curl Up: This exercise is designed to train the rectus abdominis muscles while training the maintenance of a neutral spine posture. The patient lies supine with the hips and knees flexed. It is important for the patient to maintain a neutral lordosis throughout the exercise. The patient curls up by flexing the thoracic spine while maintaining a neutral lumbar lordosis (Fig. 11-9). It is important to maintain a neutral position of the cervical spine. The patient then returns to the starting position. A more advanced version of the curl up can be performed with the hands behind the head.

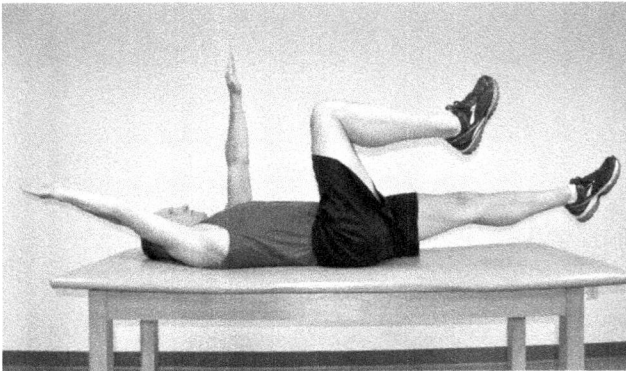

Figure 11-8. The Dead Bug Exercise.

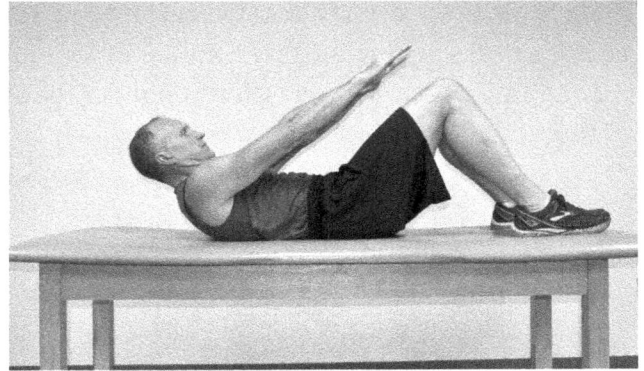

Figure 11-9. The basic Curl Up.

Quadruped track

Quadruped Single Leg Raise: The patient is in the quadruped position and performs the co-contraction maneuver. It is important that the lumbar, thoracic and cervical spine and the scapulae are in a neutral and stable position. The patient slowly and deliberately raises one lower extremity (Fig. 11-10) and returns it to the floor. The patient then raises the opposite lower extremity and returns it to the floor. This is repeated 10-20 times while maintaining the co-contraction throughout the set.

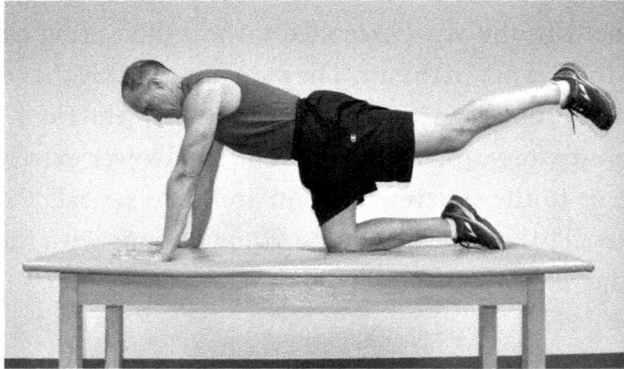

Figure 11-10. Quadruped Single Leg Raise.

Quadruped Single Arm and Leg Raise: The patient is in the quadruped position and performs the co-contraction maneuver. It is important that the lumbar, thoracic and cervical spine and the scapulae are in a neutral and stable position. The patient slowly and deliberately raises one arm overhead while at the same time raising the opposite lower extremity (Fig. 11-11) then returns them to the floor. The patient repeats this with the other upper and lower extremities. This is repeated 10-20 times while maintaining the co-contraction throughout the set.

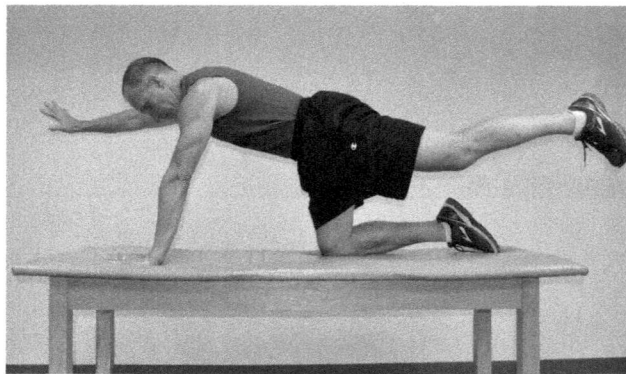

Figure 11-11. Quadruped Single Arm and Leg Raise.

Bridge Track

Basic Bridge: The patient is lying supine with the hips and knees flexed. The patient performs the co-contraction maneuver and then slowly and deliberately raises the pelvis as high as possible while

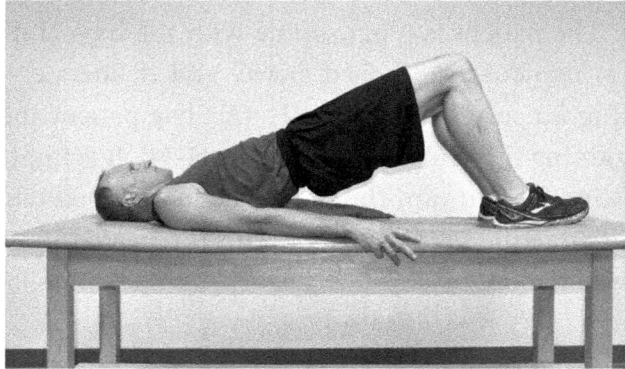

Figure 11-12. Basic Bridge.

maintaining a neutral spine (Fig. 11-12) followed by return to the starting position. This is repeated 10-20 times while maintaining the co-contraction throughout the set.

Bridge with Steps: The patient is lying supine with the hips and knees flexed. The patient performs the co-contraction maneuver and then slowly and deliberately raises the pelvis as high as possible while maintaining a neutral spine (Fig. 11- 12). The patient then slowly and deliberately raises one foot off the floor while maintaining the bridge position (Fig. 11-13). It is important that the patient does not allow the pelvis to rotate or drop toward the floor. The foot is returned to the floor and the patient raises the other foot and returns it to the floor. This is repeated 10-20 times while maintaining the co-contraction throughout the set.

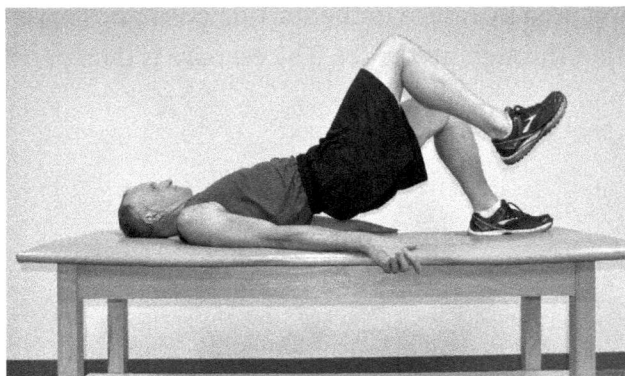

Figure 11-13. Bridge with Steps.

Bridge with Leg Extension: The patient is lying supine with the hips and knees flexed. The patient performs the co-contraction maneuver and then slowly and deliberately raises the pelvis as high as possible while maintaining a neutral spine (Fig. 11-12). The patient then slowly and deliberately extends one leg while maintaining the bridge position (Fig. 11-14). It is important that the patient does not allow the pelvis to rotate or drop toward the floor. The foot is then returned to the floor and the patient raises the other foot and returns it to the floor. This is repeated 10-20 times while maintaining the co-contraction throughout the set.

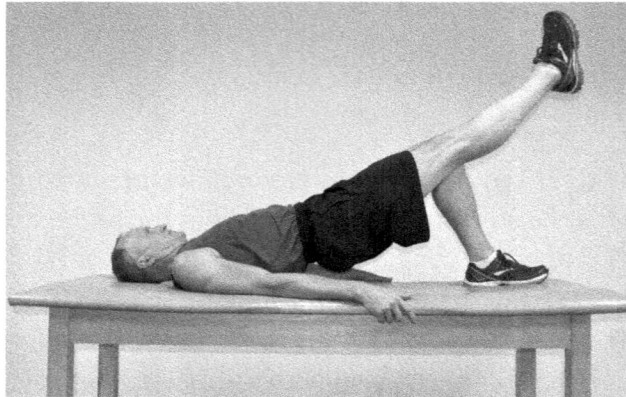

Figure 11-14. Bridge with Leg Extension.

Side Bridge with Knees Flexed: The patient is lying on one side, leaning on the elbow with the knees flexed. The patient performs the co-contraction maneuver and then slowly and deliberately raises the pelvis off the floor (Fig. 11-15) followed by return to the starting position. This is repeated 10-20 times while maintaining the co-contraction throughout the set. The exercise is then performed on the other side.

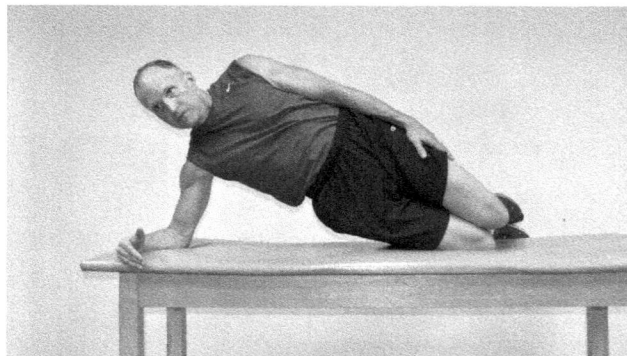

Figure 11-15. Side Bridge with Knees Flexed.

This exercise can be made more challenging by having the patient perform it with the knees extended (Fig. 11-16).

Plank: This exercise is performed in the prone position. The patient supports him- or herself on the forearms while maintaining the co-contraction maneuver and the neutral spine posture (Fig. 11-17). This is maintained as a static position. The patient should be started at a duration of time that can be held without losing the co-contraction or the neutral spine, with gradual progression to 30-60 seconds.

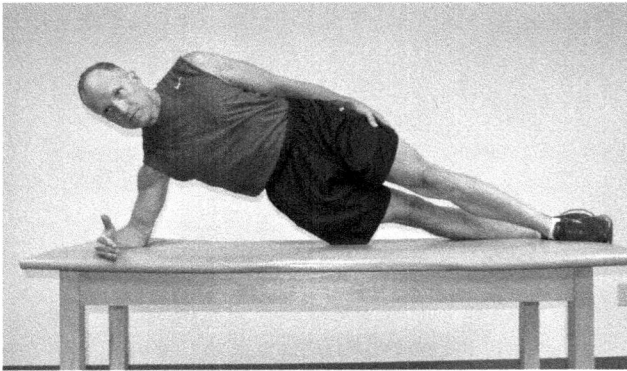

Figure 11-16. Side Bridge with Knees Extended.

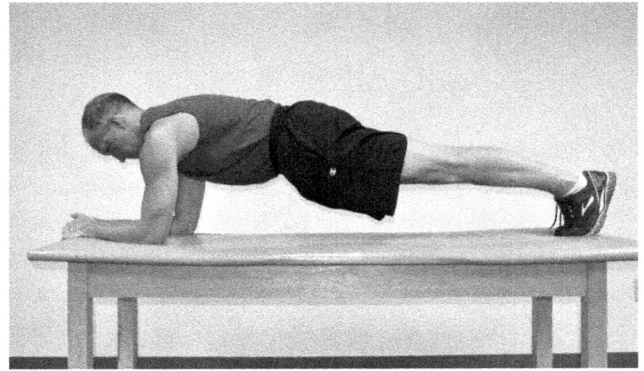

Figure 11-17. Plank.

Exercises Using a Ball

An exercise ball is less stable than the floor, thus increasing the challenge to the motor control system. Unless otherwise indicated, the ideal sized exercise ball is one in which when the patient is sitting on the ball the hips are flexed to approximately 90 degrees.

Quadruped Arm and Leg Raise: The patient is face-down in the quadruped position with the abdomen on the ball. The patient performs the co-contraction maneuver and then slowly and deliberately raise one arm and the opposite lower extremity (Fig. 11-18) followed by return to the starting position. This is repeated with the other upper and lower extremities.

Ball Curl Up: The patient is supine on an exercise ball with the lumbar spine on the ball and the feet placed approximately shoulder width apart. The patient performs the co-contraction maneuver and then slowly and deliberately curls up by flexing the thoracic spine while maintaining a neutral lumbar lordosis (Fig. 11-19). It is important to maintain a neutral position of the cervical spine. The patient then returns to the starting position. This is repeated 10-20 times while maintaining the co-contraction throughout the set.

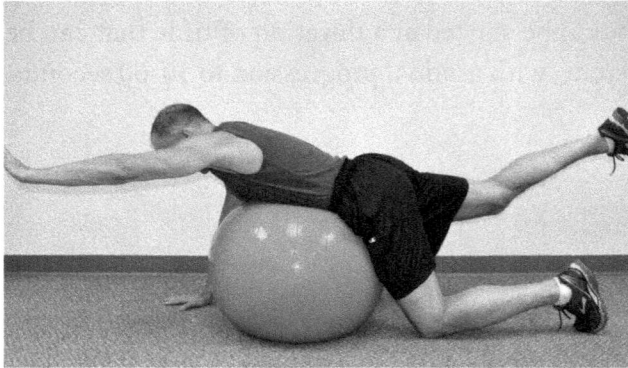

Figure 11-18. Quadruped Arm and Leg Raise on the exercise ball.

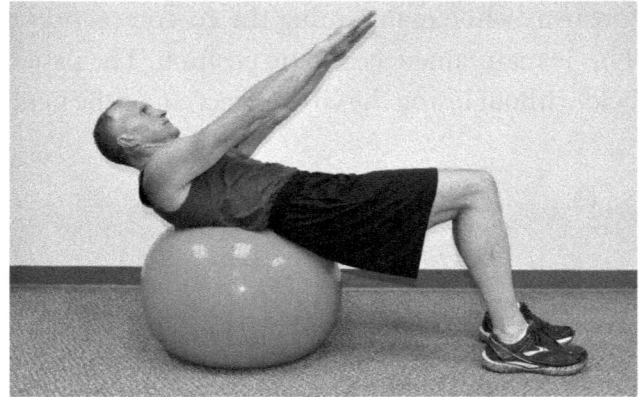

Figure 11-19. The basic Curl Up on the exercise ball.

There are a few ways to increase the challenge with the ball curl up. These include holding the hands behind the neck, performing the exercise with the feet together on the floor, and starting with the ball placed lower on the lumbar spine so that a greater portion of the trunk is behind the ball.

Bridge Track on the Exercise Ball

Basic Bridge: The patient starts by sitting on the exercise ball then slowly walks out so that the thoracic spine rests on the ball (Fig. 11-20). The patient slowly and deliberately lowers the pelvis toward the floor as far as possible without losing the lumbar lordosis (Fig. 11-21). The patient then returns to the starting position. This is repeated 10-20 times while maintaining the co-contraction throughout the set.

Bridge with Steps: The patient walks out onto the ball and into the bridge position (Fig. 11-20). The patient performs the co-contraction maneuver then slowly and deliberately raises one foot off the floor while maintaining the bridge position (Fig. 11-22). It is important that the patient does not allow the pelvis to rotate or drop toward the floor. The foot is then returned to the floor and the patient slowly and deliberately raises the other foot and returns it to the floor. This is repeated 10-20 times while maintaining the co-contraction throughout the set.

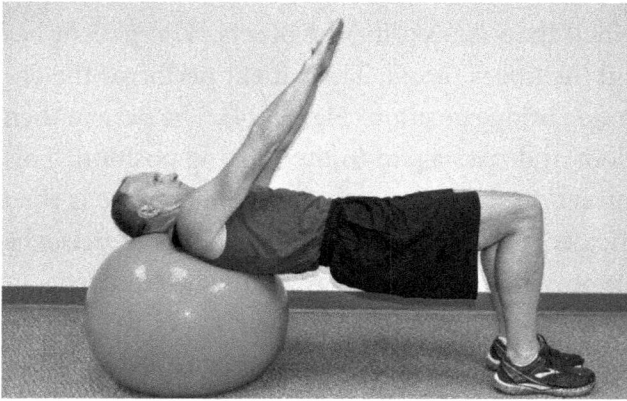

Figure 11-20. Starting position for the Basic Bridge on the exercise ball.

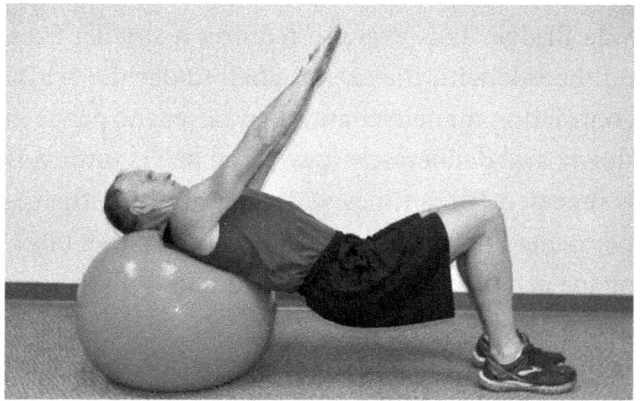

Figure 11-21. Lowering the pelvis toward the floor.

Bridge with Leg Extension: The patient walks out onto the ball and into the bridge position (Fig. 11-20). The patient performs the co-contraction maneuver and then slowly and deliberately extends one leg while maintaining the bridge position (Fig. 11-23). It is important that the patient does not allow the pelvis to rotate or drop toward the floor. The foot is then returned to the floor and the patient slowly and deliberately raises the other foot and returns it to the floor. This is repeated 10-20 times while maintaining the co-contraction throughout the set.

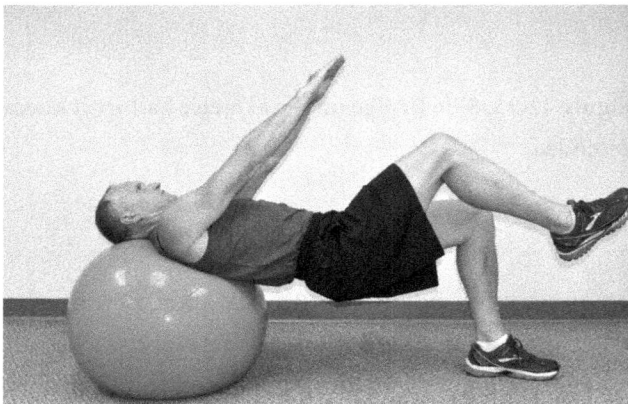

Figure 11-22. Bridge with Steps on the exercise ball.

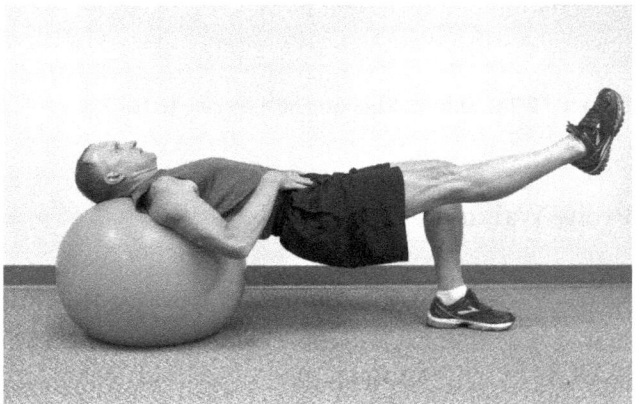

Figure 11-23. Bridge with Leg Extension on the exercise ball.

Side Bridge: This exercise requires a smaller exercise ball than is used for the others. The patient lies on the side with the exercise ball under the armpit and the knees flexed. The patient performs the co-contraction maneuver and then raises the pelvis into a side bridge position (Fig. 11-24). The patient then slowly and deliberately lowers the pelvis toward the floor and rises again to the starting position. This is repeated 10-20 times while maintaining the co-contraction throughout the set. The exercise is then performed on the opposite side. If the patient has difficulty maintaining stability with this exercise, he or she can place one hand on the ball. As the patient improves, the hand can gradually be removed.

In patients who have difficulty performing the bridge track on the ball with the arms extended as shown in Figs. 11-20 through 11-22, the exercise can be made easier by having them place the hands on the hips, as shown in Fig. 11-23.

This exercise can be made more challenging by having the patient perform it with the knees extended (Fig. 11-25).

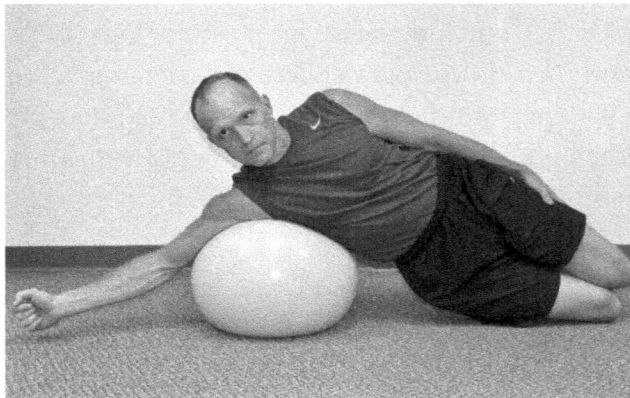

Figure 11-24. Side Bridge on the exercise ball.

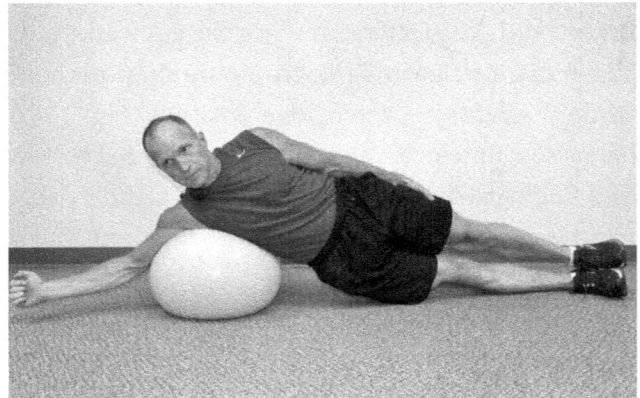

Figure 11-25. Side Bridge on the exercise ball with knees extended.

Prone Walkout Track

Basic Prone Walkout: The patient is face-down in the quadruped position with the abdomen on the ball. The patient performs the co-contraction maneuver and then slowly and deliberately walks out onto the ball until the ball is under the thighs, knees or lower legs, depending on the patient's ability (Fig. 11-26) then returns to the starting position. This is repeated 10-20 times while maintaining the co-contraction throughout the set. The exercise can be made more challenging by having the patient move farther out on the exercise ball.

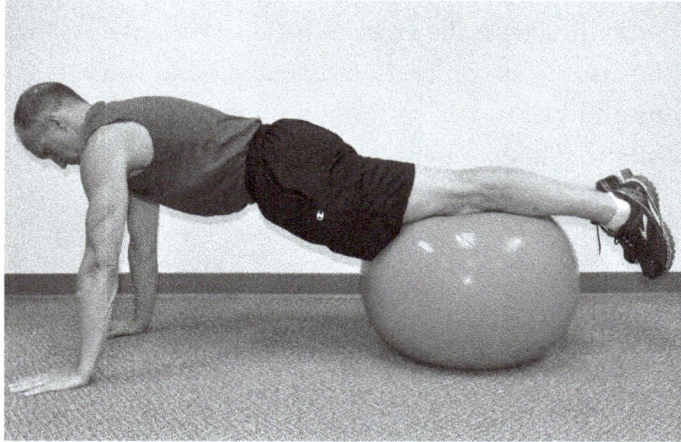

Figure 11-26. End position for the Prone Walkout.

Prone Walkout Pike: The patient is face-down in the quadruped position with the abdomen on the ball. The patient performs the co-contraction maneuver and then slowly and deliberately walks out onto the ball until the ball is under the thighs, knees or lower legs, depending on the patient's ability (Fig. 11-26). The patient then slowly and deliberately flexes the hips (Fig. 11-27). It is important to maintain the lumbar lordosis during the exercise. This is repeated 10-20 times while maintaining the co-contraction throughout the set.

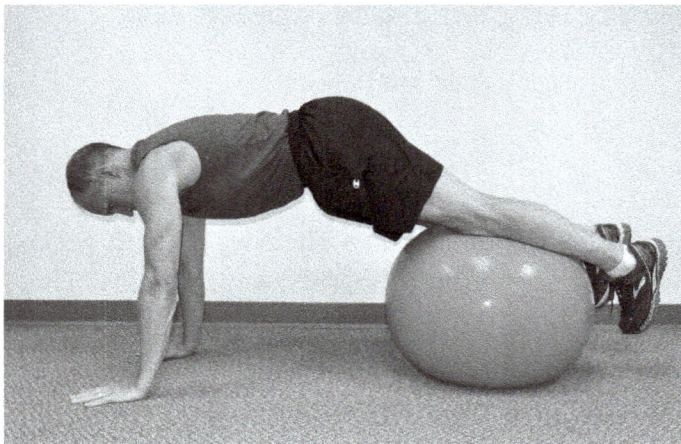

Figure 11-27. Prone Walkout Pike.

Wall Squats: The patient is standing with the exercise ball placed between a wall and the patient's lumbar spine. The patient performs the co-contraction maneuver and then slowly and deliberately squats down by flexing at the hips and knees, maintaining a lumbar lordosis (Fig. 11-28). The patient then returns to the starting position. This is repeated 10-20 times while maintaining the co-contraction throughout the set.

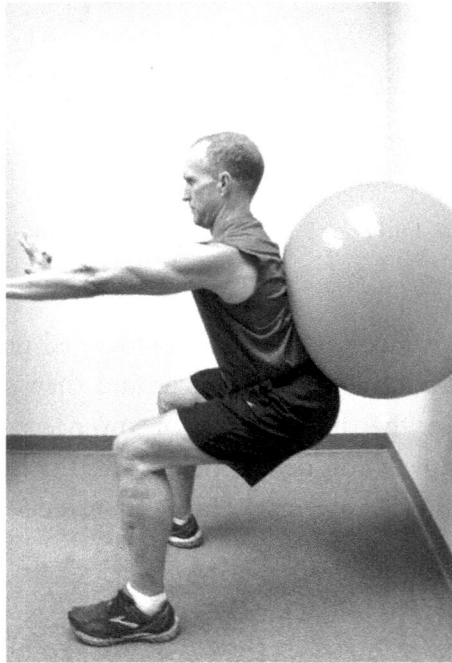

Figure 11-28. Wall Squats.

Crossed Force Couple Exercise for SI Joint Stability: The purpose of this exercise is to train the crossed force couple mechanism that is designed to increase SI joint stability. This mechanism involves the transfer of force from the latissimus dorci through the thoracolumbar fascia to the contralateral gluteus maximus and hamstrings. It requires an apparatus that allows the patient to start at approximately at a 45 degree angle. Many health clubs have such an apparatus. The pad of the apparatus should be placed at the anterior thighs to allow the patient to flex at the hips (Fig. 11-29a). The patient is holding hand weights (the amount of weight will depend on the individual patient's ability) and performs the co-contraction maneuver and then flexes forward at the hips with the arms hanging forward (Fig. 11-29b). It is important that the patient maintain the lumbar lordosis throughout the exercise. The patient

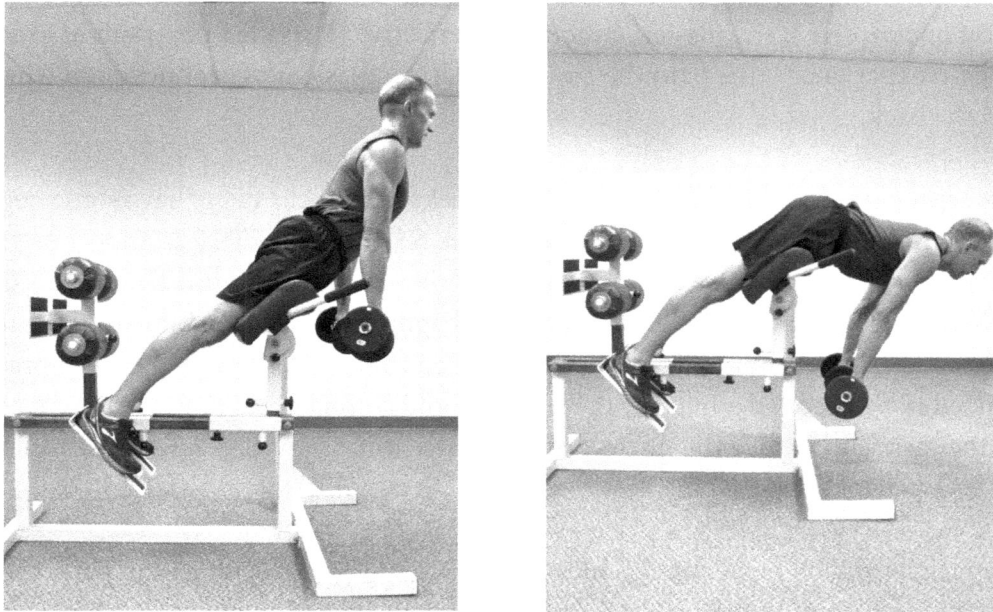

Figure 11-29a and b. Crossed Force Couple exercise for SI joint stability

should flex as far as possible without losing the lordosis. The patient then returns to the starting position. This is repeated 10-20 times while maintaining the co-contraction throughout the set.

In patients with passive instability, unless there are immediate surgical indicators (see Chapter 12) stabilization exercise is a viable option. The purpose of stabilization exercise in these cases is to attempt to train the dynamic stabilization system to compensate for the insufficient holding capacity of the passive elements. Patients with passive instability will often have to be taught to strictly limit end-range movements, particularly flexion. See Chapter 9 for specific recommendations for this.

Nociceptive System Sensitization

The management of nociceptive system sensitization (NSS) focuses on two things: education and graded exposure. As was discussed in detail in Chapter 2, NSS is a state in which the nociceptive system has become hypersensitive and, as a result, nociceptive signals that arise from the periphery have become amplified. In addition, some non-nociceptive signals, such as those from mechanoreceptors, are projected and relayed to the brain as if they were nociceptive. Finally, the central nervous system mechanisms that normally provide modulation of nociceptive signals, i.e., those mechanisms that serve to inhibit nociceptive transmission, become less effective. These factors result in exaggeration of the patient's pain experience – the pain the patient experiences is out of proportion to what is actually happening in the back.

Most patients with pain that lasts longer than a few weeks or months likely have some degree of NSS. The longer the pain lasts, the more firmly established the NSS can become. It is important to remember that NSS is a process that perpetuates the experience of *chronic* pain. So while the process of NSS starts to develop when the pain is acute, it does not take on diagnostic and therapeutic importance until the pain is in the subacute or chronic stage (other than, of course, from the standpoint of prevention). So what is discussed in this section applies to the *subacute* and *chronic* patient, *not* the acute patient. With acute LBDs, the task is to reduce the nociceptive stimulus as quickly and fully as possible in order to *prevent* the development of NSS.

The most important aspect of the management of NSS is education. That is, the patient must understand what NSS is and how it works. This does not mean the patient has to earn a PhD in pain neurophysiology. But it does mean that the patient must understand *why* the pain is so intense and so long lasting. Most important with this is the understanding that, in all likelihood, the reason is entirely different than what the patient thinks. This is the challenging part of the education process.

It is important for patients to understand that the pain they are experiencing is an exaggeration of the painful lesion in the spine. It must be made clear that *this exaggeration is occurring in the lower part of the central nervous system, below the patient's conscious awareness*. In this way it will be clear to the patient that *he or she* is *not* being "accused" of exaggerating the pain consciously.

NSS is not the patient's "fault" – it is not the *patient* who is "hypersensitive", it is the *nociceptive system* (peripheral and central). The patient is simply receiving the exaggerated information from the nociceptive system and interpreting it in the only way he or she knows – as severe pain reflective of a serious problem in the spine. The reason this is important is that many patients' response to education regarding NSS is along the lines of "oh, so you are saying that I am just being overly sensitive" or "you are saying that I am making this up." This defensive reaction is understandable and can be circumvented by a clear explanation that NSS is an *unconscious* and *involuntary* process.

Critically important in the process of educating the patient regarding NSS is for the spine practitioner to engage in the practice of acceptance that was discussed in Chapter 8. That is, the practitioner must accept the patient as he or she is. There will often be a strong temptation for the practitioner to judge the patient. The practitioner understands that the pain the patient is reporting and the pain behavior in which the patient is engaging is inconsistent with actual tissue pathology in the spine. It is often easier to label the patient a "symptom magnifier" or even a "malingerer" than it is to accept the patient and the pain, disability and suffering experience as-is. However, judgment puts up a wall between practitioner and patient and thwarts any effort to educate and empower the patient to transcend the pain and engage in a rewarding life.

For patients in whom NSS forms a prominent aspect of the diagnosis, the pain is very real. It is essential for the practitioner to connect with the patient from that frame of reference and recognize the reality of the patient's pain experience. Once this bond has been formed, the practitioner is then in a position to help the patient out of the downward spiral that can often occur during the development of chronic LBDs.

Education

The initial step in education regarding NSS is to discuss with the patient the importance of looking at and acknowledging his or her pre-conceived notions about what the pain is, what it means and how to overcome it (see the discussion of mindfulness later in this chapter and in Chapter 8). The more self-aware the patient is, the more open he or she will be to challenging those notions that are inaccurate and incompatible with recovery. This is followed by an explanation about pain as a "warning signal."

Most people see pain as a sign that "something is wrong in the body" and, more specifically, that a tissue is "damaged." With this thinking, the sensation of pain serves to warn the person that he or she must avoid any movement, position or activity that is painful, as pursuing these things will "worsen" the "damage." The natural conclusion one draws from this is that any activity that provokes pain must be avoided. Failure to heed the body's warning will lead to further injury. This is a reasonable approach to take with acute pain. Acute pain typically results from injury and acute inflammation of a tissue. When the involved tissue is stretched, compressed or contracted, further inflammation and worsening pain can result. So while complete avoidance of movement and activity is not necessary or beneficial in most cases of acute pain, temporarily modifying activities is often useful. However, chronic pain is different. In most cases, as pain becomes chronic, central nervous system processes gradually come to play a more prominent role and peripheral processes a lesser role. Acutely injured tissues eventually heal and the acute inflammation reduces. So if pain persists and becomes chronic, a different interpretation – and a different approach – must apply.

The spine practitioner might want to engage directly in an education process with the patient regarding the mechanisms of NSS. Or the spine practitioner might choose to point the patient to educational resources for such an understanding. Some examples of this are Explain Pain by Butler and Moseley (see Recommended Reading list) and the simple video entitled "Understanding Pain: What to do about it in less than five minutes." This can be found at:

http://www.the practitionertube.com/watch?v=4b8oB757DKc [accessed 18 July 2013].

Because of the well-engrained notions that most people have about pain, many patients will have a very difficult time accepting an accurate explanation as to the reality of chronic pain. As was stated earlier it is important for the spine practitioner to be mindful of his or her own tendency to judge the patient because of this resistance, and to try to force the patient to understand. The spine practitioner must accept the patient and the resistance. The patient does not *have to* accept an accurate explanation of pain. In fact, the patient does not *have to* overcome the pain at all. Overcoming the pain or holding onto the pain is the patient's choice and this must be respected. Here is where the principles of Motivational Interviewing (see Chapter 9) can come in handy in allowing the patient come to the realization him- or herself that rethinking the nature of chronic pain is beneficial.

The explanation as to the reality of chronic pain is provided purely to help the patient more effectively transcend the pain and return to a productive, fulfilling life. It is useful in this situation to remember that the purpose of the practitioner is as "helper", "coach" and "guide" rather than "dictator" or "authoritarian." In addition, helping the patient understand the pain and to thus start on the road to recovery does not require the patient to fully embrace this new understanding of pain; just being open to the possibility that this is accurate is enough to start taking the next step. "A little willingness" is often all that is needed to start the process.

In many cases of NSS, treating the primary pain generator, addressing dynamic instability with stabilization exercise, educating the patient with regard to the nature of spinal pain and NSS and encouraging the patient from the very start to gradually return to normal activities will be enough to adequately desensitize the nociceptive system and bring about recovery. However, there will be some patients in whom activity intolerances will remain. In these patients, graded exposure is often helpful.

Graded exposure

Graded exposure is the process of introducing movements, positions and activities that provoke the pain to a level that the patient finds unpleasant but tolerable. Particularly useful is an activity that the patient also fears. The best activity to use is one that provokes pain and fear but that the patient is very enthusiastic about returning to. Important however, is to choose an activity that provokes the pain and fear *only to a level that the patient finds unpleasant but that does not provoke severe pain and fear.* This provides the patient an opportunity to use mindfulness techniques (see below and Chapter 8) to fully experience the actual sensation of pain in a non-judgmental way. In addition, it allows for the utilization of the principle of *habituation.*

Habituation is the process by which repetition of a painful stimulus gradually results in modulation of the central nervous system's response to subsequent nociceptive input. What gets many patients with LBDs in trouble is that they try to avoid painful activities. Again, this is certainly sensible in the acute stage of a tissue injury and is a natural tendency in the face of any unpleasant, painful and frightening experience. However, as pain becomes chronic, avoiding painful stimuli actually serves to reinforce the pain experience. Graded exposure allows for gradual introduction of painful stimuli that, first, gives the patient an opportunity to mindfully experience the pain stimulus as an objective, non-judgmental observer and, second, gives the central nervous system an opportunity to habituate to the stimulus.

Often with activities that provoke pain the patient does not experience the actual pain provocation until later in the day or the next day. So when applying graded exposure it is important to monitor the pain provocation over time. If the patient engages in an exercise or activity and reports mild to moderate increase in pain later in the day or the next day it is useful to have the patient try that exercise or activity again and observe the degree of pain provocation that results from that exposure. If the pain is of the same or lesser intensity as after the first application of the exercise or activity, the patient should continue a few more times, always monitoring the degree of discomfort that occurs afterward. As habituation takes place the patient experiences a gradual decrease in discomfort with each application.

The process of graded exposure:

1. Choose an exercise or activity that is most likely to provoke mild to moderate pain. As stated earlier, it is best to choose an activity that the patient enjoys but has been avoiding because of pain. The patient's motivation to go through the graded exposure process is perhaps the most important factor in the success of the effort. It is also best if the activity chosen is one that involves movement (such as jogging or exercising in a gym) rather than a static posture (such as gardening).

2. Explain to the patient the graded exposure process, its purpose and the expected result. It is important to make it clear ahead of time that increased pain during, immediately after, later in the day or the next day is expected, but that it is not expected that this pain will be severe. And it is expected that this increased pain will be short-lived. It is also expected that the second

application of the activity will again provoke pain but of a lesser intensity than was provoked on the first application.

3. Instruct the patient to *observe* what happens during and immediately after the activity as well as later that day and the next day. It is essential that the patient is simply asked to *observe* and not to *evaluate, analyze* or *attempt to interpret* what happens. The patient should observe and experience the actual sensation of pain itself, in isolation of any opinion, judgment or evaluation of the pain. If such opinions, judgments or evaluations should arise, the patient should not try to cease judging or to shut out those thoughts. Rather the patient should observe the thoughts, as well as his or her reactions to the thoughts. This will help the patient develop into a detached, objective observer of the pain stimulus itself as well as of the entire pain, disability and suffering experience. If the patient has difficulty with this, it is often useful to give the sensation of pain non-judgmental characteristics. For example, the patient can be instructed to think about what color the pain would be if it had a color or what the pain would sound like if it had a sound.

4. When applying graded exposure the "green light, yellow light, red light" approach is useful (see Table 11-1). That is, once an exercise or activity is identified that provokes mild to moderate pain and/or fear to a level that somewhat disturbs the patient but is well tolerated, this should be pursued, with careful monitoring as to how the patient feels during and immediately after the exercise or activity, later that day and the next day. If the exercise or activity does not cause any pain at any point between the application and the following day this is a green light to increase the intensity of the stimulus. This can be done by increasing the weight that is lifted during an exercise, increasing the challenge of an exercise or increasing the duration or intensity of the activity. If the initial application of the exercise or activity causes a mild to moderate increase in pain later in the day or the next day to a level that the patient can reasonably tolerate, this is a yellow light, which means the exercise or activity should be applied again with careful monitoring of the result. If the initial application of the exercise or activity markedly increases the pain (or fear), this is a red light which may mean that that exercise or activity should be repeated at a lesser intensity or that the patient is not yet ready for that particular exercise or activity and another should be chosen.

5. On the next office visit (which can be scheduled a few days after the beginning of the process if the patient requires close monitoring or a week after if the practitioner feels the patient can get started on the process him- or herself) the patient and practitioner should discuss the result of the initial steps in the process and plan for further steps.

6. When the patient reaches the point at which the exercise or activity that was used to initiate the graded exposure process can be carried out with little or no pain, the intensity should be increased to a point at which mild to moderate pain is again provoked. As always this should be pain that is unpleasant to the patient but is well tolerated. Then, the same process should be followed, in which the exercise or activity is continued, with observation of the result. This should again be guided by the "green light, yellow light, red light" principle.

7. If a point is reached at which a certain exercise or activity provokes mild to moderate pain, and habituation does not occur with repeated exposure, the patient should be reassessed and an attempt should be made to determine the reason. Diagnosis question #2 can be re-investigated to determine whether there is a residual pain generator that has not been fully resolved (see Chapters 5 and 10). The patient's posture and body mechanics while engaging in the exercise or activity should be assessed to determine whether it is being performed properly. It may well be that a limit has been reached at which the nociceptive system is not willing to habituate further. Obviously this needs to be evaluated on a case-by-case basis.

Table 1. The "green light, yellow light, red light" approach to graded exposure.

Result of exposure to an exercise or activity	Light	Action to be taken
No increased pain during or immediately after the activity No increased pain later that day or the next day	Green	Perform the same exercise or activity again but with greater intensity or duration (e.g., increase weight or challenge of the exercise, increase duration or intensity of the activity)
Mild to moderate pain during or immediately after the activity Mild to moderate pain later in the day or the next day	Yellow	Perform the same exercise or activity again and monitor the result during and immediately after as well as later that day and the next day
Severe pain during or immediately after the activity Severe pain later in the day or the next day	Red	Allow the pain to return to baseline and then decide whether to try a different exercise or activity or the same exercise or activity but at reduced intensity

In the case of a red light situation it is important to make it clear to the patient that the worsening of the pain likely does not reflect "increasing the tissue damage" but rather represents provocation of the nociceptive system to a level that the system is not yet ready to handle. Of course, careful monitoring of potential tissue injury must be carried out throughout the process. However it is very unlikely that mild exercise or normal activity will cause actual tissue damage in a spine that does not currently have an acute injury.

For the primary spine practitioner, exercise can be used for graded exposure. Weight training or even basic floor exercises are useful for this purpose. If a certain exercise causes mild pain, the exercise can be continued as discussed here to see if the pain habituates. This may occur gradually over the course of days or a week.

Also, manipulation and other forms of manual therapy can have a habituating effect on the nociceptive system. It is well known that approximately 1/3 to 1/2 of patients who are treated with manipulation will experience increased pain after the first and/or second treatment session. The pain almost always resolves within 24-48 hours. This is likely a habituation response and should not be considered an "adverse reaction" but a necessary and therapeutic response on the part of the nociceptive system.

The end range loading protocols discussed in Chapter 5 and 10 also likely involve graded exposure and desensitization of the nociceptive system. Typically, the direction of movement that leads to centralization and abolishment of the pain is one that initially *provokes* the pain. With repeated movements the pain gradually centralizes and/or decreases in intensity. It is likely that part of the mechanism of this response is habituation. Worth noting here is that, if these movements were to be avoided in order to avoid "provoking" the pain, the patient would be denied the very maneuver that would bring about resolution of the pain!

It is important for the practitioner to take great care during the graded exposure process not to exacerbate the NSS. Three important principles apply to this:

1. It must be clear to the patient that in the chronic stage pain provocation as a result of movement or positioning is almost always a result of facilitation of the already-sensitized nociceptive system and is not reflective of "tissue "damage" (however, *it is always up to the practitioner to distinguish between pain from NSS and true tissue-related pain*). If the patient does not "get it" and has a strong belief that pain is reflective of "damage" the graded exposure approach is likely to worsen both pain and emotional distress. Therefore it should *not* be pursued until and unless the patient is ready.

2. Pain that is provoked during the graded exposure process must be mild or moderate and well-tolerated by the patient. There is nothing to be gained by "working through" severe pain, even if the patient desires to do this.

3. It must be clear to the patient that the purpose of graded exposure is to de-sensitize the nociceptive system in order to promote greater activity tolerance. The purpose is *not* to "make the pain go away." Focusing on "making the pain go away" will tend to *increase* NSS rather than promote desensitization and improved activity tolerance.

Psychological Factors

For the primary spine practitioner the management of psychological factors is more contextual than it is literal. It does not involve engaging in detailed and time-consuming psychotherapy sessions. It involves creating a relationship-centered environment that focuses on the principles of Cognitive-Behavioral Therapy and Acceptance and Commitment Therapy, which includes Mindfulness. These principles were discussed in detail in Chapter 8. While there are specific techniques that are useful to the spine practitioner in addressing psychological factors, most important is the *context in which the entire management strategy is employed*. In other words, as was discussed in chapter 8, all communication, verbal and non-verbal, explicit and implicit, between the practitioner and the patient, should occur in a context in which messages that promote recovery permeate the entire management process. These messages should revolve around:

1. Acceptance: First and foremost this means the practitioner accepting the patient as-is and then helping the patient accept the present situation as a starting point for overcoming the LBD.

2. The realities of LBDs: That is, LBDs can be very painful and can be *temporarily* disabling but the problem does not have to be a fearsome catastrophe. In the vast majority of cases the pain, as severe as it appears to be, is not reflective of serious spine pathology and in almost all cases can be effectively managed.

3. There is a great deal the patient can do to overcome the problem as well as to lessen the likelihood of recurrence. And there is much the patient can do to deal with recurrences if they do arise.

4. Developing severe emotional reactions to the problem is very understandable. This is a common process that we all go through in the face of painful or frightening experiences. This is *not* an indication that the patient is "weak"; it is an indication that the patient is a normal human being.

5. However some emotional reactions can interfere with recovery. Together the spine practitioner and patient can identify and address these.

6. NSS can cause the problem to *appear to be* more severe than it actually is. Understanding this will aid in recovery.

7. The best way deal with a LBD is to place the focus on *overcoming* the problem as opposed to trying to *get the pain to go away*. In fact, focusing on *getting the pain to go away* actually perpetuates the pain, disability and suffering experience.

8. However it is common for people, in the face of any problem, to want the problem to "just go away." This is normal. But because this desire can interfere with recovery it is important to acknowledge it and then get on with the business of overcoming the problem.

Again, these concepts were covered in greater detail in chapter 8. They are reiterated here as a reminder that these messages must permeate everything the spine practitioner does and must inform all communication between practitioner and patient.

Acceptance and transcendence *versus* "control"

A great deal of emphasis in spine care is placed on "pain control." The focus of pain control is the practitioner applying methods and techniques to "control" the pain or teaching the patient ways in which he or she can "control" the pain. This is not a problem *per* se. As has been discussed throughout this book, teaching the patient methods of decreasing pain intensity is a very powerful means by which self-efficacy can be promoted. However, the practitioner has to be careful about how this is communicated to the patient. It is critical to remember that the primary focus of spine care is not *pain*, it is *suffering*. That is, the reason patients seek care for a LBD is not because of they have a focus of nociception somewhere in the spine, it is because they are *suffering*, partly as a result of that nociceptive focus. So while engaging in processes that reduce the intensity of the nociceptive focus (i.e., that address the findings of diagnostic question #2 – see Chapter 10) is appropriate and useful these methods must be applied in the context of *acceptance*. The way to truly overcome a LBD is to accept its presence (as opposed to wishing it would go away) and then to engage in the process of treating it and limiting the likelihood of recurrence. By focusing on "control" in isolation from "acceptance" the spine practitioner runs the risk of reinforcing the thinking that a LBD is a fearsome catastrophe, a vicious monster that must be "controlled" or else it will become "out of control." On the other hand, through acceptance the patient can relax and let go of the need to "make the pain go away" and calmly go about the process of rising above the pain and taking charge of his or her life, rather than allowing the pain to be in charge. Then, given the fact that the pain itself is an unpleasant sensation, the patient can go about reducing its intensity through self-care strategies.

The proper communication of acceptance

It is important that acceptance is communicated to the patient as it relates to the present moment. It is common for patients' reaction to the concept of acceptance to be along the lines of "OK, so you are saying that I have to accept that I will be in pain the rest of my life." This is *not* what acceptance is. Acceptance applies only to *right now*. That is, if the patient is going to successfully overcome the LBD, it is essential that he or she accept the presence of the pain *now, in this moment*, to acknowledge the pain and even to fully experience the pain. Only then will the patient be in the position to, not "defeat" the pain but transcend it, move beyond it and become independent of the presence or absence of pain at any given time. Thus it is essential that the practitioner help the patient make the distinction between accepting the pain in the present moment and "accepting that this pain is never going to go away." As is discussed throughout this book, "making the pain go away" is not the focus of quality spine care. The focus of quality spine care is helping the patient move beyond the presence or absence of pain to live according to his or her values. Reducing pain intensity, and even eliminating pain for extended periods of time, is certainly possible in the majority of patients. But it is critical that the principle of "overcoming" as opposed to "getting rid of" the pain informs the patient management process in order to avoid the emotional roller coaster ride that can result from the natural fluctuations that occur with pain.

Acceptance is particularly important in patients in whom perceived injustice is a major perpetuating factor. As was discussed in Chapter 2, this is particularly important in patients whose LBD began following a work-related incident, a motor vehicle collision or a slip-and-fall incident in which someone else is perceived to be "at fault." Thoughts related to "if he (or she) only knew how much I am suffering", "that person has ruined my life" and (usually unconscious) "I will show them by remaining disabled" can be pervasive in these patients. Acceptance is critical if these patients are going to overcome the pain, disability and suffering.

As is always the case, helping a patient affected by perceived injustice to accept starts with the *practitioner* accepting the *patient* and all his or her perceptions and judgments. Then, it is important for the practitioner to make it clear to the patient that he or she has the right* to hold on to the pain, disability and suffering experience. The patient is allowed to continue suffering and the practitioner will not judge the patient as "right" or "wrong", "good" or "bad." Next, an exploration can take place of *what* the patient is suffering *from*. In most cases it is not the *pain* it is the *blame* that is contributing greatest to the suffering. The question then should arise, "What is most important to you in your life?", "What are your deepest held values?" and "Does blaming the perceived perpetrator *enhance* or *interfere with* your ability to live your life according to your values?" Care should be taken to keep this conversation on the patient's suffering and its true causes as there will be a tendency for some patients to respond first with the thought "Yes, I want to live my life according to my values but because of that person's negligence, now I can't!" Again, redirecting the conversation to what is truly causing the patient's suffering will help him or her see that it is not the "injury" that is the problem (injuries heal in a relatively short period of time) but the perpetuating factors, one of the most important of which is the perceived injustice. This is under the patient's control and the patient has the ability to make a different choice. However, again, the patient does not "have to" make a different choice. He or she can remain in suffering. But the patient may want consider whether making a different choice (e.g., to let go of blame) might lead to a more fulfilling life.

*This "right" is a personal "right" and not necessarily a legal one. Whether the patient has the "right" to collect disability payments or awards is a completely separate issue from the practitioner's communication with the patient with regard to acceptance. These concepts should not be confused and because the practitioner is taking this approach does not mean that he or she is bound to sign disability statements.

Techniques of mindfulness that can be applied in primary spine care

Mindfulness is a method by which the patient is taught to become an objective observer of the pain. This allows the patient to "look at" his or her suffering. Usually the patient discovers that what is causing the suffering is much different than what he or she thought. A good way to start this process is by encouraging the patient to experience the actual sensation of nociception. That is, to fully experience the sensation itself, independent of any thoughts, beliefs, judgments or cognitions about the pain.

This is one of the powerful mechanisms behind the McKenzie approach (i.e., end range loading looking for centralization or reduction of pain – see Chapters 5 and 10). During the process of the end range loading examination the patient is asked to *observe* the pain and to *report what it is doing*. The process does not involve asking the patient to report all of the things he or she thinks the pain means. The patient is simply asked to observe the actual sensation itself. This can be done not only during the end range loading portion of the examination but during the entire part of the examination that seeks an answer to diagnostic question #2. That is, as pain provocation maneuvers are applied, the patient is asked to observe the symptomatic response to the maneuver. The practitioner can identify whether the patient is actually doing this or is engaging in a response pattern that clearly indicates *judgments about* the pain rather than *observation* of the actual sensation. When this occurs the practitioner can gently and non-judgmentally listen to the patient and then ask "what do you feel when I do this?", "where do you feel it?" and "is this a familiar sensation – does it reproduce the pain you are seeing me for?" This is the first step toward teaching the patient mindfulness. It is an example of what was stated earlier regarding the fact that it is not necessary for the spine practitioner to undergo a detailed and time-consuming education or psychotherapy process. Addressing the psychological factors that perpetuate suffering in patients with spine related disorders (SRDs) can be done quite effectively by incorporating simple but consistently applied methods during the normal course of examination and treatment.

It may appear that the process of addressing the psychological factors that perpetuate LBDs is too time-consuming for application in a primary spine care setting. However this need not be the case. As has been emphasized throughout this book, the messages of Cog-B and ACT should permeate all communications between the spine practitioner and the patient. There is no need to spend a great deal of time with patients who have difficulty understanding the concepts. In these cases there are many resources available to which the spine practitioner can direct the patient for more intensive coverage of these topics. Some examples are provided in the Recommended Reading list as well as in Table 11-2.

Table 2. Resources to which the spine practitioner can direct the patient for education regarding pain and psychological methods for overcoming LBDs

Resource	Purpose
Butler DS, Moseley GL. Explain Pain. Adelaide, Australia: Noigroup Publications, 2003.	Understanding pain physiology and psychology, particularly with regard to central pain hypersensitivity.
Hayes SC, Smith S. Get Out of Your Mind and Into Your Life. The New Acceptance and Commitment Therapy. Oakland; New Harbinger Publications, 2005.	Practical workbook on the general application of principles of Acceptance and Commitment Therapy.

Dahl J, Lundgren T. Living Beyond Your Pain. Oakland; New Harbinger Publications, 2006.	Practical workbook on the application of principles of Acceptance and Commitment Therapy for chronic pain.
Kabat-Zinn J. Mindfulness Meditation for Pain Relief: Guided Practices for Reclaiming Your Body and Your Life. Audio CD, 2009.	Application of principles of mindfulness for pain.
If Opioids Have Not Relieved Your Chronic Pain. Webility [www.webility.md]	Information on opioid medications and chronic pain.
Hanscom, D. Back in Control: A Spine Surgeon's Roadmap Out of Chronic Pain. Seattle, WA: Vertus Press, 2012.	Helping patients understand how people fall into the chronic pain trap and how to navigate the way out.
Schubiner H, Betzold M. Unlearn Your Pain, 2nd ed. Pleasant Ridge, MI: Mind Body Publishing, 2012.	Discussion of the "Mind-Body Syndrome" with instruction for patients on how to reprogram the central nervous system to "unlearn" the chronic pain cycle.
Thernstrom, M. The Pain Chronicle: Cures, Myths, Mysteries, Prayers, Diaries, Brain Scans, Healing and the Science of Suffering. New York: Farrar, Straus and Giroux publishers, 2010.	Information for patients with chronic pain as well as their loved ones.
Botehlho, Rick. Motivate Healthy Habits: stepping stones to lasting change. Rochester, NY: MHH Publications, 2000.	Information and methods for making positive behavioral change.

In cases in which the psychological processes that perpetuate LBDs are so well established that the basic primary-level approaches discussed here are not effective in helping the patient overcome the problem, it is best to refer the patient for more intensive intervention. This may involve referral to a psychologist trained the application of Cognitive Behavioral Therapy and/or Acceptance and Commitment Therapy. Or it may involve referral to a reputable facility for intensive multidisciplinary chronic pain management (see Chapter 12). It is important in these situations for the primary spine practitioner to follow up periodically with the patient to monitor his or her progress and to troubleshoot any problems that arise.

As discussed in Chapter 2, depression can be a maladaptive psychological response to a LBD or it can be a diagnosable condition that is often part of a generalized pattern of ill-health that can include obesity, metabolic syndrome, type II diabetes, hypertension and other risk factors for stroke, and chronic LBD. In this case, more comprehensive management may be required. Much of the management can be provided directly by the spine practitioner, through effective treatment for the LBD as well through facilitating diet and lifestyle changes known to address inflammation and mood disturbance (see Chapter 9). However it is important for the spine practitioner to coordinate with the patient's primary care practitioner with these patients.

Diagnostic question #3 allows the practitioner to look at the patient as a whole and identify the neurophysiological and psychological factors that contribute to the pain, disability and suffering experience. Of utmost importance is helping patients find the inner ability to overcome these factors themselves through exercise, gradual return to normal activities, healthy psychological practices and a greater understanding of pain.

Recommended Reading

Butler DS, Moseley GL. Explain Pain. Adelaide, Australia: Noigroup Publications, 2003.

Dahl J, Lundgren T. Living Beyond Your Pain. Oakland; New Harbinger Publications, 2006.

Lee D. The Pelvic Girdle. 4th Ed. Edinburgh, Churchill Livingstone, 2011.

Liebenson, C. (Ed.), Rehabilitation of the Spine: a Practitioner's Manual, 2nd Ed. Baltimore, Lippincott/Williams and Wilkins, 2006.

McGill S. Low Back Disorders. Evidence-Based Prevention and Rehabilitation. Champaign, IL: Human Kinetics; 2002.

Rennefeld C, Wiech K, Schoell ED, Lorenz J, Bingel U. Habituation to pain: further support for a central component. Pain 2010;148(3):503-8.

Richardson C, Hodges P, Hides J. Therapeutic Exercise for Lumbopelvic Stabilization. A Motor Control Approach for the Treatment and Prevention of Low Back Pain. 2nd Ed. Edinburgh, Churchill Livingstone, 2004.

• CHAPTER 12 •

Maximum Medical Improvement, Aftercare and Clinical Decisions Regarding Patients Who Do Not Improve

Maximum Medical Improvement

"Maximum Medical Improvement" is defined by the 6th Edition of the AMA Guides for Permanent Impairment (see Recommended Reading list) as "a status where patients are as good as they are going to be from the medical and surgical treatment available to them. It can also be conceptualized as a date from which further recovery or deterioration is not anticipated, although over time (beyond 12 months) there may be some expected change." Making this official determination is important in medicolegal circumstances such as with auto accident, slip-and-fall and work-related low back disorders (LBDs). But even in patients with no medicolegal involvement, it is important to determine the point at which structured clinical care should stop. This is not always straightforward and is highly individual. There are some patients in whom periodic follow-up visits may be required over the course of a few months to reinforce the home exercise program and self-care strategies as well as to maintain healthy cognitions and beliefs.

Nonetheless, in the vast majority of cases there reaches a point at which no further treatment is necessary or at which no further treatment can be expected to bring about additional functional improvement. Many times this results from the patient having become symptom-free and/or having returned to all usual activities of daily living. In other cases there may be a point at which the patient is still symptomatic and/or has not reached a level of functional improvement that is satisfactory (at least at present) but that further improvement or deterioration in the condition is not going to occur for the foreseeable future. In still others there may be residual symptoms, but the patient has reached a point at which the achieved functional level can be maintained and the symptoms self-treated with exercises and other strategies. Of course, variations of these situations are often seen. In any case, this is the point at which practitioner-generated treatment should cease.

The determination of the endpoint of care is an art and there are no hard-and-fast rules in making this determination. At times a "trial and error" process may be required. However there are some general principles that can provide guidance:

1. The endpoint of clinical care should not be determined solely on the basis of the presence or absence of symptoms. In many cases patients with LBDs are able to reach a point of being symptom-free. However there are some cases in which being symptom-free is not possible, but is also not necessary in order for the patient to live a fulfilling life according to his or her values. In most patients it is not necessary to continue to apply practitioner-driven treatment until the patient is completely free of symptoms. From the initial patient-practitioner encounter patients should be taught exercises and self-care strategies that are designed to reduce symptoms and improve functional abilities. The patient should be prepared to be released from care even if there are residual symptoms, provided the patient is appropriately educated.

2. The patient's functional abilities should be the primary determiner of improvement. Whether the patient is ready to be released from care should be determined primarily by the extent to which he or she has successfully returned to a productive and fulfilling life. Of course, as was discussed regarding symptoms, in many cases the patient can be appropriately released from care before this goal has been completely met. In most cases, once a certain level of functional improvement has occurred, patients can continue the improvement on their own with the exercises and self-management strategies they have been taught and with the sense of empowerment and self-efficacy they have gained. In determining the endpoint of care, it is important to consider not only the degree to which the patient has returned to normal activities but also the likelihood of continued improvement with self-care.

3. Often the most critical functional activity is work. Therefore, whether the patient has returned to meaningful employment is one of the most important factors in determining readiness for release from care. This does not mean that care should automatically cease once return to work has been achieved. As discussed in Chapter 8 it is common for symptoms to worsen upon initial return to work, particularly in patients whose LBD began at work. Therefore, most patients need to be guided through this process. A transition period between successful return to work and release from a formal practitioner-driven care is important for this purpose.

4. Shared decision making should be utilized in determining the endpoint of care. This arises from discussion between the spine practitioner and the patient, always keeping in mind the goal of maximizing patient empowerment and self-efficacy and minimizing patient dependency.

Some patients are fearful of having care cease while others will be enthusiastic about moving on to self-care. While the patient's perceived readiness should be strongly considered, it is essential that the practitioner provide leadership in making this determination. This means understanding and acknowledging the patient's fears, uncertainties, confidence level and expectations regarding being released from care. Oftentimes the practitioner has to challenge the patient's beliefs in this regard.

5. The concept of "begin with the end in mind" (to quote Steven Covey) is useful. All communication with the patient, from the very first encounter, should be in preparation for release from practitioner-driven care. This is part of self-efficacy building as it places in the patient's mind the expectation that, ultimately, everything that is required to overcome the problem is within the patient's capability.

6. Patient empowerment should always be the top priority. As has been discussed throughout this book, the primary goal in the management of all patients with LBDs should be to help the patient return to as productive and fulfilling a life as possible, a life that is consistent with his or her core values. This means empowering the patient to take charge of the problem and raising the patient's confidence (i.e., self-efficacy). Therefore, the determination of the endpoint of practitioner-driven care should be made on the basis of how well the patient is able to self-manage any remaining symptoms and engage in normal activities.

7. Some spine practitioners regularly place patients on "maintenance care", i.e., a routine schedule of treatments in the absence of symptoms or disability for the purpose of "maintaining" the pain-free and disability-free state. This should be avoided. Again, as has been emphasized throughout book, the essence of effective primary spine care is patient empowerment and the bolstering of patient self-efficacy. Most patients can "maintain" their own improvement through simple things they can do for themselves, without dependency on practitioners to "maintain" their improvement for them. It is important for the practitioner to set aside his or her "philosophy" or self-interest and to always hold patient welfare first and foremost.

8. There are times in which continuing to see doctors and therapists in search of a solution to the LBD actually perpetuates the patient's ongoing pain, disability and suffering experience. It is essential for the spine practitioner to recognize this and to communicate with the patient that it may be best to stop receiving care and to move on with life. Having created an environment of acceptance, mindfulness and self-care from the beginning makes this far easier in most cases. Nonetheless, ceasing treatment of a patient who continues to experience pain is one of the most

difficult things for a caring clinician to do. Naturally, health practitioners see themselves as being in the business of "helping sick people get well" and the natural inclination is to continue seeking to end the patient's suffering, taking as much time and effort (and expense, as it turns out) as necessary. However, there are times when the most compassionate thing is teach the patient how to best cope with condition and allow the patient to detach from the treatment process. Any management strategy naturally places a certain degree of focus on the patient's pain and, as a result, can reach a point at which the process merely reinforces the pain experience and pain behavior, leading to dependency and despair. Knowing when to end treatment in this situation is a fine art and one that requires a great deal of compassion and courage on the part of the clinician.

Aftercare

Once the endpoint of care has been determined it is important that the patient is left with home exercises, ergonomic and postural advice, self-care strategies and an understanding of the nature of LBDs. LBDs tend to recur over time, though in most instances there are actions the patient can take to limit the frequency of recurrences. Stabilization exercises, if continued after resolution of the LBD, are useful for this. All patients should be left with at least a basic stabilization exercise program. Those in whom diagnostic question #3 revealed significant signs of dynamic instability should be on a more extensive stabilization program. The prone extension exercise (see Chapter 5 and Figure 5-7) is also useful to limit the frequency of recurrences, provided it does not cause peripheralization of symptoms. One set of 10-15 repetitions is adequate for this purpose. Also, teaching patients to limit end range flexion (see Chapter 9) can reduce the frequency of recurrences.

Most important is for the patient to leave the active management process with confidence in his or her ability to effectively deal with any recurrence that may arise. To maximize this confidence it is important that the patient:

1. Has a clear understanding that a LBD is not a fearsome catastrophe but rather a painful inconvenience that can be overcome.

2. Has been taught self-care strategies to employ if and when recurrence of pain arises. These strategies should be designed to resolve the problem relatively quickly without the need for

professional care. In patients with disc derangement (diagnostic question #2) this is particularly easy as they will have already been taught exercises in the Direction of Benefit that had been determined by the end range loading exam (see Chapter 5). If disc derangement recurs, often the same exercise that resolved the problem the first time will be useful for recurrence. Patients with joint dysfunction (diagnostic question #2) should be instructed to use the self-mobilization exercises they were taught at the beginning of the management process to self-treat recurrences (see Chapter 10).

3. Knows to return to the spine practitioner if a recurrence develops that he or she is not able to resolve with self-care. Typically acute recurrences are relatively easy to self-treat. However if the patient is not able to take care of the problem within a few days to a week, particularly if the problem is interfering with important and valued activities, a return visit to the practitioner is indicated.

What if the patient does not respond to an adequate trial of treatment?

If clinically meaningful improvement has not occurred by the re-examination, the practitioner should re-think the diagnosis as well as the management strategy and consider a change. This thought process should consider the following possibilities:

1. The diagnosis is not correct.

2. The diagnosis is partly correct but there are factors contributing to the patient's pain, disability and suffering experience that had not previously been detected or addressed.

3. The diagnosis is correct but the treatment being applied is not the best one in that particular case.

4. The diagnosis and treatment are appropriate but there are perpetuating factors, involving activities of daily living, ergonomics, "stress" or other issues that are interfering with recovery.

5. The patient has not been compliant with exercise and self-care recommendations.

Therefore, the re-examination process should focus on investigating these possibilities and making alterations accordingly. This involves:

1. Re-applying the CRISP™ protocols by repeating the history and examination to confirm or revise the diagnosis.

2. If the diagnosis appears to be correct, considering alternate treatments designed to address that diagnosis.

3. Discussing with the patient work, home and recreational behavior (or beliefs) to determine whether potential perpetuating factors can be uncovered.

4. Reviewing the exercise and self-care strategies to determine the patient's level of compliance or whether they are being performed as directed.

5. Asking the patient if he or she has any ideas as to why improvement has not occurred.

In most patients, making alterations in the management strategy will successfully put them on the path to recovery. However there will be some patients whose pain, disability and suffering experience remains recalcitrant. The CRISP™ protocols provide guidance in making decisions in these cases. There are various referral channels that can be considered depending on the specific findings in each patient. The answers to the three questions of diagnosis can help guide decision making.

Further diagnostic evaluation

Diagnostic question #1 (Do the presenting symptoms reflect a visceral disorder, or a serious or potentially life-threatening illness?):

If upon repeating the history and examination there appear to be significant signs and/or symptoms that may suggest a visceral disorder or a potentially serious or life-threatening condition, investigation should be carried out or referral should be made either to the patient's primary care practitioner or to an appropriate specialist. The specific actions that are taken will depend on the case, but the reader should refer to Chapter 4 for particulars regarding further investigation. Even in the absence of specific findings related to diagnostic question #1, MRI should be considered in a patient who does not respond within 4-6 weeks of care.

As was discussed in Chapter 4, just prior to the writing of this book information came to light suggesting that certain individuals with chronic LBDs may have infection within the disc, most commonly involving the anaerobic bacterium *Propionibacterium acnes* that leads to inflammation of the vertebral bodies (see Albert, et al in Recommended Reading list). In these patients, Modic type 1 change can be seen on MRI (see Fig. 4-1). However, many asymptomatic individuals have Modic type 1 change on MRI and clinical experience suggests that many patients with LBDs who have Modic type 1 change seem to respond quite well to management according to the CRISP™ protocols. So it should not be assumed that Modic type 1 change is necessarily reflective of symptomatic infection, or that this finding has any particular clinical relevance. It is not known whether there are historical or examination findings that can help determine the clinical relevance of Modic 1 change in any individual patient.

Diagnostic question #2 (Where is the pain coming from?):

In patients with suspected disc pain, discogram is considered by many to be the gold standard for diagnosis however it must be noted that false positives are common, particularly in patients with significant psychological distress. In addition, discogram can accelerate disc degeneration or disc herniation in some individuals. So this test is not recommended for use by the primary spine practitioner.

As discussed in Chapter 5, discoblock shows promise as a test to confirm the presence of disc pain, however further research is needed before it can be considered a viable option.

In patients in whom lumbar facet or sacroiliac joint pain is suspected, diagnostic joint injection (joint block) is a consideration. Significant pain improvement following injection suggests that the injected joint is the pain generator. The ideal utilization of diagnostic blocks is one in which a double block approach is taken. With this, a short-acting analgesic substance, such as lidocaine, is injected and if this is followed by short-term pain improvement, a longer acting analgesic substance, such as bupivacaine, is used. If this injection is then followed by longer-duration relief, the painful joint has been identified. This double-block approach is not always practical, however. A single block approach is more time- and cost-effective. To have confidence that the pain-generating joint has been identified, there should be at least 80% improvement in pain intensity. This should be measured with a Numeric Rating Scale (see Chapter 7) that the patient completes just prior to the injection, then again within a day or two after the injection. Relying on recall (i.e., "please rate the intensity of your pain now as compared to before the injection" or "how much has your pain improved since receiving the injection") is not recommended.

As discussed in Chapter 5, epidural steroid injection (ESI) or nerve root block can sometimes be useful to identify whether the nerve root is the primary pain generator. As with other diagnostic injections, at least 80% improvement in pain, as measured with pre- and post-procedure pain scales, should be the criterion for a positive test.

There is currently no objective test that allows for the confirmation of myofascial pain.

Diagnostic question #3 (What is happening with this person as a whole that would cause the pain experience to develop and persist?):

There is no objective test that identifies the presence of dynamic instability. In patients who do not respond to primary spine care and have clinical indications that suggest the possibility of passive instability (trauma severe enough to cause ligamentous disruption or who have degenerative spondylolisthesis – see Chapter 6), flexion-extension radiographs are indicated.

With suspected nociceptive system sensitization (NSS), functional magnetic resonance imaging (fMRI) holds promise as a confirmatory test in patients. This imaging technique allows visualization of blood flow in areas of the brain that are involved in the experience of pain. In the vast majority of patients, NSS can be suspected clinically without the need for advance testing. Currently fMRI is a useful research tool and further investigation will be helpful in identifying those circumstances in which this tool can be helpful diagnostically.

In patients in whom it is suspected that the psychological factors are the most important features interfering with recovery, it is best to refer the patient to a psychologist or other behavioral health practitioner. This should preferably be one trained and experienced in Cognitive-Behavioral Therapy and/or Acceptance and Commitment Therapy and who has experience evaluating pain patients.

Clinical Decision Making Regarding Invasive Procedures

The majority of patients with LBDs can be managed at the primary spine care level without the need for referral. However, a small percentage requires testing and/or treatment beyond primary spine care. It is important for the primary spine practitioner to have an evidence-based clinical reasoning process by which to make referral decisions. As with primary spine care, the CRISP™ protocols provide guidance with these decisions.

Diagnostic question #1 (Do the presenting symptoms reflect a visceral disorder, or a serious or potentially life-threatening illness?)

In patients with Modic type I change on MRI who do not respond to an adequate trial of management and in whom the practitioner has gone through the steps discussed previously regarding reconsideration of the diagnosis and management strategy, antibiotic therapy may be one consideration (see Albert, et al in Recommended Reading list). At the time of this writing, additional research is needed to clarify whether this is a useful management option. If further investigation confirms the usefulness of antibiotic therapy in this select group of patients, this will be of benefit in the primary care of LBDs as these patients are often considered candidates for fusion surgery. Therefore, referral for antibiotic therapy may prove to be a viable alternative to fusion.

Diagnostic question #2 (Where is the pain coming from?)

Disc derangement

It is extremely uncommon for patients who exhibit clear centralization or improvement in symptoms with a detailed end range loading examination (see Chapter 5) to fail primary management. In those few whose problem does not resolve on the primary level, perpetuating factors (i.e., factors related to diagnostic question #3) should be examined carefully. However patients with chronic, nonresponsive pain that is thought to be arising from the disc are often considered fusion candidates.

Fusion surgery in this patient population is controversial. Whereas in patients who exhibit clear evidence of passive instability the need for fusion is more straight forward, it is not known whether and in whom fusion is indicated in patients without frank passive instability. Further, the complication and reoperation rates can be as high as 18% and 22%, respectively (see Airaksinen, et al in Recommended Reading list). Patients who benefit often have lasting improvement but those who do not are often left with severe pain, disability and suffering well beyond pre-surgical levels. Therefore, referral for consideration of fusion should be made only after non-surgical management has been completely exhausted. Further it is often useful for a shared decision making process to take place between the patient, the primary spine practitioner and the surgeon prior to consideration of fusion.

Joint dysfunction

In patients with confirmed facet or sacroiliac pain who do not respond to primary spine care, therapeutic injections or radiofrequency neurotomy can be considered (see Chapter 10). It is uncommon for patients to experience long-term relief with joint injections, however occasionally certain patients do experience extended benefit. In patients with confirmed facet pain who do not experience long-term benefit to joint injection, medial branch block should be performed (see Chapters 5 and 10). If this is positive, radiofrequency neurotomy can be considered. As with injections, radiofrequency neurotomy is "hit or miss", that is, some patients experience benefit and others do not. In addition, the duration of improvement is variable and is not usually permanent. Therefore, careful clinical reasoning and shared decision making, in light of the entire clinical picture presented by the CRISP™ protocols as well as the patient's values, should be used in making the recommendation.

Radiculopathy

As discussed in Chapter 10, ESI is a therapeutic option in patients with painful radiculopathy. The majority of patients with radiculopathy do not need ESI but there are certain circumstances in which this method is very useful.

ESI is most beneficial in patients with acute radiculopathy, as this is when nerve root inflammation plays the most prominent role in pain generation. In general, the more chronic the radicular pain, the less beneficial ESI becomes. Therefore, ESI should be considered in patients with acute radiculopathy that is so painful and immobilizing that active treatment cannot be instituted. The purpose of ESI (or NSAIDs and oral steroids) in patients with acute radiculopathy is to rapidly reduce inflammation and thus to reduce pain. This effect is temporary. However, the temporary reduction of inflammation and pain allows the spine practitioner to more rapidly transition the patient to more active treatments that are designed to bring about lasting benefits in terms of symptom reduction, coping, self-efficacy and functional restoration.

There are some patients in whom ESI is sufficient to resolve the radicular pain with very little need for any other treatment. In others, ESI can reduce the radicular pain enough to allow the primary spine practitioner to apply treatment to other possible pain generators, such as the disc, and/or to more expeditiously start addressing issues related diagnostic question #3, such as dynamic instability or psychological processes.

It is common for practitioners who perform ESIs to recommend a "series of three", i.e., to recommend pre-scheduling three injections over a period of days, weeks or months. This is not supported by the evidence. It is important for the primary spine practitioner to utilize ESI referrals properly. This means obtaining one ESI and then following up with the patient a few days to a week later. The practitioner should evaluate the patient's symptomatic response to this injection, particularly in light of whether sufficient pain improvement has occurred that allows transition to more active treatments. If such a response has occurred, no additional injections need be performed. If partial improvement has occurred after the initial injection, but not enough to allow transition to more active treatments, a second injection should be considered and the practitioner should again follow up with the patient to determine readiness for active treatments. If no improvement occurs after the initial injection, the practitioner should have a discussion with the patient regarding the possibility of obtaining a second injection. There are some cases in which no improvement occurs after the first injection but improvement does occur after the second. If a second ESI is obtained and there is no additional benefit, no further ESIs are indicated.

It is generally recommended that an individual not have more than three ESIs in a 12 month period.

ESI is occasionally helpful in patients with chronic radiculopathy but this is highly variable. Unlike acute radiculopathy, in which the pathophysiologic picture is dominated by acute inflammation of the nerve root, chronic radiculopathy primarily involves fibrosis, congestion and hypersensitivity of the nerve root (more accurately, hypersensitivity of the nociceptive system in relation to the nerve root - see Chapter 2). As a result, ESI is often not effective in patients with chronic radiculopathy. However, in the patient with nerve root pain in whom surgery is being considered, it is reasonable to try ESI to see if sufficient relief can be achieved for the purpose of delaying or avoiding surgery (provided the patient does not have cauda equina syndrome or rapidly progressive motor loss – see below). However, caution must be taken because in some cases ESI may negatively impact long-term outcome and increase the recovery time from surgery. As discussed earlier, ESIs should be used judiciously and a rigorous shared decision-making process should be employed.

As presented in Chapter 2, the most common causes of radiculopathy are spinal stenosis and disc herniation. The vast majority of patients can be taken care of quite well with non-surgical management. However patients whose radiculopathy does not resolve with non-surgical management are candidates for surgery.

The general indications for surgical consult in patients with radiculopathy are:

- Progressive neurologic deficit that does not improve with an *adequate* trial of nonsurgical management

- Intractable nerve root pain that does not improve with an *adequate* trial of nonsurgical management

- Severe motor loss, even of recent onset

- Cauda equina syndrome

As can be seen from these indications, there are two factors that dictate the referral decision – neurologic deficit and pain. With regard to neurologic deficit, it is primarily motor findings that drive the decision (with the exception of patients with cauda equina syndrome, who should be referred for immediate surgical consult). It is common for patients with radiculopathy to experience some degree of neurogenic weakness. In most cases, this will improve without surgery. However, motor strength must be carefully monitored in these patients because if progressive loss of strength occurs during the course of non-surgical management, the patient may be at risk of permanent motor loss. Little is known about the time frame involved in the development of permanency. That is, it is not known how long it takes for motor loss to become permanent. Likewise, it is not known how profound motor loss must become before it becomes permanent. A good general rule of thumb is the "3/5 rule" (i.e., the point at which motor loss reaches the 3/5 level, using the scale presented in Chapter 4 regarding the clinical evaluation of muscle strength). If a patient with radiculopathy develops motor loss (or has motor loss upon initial presentation) and this motor loss progresses to the point of being graded 3/5, surgical consult should be considered. If the patient initially presents with motor loss that is already at the 3/5 level, surgical consult should be considered from the start. This does not necessarily mean that non-surgical management should be avoided in these cases. Many patients with weakness graded 3/5 will improve. It simply means that the practitioner should strongly consider initiating the surgical referral process at the 3/5 point. There are a number of factors that go into this decision, including how soon the patient is likely to be able to get to see the surgeon, how quickly the motor loss developed (the more quickly, the more urgent the referral) and how long the weakness has been present

Sensory loss is less of an urgent matter when it comes to progression because, whereas permanent motor loss can be a major impairment, permanent sensory loss has a far less profound impact on function. In the patient with progressive sensory loss without motor loss, it is important to counsel the patient in this regard, making it clear as to the implications of the condition and shared decision making should be pursued.

In the case of intractable nerve root pain, shared decision making is essential. In these cases, surgical consult should be discussed however, there is more flexibility regarding how quickly, if at all, surgical consult should be pursued. In many cases, time is on the patient's side. Many patients will improve without the need for surgery. However, improvement will typically occur more quickly with surgery.

Again, shared decision making between the primary spine practitioner and patient, often with the inclusion of the surgeon, should take place, considering the risks, benefits and alternatives to surgery in that particular patient's case.

Myofascial pain

As discussed in Chapters 5 and 10, treatment of trigger points (TrPs) is usually not necessary, as they tend to develop in response to one of the other pain generators and thus tend to resolve when the primary pain generator is addressed. However, in some patients myofascial therapy is necessary. When treatment of TrPs is deemed necessary but manual and/or muscle lengthening techniques are not successful, TrP injection should be considered. As manual myofascial treatments are usually quite effective, TrP injections are rarely necessary.

Diagnostic question #3 (What is happening with this person as a whole that would cause the pain experience to develop and persist?)

Passive instability

As discussed in Chapter 11, patients with passive instability should be provided with a spinal stabilization exercise program and instructions to strictly limit end-range movements, particularly flexion (see Chapter 9). In these patients, it is particularly important that they are diligent about staying with the home exercise program and postural advice. In those who develop ongoing pain and disability attributable to the passive instability, or who have the surgical indicators discussed in this chapter, surgical referral should be considered.

Nociceptive system sensitization and psychological factors

In the vast majority of patients with LBDs the development of chronic pain can be avoided with appropriate evidence-based, relationship-centered primary spine care. However there is a subset of patients who become chronic despite appropriate primary spine care. In some of these patients the problem is that the psychological perpetuating factors are such that they are not manageable at the primary spine care level. In these patients, referral to a psychologist or other behavioral health practitioner, preferably one trained in Cognitive-Behavioral Therapy or Acceptance and Commitment Therapy, is indicated. Often this is the only addition to the primary spine care presented in this book that is needed to help the patient on the path to recovery.

In some patients, NSS and psychological factors combine to produce a recalcitrant chronic pain state. Other perpetuating factors, such as dynamic instability or deconditioning, chronic opioid use and an overall pattern of ill health, can contribute to the clinical picture. In patients in whom the combination of NSS, psychological factors and other contributing factors is so well established that primary spine care is unsuccessful in bringing about resolution, a comprehensive multi-disciplinary chronic pain management program may be helpful.

Chronic Pain Management Programs

Various programs have been developed that bring professionals of various disciplines together to take a team approach to helping the patient overcome chronic pain. These are usually referred to as "Chronic Pain Management" programs (CPMP) or "Functional Restoration" programs. The approach taken in these programs vary and it is important for the primary spine practitioner to know what to look for in a high-quality program. There is a great deal of overlap in approach between CPMP and Work Hardening (WH) programs (see below) the primary difference being the emphasis of WH on return to occupational activities.

There are a variety of centers that claim to specialize in "pain management." Some "pain management" facilities focus primarily on various types of injections, and little else. Injections are generally of very limited to no benefit in the chronic LBD patient and should be avoided unless there are specific indications for injection in a particular individual, and the injections are utilized as part of the overall management strategy aimed at promoting functional independence. So "pain management" facilities that focus primarily on injections should be avoided.

The term typically used for the condition in which a patient does not successfully recover is "chronic pain" but, as has been emphasized throughout this book, it is not the pain itself that is the only, or even the primary, issue. The problem is that the patient's life is being dominated by the pain, disability and suffering experience. A quality chronic "pain" management program must recognize this and take a multidisciplinary approach to the assessment and management of patients. This has to consider the psychological, behavioral, functional and medical aspects of the chronic pain, disability and suffering experience. The emphasis should be on helping the patient understand the nature of pain, particularly in light of NSS and the role cognitions and beliefs play in perpetuating the problem. Essential is an approach that focuses on helping patients learn to conduct and enjoy life *independent of the pain.* This, of course, is the emphasis of primary spine care, as has been discussed throughout this book. This has to be carried forward in a multidisciplinary fashion in a quality CPMP.

The characteristics of an effective chronic pain management or functional restoration program that the primary spine practitioner should look for are:

1. A multidisciplinary approach to both assessment and management, including psychological, behavioral, physical and medical involvement.

2. A baseline assessment that determines the patient's current functional level, psychological barriers to recovery, medication usage, disability status and motivation for change.

3. Assessment of current opioid/ narcotic usage with a clear plan for decreasing medication dependence. Often a trained addiction specialist is necessary.

4. Evaluation and management by a psychological or behavioral specialist. This should *not* involve the patient simply being given a few psychological questionnaires but rather should involve one-on-one interaction between the patient and a trained professional.

5. Evaluation of social and vocational issues, with a clear plan to help the patient restore normalcy in these areas. Although CPMP generally do not have the return-to-work focus that are characteristic of WC and WH programs, chronic work disability must be addressed and there should be recognition of the important role that meaningful work plays in recovery.

6. Progressive physical rehabilitation, reconditioning and desensitization that involves a graded approach to exercise and restoration of physical function.

The primary spine practitioner should reassess the patient after two weeks or 10 days in the program. It should be expected that a good CPMP will perform such an assessment and provide the referring practitioner with data regarding the patient's progress in the program. This progress report should include physical functional capacity, medication usage, psychological factors and social and vocational functioning. The program should generally be expected to last a total of four weeks or 20 days. A good CPMP will provide the referring practitioner with recommendations for post-program monitoring and care.

Chronic Work Disability

Patients whose LBD began during the course of employment (i.e., workers' compensation patients) and who are not able to successfully return to work in a reasonable amount of time should be considered for a Work Conditioning (WC) or Work Hardening (WH) program. While definitions of WC and WH vary somewhat, in general WC involves intensive physical training that places emphasis on work simulation, i.e., graded activity that is specific to the patient's work requirements. WH also involves physical training and work simulation but also typically has a psychological and behavioral component that addresses fear-avoidance, catastrophizing, depression, poor self-efficacy and the other psychological perpetuating factors discussed throughout this book. The emphasis is on implementing and facilitating an aggressive return-to-work program. Sessions are typically three to five times per week and can last from a few hours (for WC) to eight hours (for WH) per day.

Prior to the commencement of a WC or WH program it is important that a Functional Capacity Evaluation (FCE) is performed. This is an intensive evaluation of the patient's current functional abilities that allows the calculation of a Physical Demand Level (PDL), i.e., the level at which the patient is currently able to function. A good FCE will evaluate the patient's ability in dynamic (*not* static) lifting activities and will include sincerity of effort checks. With a properly conducted FCE the patient's current PDL can be compared to the PDL that is required of his or job. A quality facility that performs WC and/or WH will include an FCE in its assessment process and will not only determine the patient's current PDL but will also determine the required PDL for return to work. The required PDL is best obtained from the employer via a job description but in lieu of this can be estimated from the Dictionary of Occupational Titles. In general, WC or WH should only be considered for patients whose occupational PDL requirement is at least at the level of Medium. The Dictionary of Occupational Titles can be found at:

www.occupationalinfo.org [accessed 18 July 2013]

If possible, it is often useful for the primary spine practitioner to obtain an FCE from a different facility than the one at which the patient will be participating in WC or WH, to have an independent assessment of the patient's functional PDL. Once the patient has begun WC or WH, it is important that the primary spine practitioner reassess the patient after two weeks or 10 sessions to determine whether significant functional progress is being made toward successful return to work. It should be expected that the WC/ WH facility will reassess the patient's PDL during this time period, either through repeat FCE or through documentation of the patient's dynamic lifting ability while in the program. Psychological measures in patients in a WH program should also be repeated at regular intervals.

WC/ WH programs should be considered for patients who have failed to successfully return to work after six weeks or more of continuous disability, despite appropriate primary spine care. However, patients who have been out of work for greater than two years have a negative prognosis with regard to

WC/ WH (though there are notable exceptions). In these patients, the practitioner may consider CPMP or functional restoration rather than WC/ WH.

For further guidelines regarding WC/ WH programs and CPMP the reader is directed to the American College of Occupational and Environmental Medicine:

http://www.acoem.org/practiceguidelines.aspx [accessed 9 August 2013]

and the Official Disability Guidelines of Work Loss Data Institute:

http://www.worklossdata.com/ [accessed 9 August 2013]

It has been emphasized throughout this book that effective primary spine care involves *management* of the condition in helping the patient *overcome* the problem. This involves the application of specific procedures for diagnosis and treatment, but the power of primary spine care comes from the *relationship-centered process* of management rather than from the application of particular procedures. There are a number of diagnostic and therapeutic procedures that require great skill and play important individual roles but it is the overall process, not the procedures, that is the essence of effective care.

Because of the multifactorial nature of LBDs, and the subjectivity of the LBD experience, primary spine care can be quite challenging at times. High-quality primary spine care requires a practitioner who is highly skilled and knowledgeable and who can be comfortable in wading through the "gray areas" of non-surgical spine problems. The primary spine practitioner also must be able to recognize and appreciate the subtleties of the spine related disorder SRD experience and empower patients to rise above the pain, disability and suffering experience to return to a happy and productive life.

The authors of this book encourage practitioners who have the appropriate background to seek credentials as primary spine practitioners. In addition, the authors encourage others to support the primary spine care movement and do play whatever role they can in helping patients with SRDs.

Further information about the credentialing process to become a primary spine practitioner can be found at:

www.primaryspineprovider.com

Recommended Reading

Airaksinen O, Brox JI, Cedraschi C, et al. Chapter 4. European guidelines for the management of chronic nonspecific low back pain. Eur Spine J 2006;15(Suppl 2):S192e300.

Albert HB, Lambert P, Rollason J, Sorensen JS, Worthington T, Pedersen MB, et al. Does nuclear tissue infected with bacteria following disc herniations lead to Modic changes in the adjacent vertebrae? Eur Spine J. 2013 Feb 10.

American College of Occupational and Environmental Medicine Occupational Medicine Practice Guidelines Chronic Pain chapter, 2008.

Chou R, Loeser JD, Owens DK, Rosenquist RW, Atlas SJ, Baisden J, et al. Interventional therapies, surgery, and interdisciplinary rehabilitation for low back pain: an evidence-based clinical practice guideline from the American Pain Society. Spine. 2009 May 1;34(10):1066-77.

Hides JA, Jull GA, Richardson CA. Long-term effects of specific stabilizing exercises for first-episode low back pain. Spine (Phila Pa 1976) 2001;26(11):e243-e8.

Larsen K, Weidick F, Leboeuf-Yde C. Can passive prone extensions of the back prevent back problems? A randomized, controlled intervention trial of 314 military conscripts. Spine (Phila Pa 1976) 2002;27(24):2747-52.

Work Loss Data Institute. Official Disability Guidelines Pain chapter, 2013.

• ABOUT THE AUTHOR •

Dr. Donald R. Murphy is a chiropractic physician and holds a Diplomate from the American Chiropractic Academy of Neurology. He is the Clinical Director of the Rhode Island Spine Center in Pawtucket, RI as well as Clinical Assistant Professor in the Department of Family Medicine at the Alpert Medical School of Brown University. He has been on the Expert Panel for several spine care guidelines and lectures all over the world on various topics related to spine disorders. Dr. Murphy has published dozens of articles in numerous peer-reviewed scientific journals and trade publications.

Dr. Murphy is also the lead instructor for the postgraduate certificate course in Primary Spine Care given by the Primary Spine Practitioner Network. Information on this course can be found at www.primaryspineprovider.com.

Dr. Murphy lives in Cranston, RI with his wife Laura and his three daughters Jessica, Alison and Melissa.

www.ingramcontent.com/pod-product-compliance
Lightning Source LLC
Chambersburg PA
CBHW080926220326
41598CB00034B/5695